Advances and Controversies in Hematopoietic Transplantation and Cell Therapy

Series Editors

Syed A. Abutalib
Deerfield, Illinois, USA

James O. Armitage
Omaha, Nebraska, USA

Each volume will focus on different aspects of blood and marrow transplantation or cellular therapy and presents up-to-date data and concepts as well as controversial aspects.

More information about this series at http://www.springer.com/series/13907

Miguel-Angel Perales
Syed A. Abutalib • Catherine Bollard
Editors

Cell and Gene Therapies

Springer

Editors
Miguel-Angel Perales
Adult Bone Marrow Transplant Service
Memorial Sloan Kettering Cancer Center
New York, NY
USA

Syed A. Abutalib
Cancer Treatment Centers of America
Deerfield, IL
USA

Catherine Bollard
Center for Cancer and Immunology
Research Children's National and The
George Washington University, Division
Allergy and Immunology
Washington, DC
USA

ISSN 2569-1376 ISSN 2569-135X (electronic)
Advances and Controversies in Hematopoietic Transplantation and Cell Therapy
ISBN 978-3-319-54367-3 ISBN 978-3-319-54368-0 (eBook)
https://doi.org/10.1007/978-3-319-54368-0

Library of Congress Control Number: 2018957701

This Springer imprint is published by the registered company Springer Nature Switzerland AG
The registered company address is: Gewerbestrasse 11, 6330 Cham, Switzerland

Contents

Historical Perspective and Current Focus 1

Miguel-Angel Perales and Catherine Bollard

In the beginning days of blood banking, surgeons would call imperiously for "fresh whole blood" recognizing its superior restorative properties over banked blood. Since then technological advances have made it possible to break down the therapeutic elements of fresh blood into their constituent platelets, red cells, plasma, and clotting factors, and through apheresis, blood bankers can even provide granulocytes, lymphocytes, progenitors, and stem cells. The component therapy concept is so widely accepted that we cease to think it as being unusual. Curiously, and in contrast, transplant physicians have been slower to apply a component therapy approach to their practice. Even today the majority of hematopoietic cell transplantation (HCT), whether from the bone marrow, peripheral blood, or cord blood, is as unmanipulated as the "fresh whole blood" beloved of our surgeons of the past. Nevertheless, the attractions of a component therapy approach to HCT are many including but not limited to (1) T-cell depletion by selection of $CD34^+$ cells, which can reduce GvHD, and (2) infused donor lymphocytes which can improve engraftment and treat leukemic relapse. Careful studies in the 1990s determined the doses

M.-A. Perales
Adult Bone Marrow Transplantation Service, Department of Medicine, Memorial Sloan-Kettering Cancer Center, New York, NY, USA

Weill Medical College of Cornell University, New York, NY, USA
e-mail: peralesm@mskcc.org

C. Bollard (✉)
Center for Cancer and Immunology Research Children's National and The George Washington University, Division Allergy and Immunology, Washington, DC, USA
e-mail: CBollard@childrensnational.org

M.-A. Perales et al. (eds.), *Cell and Gene Therapies*, Advances and Controversies in Hematopoietic Transplantation and Cell Therapy,
https://doi.org/10.1007/978-3-319-54368-0_1

of $CD34^+$ cells and lymphocytes in the graft that led to the best outcomes, and donor lymphocyte infusion doses were calibrated to achieve graft-versus-leukemia effects with minimal graft-versus-host disease.

These initial graft manipulations contributed to steady progress to improving HCT outcome, extending the upper age limit of HCT recipients and paving the way for successful transplants from HLA-haploidentical mismatch donors. However, we now see these advances as merely a prelude to the full realization of the component therapy approach through modern cell and gene therapies. Advances in technology in translational research have opened up exciting and powerful new cell-based treatments which promise to dramatically transform the way we perform allogeneic HCT and eliminate the obstacles of GvHD, relapse, and transplant-related mortality (TRM).

In this volume, we review the exciting developments in cell and gene therapy as it relates to HCT. From blood or marrow, a diverse repertoire of cell products are now manufactured including mesenchymal stromal cells (Chap. 12), dendritic cell vaccines (Chap. 11), and NK cells (Chap. 10). Gene-modified T cells can potentially control GvHD through inserted suicide genes. T cells can be targeted to neoplastic cells by transducing them with chimeric antigen receptors (CAR T cells) or artificial receptors (α/β TCRs) (Chaps. 2, 3, 4, 5, 6, and 7). The ultimate goal of cell and gene therapy is to provide remedies for all the major obstacles to successful outcomes of HCT. Regulatory T-cell (Chap. 9) or mesenchymal stromal cell infusions aim to prevent or treat GvHD. Tumor antigen-specific T cells, CAR T cells, α/β TCR T cells, and NK cells can prevent or treat leukemic relapse, and T cells targeting multiple viruses (Chap. 8) can reduce transplant morbidity and mortality. Finally, gene therapy is being used not only in malignant but also in nonmalignant hematologic disorders (Chaps. 13 and 14).

With the rapid advances in treatments of neoplastic disease and the prospect of continuing breakthroughs in treatments, as we have seen with the introduction of tyrosine kinase inhibitors and recently checkpoint inhibitors, we should be wary about predicting where HCT will be by the next decade. However, the rapid advances in cell therapy show a growing ability to render HCT safer and more effective. The progress documented with cell and gene therapy ensures that HCT will continue to remain central to the treatment of neoplastic and nonmalignant disorders for the foreseeable future.

Most Recent Clinical Advances in CAR T Cell and Gene Therapy 2017/2018

2

Syed A. Abutalib and Saar I. Gill

2.1 Introduction

Adoptive cell therapy with gene-engineered T cells bearing antitumor-reactive T-cell receptor or chimeric antigen receptor (CAR) is a promising and rapidly evolving field of translational medicine. This approach has delivered exciting responses for some patients with lymphoid hematologic neoplasms, leading to recent US Food and Drug Administration approvals. Hematopoietic stem cellular gene therapy has also shown promising advances, with durable and potentially curative clinical benefit and without the potential toxicities of allogeneic hematopoietic cell transplant. However, for both of these novel strategies, many questions remain unanswered. Compared to synthetic viral gene addition therapy (e.g., CAR T-cell engineering), translation of gene-editing technologies to patient care is in its infancy. Multiple clinical trials are ongoing or expected to open for CAR T cell and inherited monogenic disorders (Gardner et al. 2017) (refer to subsequent disease-specific chapters in the book). In this chapter, we will highlight the most recent and clinically relevant developments in the arena of gene-modified T-cell-based therapies and hematopoietic stem cellular gene therapy specifically focusing on hematologic disorders. We will conclude the chapter by summarizing the apparent challenges and directions for the future.

S. A. Abutalib (✉)
Cancer Treatment Centers of America, Zion, IL, USA

Chicago Medical School, Rosalind Franklin University of Medicine and Science, North Chicago, IL, USA

S. I. Gill
Division of Hematology-Oncology, Department of Medicine, University of Pennsylvania, Philadelphia, PA, USA

Smilow Translational Research Center, Philadelphia, PA, USA
e-mail: saar.gill@uphs.upenn.edu

M.-A. Perales et al. (eds.), *Cell and Gene Therapies*, Advances and Controversies in Hematopoietic Transplantation and Cell Therapy,
https://doi.org/10.1007/978-3-319-54368-0_2

2.2 Relapsed/Refractory B-Lineage Acute Lymphoblastic Leukemia

2.2.1 Children and Young Adults: CAR T Cells Show Promising Results

Transitioning CD19-directed CAR T cells from early-phase trials to a viable therapeutic approach with predictable efficacy and low toxicity for broad application is currently complicated by product heterogeneity resulting from (a) transduction of T cell of undefined subset composition, (b) variable efficiency of transgene expression, and (c) the effect of ex vivo culture on the differentiation state of the manufactured cells (Gardner et al. 2017; Rouce and Heslop 2017). Gardner et al. (2017) enrolled 45 children and young adults in PLAT-02 phase I trial with $CD19^+$ relapsed or refractory B-lineage acute lymphoblastic leukemia (ALL). They used CD19 CAR product of defined $CD4^+/CD8^+$ (1:1 ratio) composition with uniform CAR expression and limited effector differentiation (described later). The rationale for this strategy comes from preclinical studies that suggest that a 1:1 ratio of $CD4^+$ to $CD8^+$ cells and culture with appropriate homeostatic cytokines would ensure maximum effectiveness of both T-cell subsets and would yield a less terminally differentiated T-cell population with maximum tumor killing capacity, prolonged CAR T-cell persistence, and the ability to retain memory and self-renewal capacity (Gardner et al. 2017; Rouce and Heslop 2017; Riddell et al. 2014). Products meeting all defined specifications could be manufactured in 93% of enrolled patients. The maximum tolerated dose (MTD) was $1\text{x}10^6$ CAR T cells/kg (doses ranged from 0.5 to 10×10^6 cells/kg), and there were no deaths or instances of cerebral edema attributable to the product toxicity. The overall intent-to-treat minimal residual disease-negative (MRD-negative) remission rate was 89%. The MRD-negative remission rate was 93% in all patients who received a CAR T-cell product and 100% in the subset of patients who received fludarabine (Flu) and cyclophosphamide (Cy) lymphodepletion. Twenty-three percent of patients developed reversible CRS and/or reversible but severe neurotoxicity. No deaths resulting from toxicities were reported. These data demonstrate that manufacturing a defined composition CD19 CAR T cell identifies an optimal cell dose with highly potent antitumor activity and a tolerable adverse effect (AEs) profile in a cohort of patients with an otherwise poor prognosis. This manufacturing platform therefore provides a significant advantage over prior reported trials (see Chaps. 4 and 5). The observation that 100% of patients receiving Flu/Cy lymphodepletion had an MRD-negative remission further reinforces the importance of lymphodepletion regimens that include Flu, as opposed to Cy alone (Gardner et al. 2017; Turtle et al. 2016) (see Chap. 4).

2.2.2 Children and Young Adults: Tisagenlecleucel (CTL019) and Its US FDA Approval[1] (2017)

On August 30, 2017, the US FDA granted approval to tisagenlecleucel for the treatment of patients up to age 25 years with B-cell precursor ALL that is refractory or in second or later relapse (see footnote 1). Approval of tisagenlecleucel was based on a phase II single-arm trial (ELIANA; NCT02435849) of 63 patients with relapsed or refractory pediatric precursor B-cell ALL, including 35 patients who had a prior hematopoietic cell transplantation (Buechner et al. 2017). Median age of the participants was 12 years (range, 3–23 years). Noteworthy, during the presentation of updated results of this global multicenter ELIANA trial at European Hematology Association (EHA®) 2017, it was reported that as of November 2016, 88 patients were enrolled. There were seven (8%) manufacturing failures, nine (10%) patients were not infused due to death or AEs, and four patients (5%) were pending infusion at the time of data cutoff. All patients received a single dose of tisagenlecleucel intravenously within 2–14 days following the completion of lymphodepleting chemotherapy. Of the 63 patients who were evaluable for efficacy, the confirmed overall remission rate as assessed by independent central review was 82.5% (95% CI 70.9, 91.0), consisting of 63% of patients with complete remission (CR) and 19% with CR with incomplete hematological recovery (CRi). All patients with a confirmed CR or CRi were MRD-negative by flow cytometry (FC) method. Median remission duration was not reached (range: 1.2 to 14.1+ months). Grade III or IV AEs were noted in 84% of patients. Serious adverse reactions such as CRS, including fatal CRS and CRS-associated disseminated intravascular coagulation with intracranial hemorrhage, prolonged cytopenias, infection, cardiac failure, and cardiac arrest occurred in patients receiving tisagenlecleucel. FDA approved tisagenlecleucel with a Risk Evaluation and Mitigation Strategy (see footnote 1). The recommended tisagenlecleucel dose is one infusion of $0.2–5.0 \times 10^6$ (CAR)-positive viable T cells/kg body weight intravenously for patients who are less than or equal to 50 kg and $0.1–2.5 \times 10^8$ total CAR-positive viable T cells intravenously for patients who are >50 kg, administered 2–14 days after lymphodepleting chemotherapy (see footnote 1) (Buechner et al. 2017) (see Chap. 4).

2.2.3 Adults with Relapsed/Refractory B-ALL: Phase I Trial from Memorial Sloan Kettering Cancer Center (MSKCC)

Park et al. (2018) enrolled 83 adult (age range, 23–74 years) patients with relapsed B-cell ALL, of whom 53 who received an infusion of anti-CD19 autologous T cells costimulated with CD28. A total of 78 patients underwent leukapheresis, 11 of

[1] https://www.fda.gov/downloads/BiologicsBloodVaccines/CellularGeneTherapyProducts/ApprovedProducts/UCM573941.pdf. Accessed July 4, 2018.

whom did not undergo an attempt at cell production (owing to death or the receipt of alternative treatment), and 13 did not have cells infused (2 because of production failure and 11 owing to infection, alternative treatment, or death). A total of 36 patients (68%) received CAR T-cell therapy as a third or later salvage treatment, 12 (23%) had primary refractory disease, 19 (36%) had undergone allogeneic hematopoietic cell transplantation (allo-HCT) previously, and 13 (25%) had received blinatumomab previously. A total of 16 patients (30%) had Philadelphia chromosome-positive ALL, including 5 patients with the T315I ABL kinase mutation. Safety and long-term outcomes were assessed, as were their associations with demographic, clinical, and disease characteristics. After infusion, severe CRS occurred in 14 of 53 patients (26%; 95% confidence interval [CI], 15–40); 1 patient died. CR was observed in 83% of the patients. At a median follow-up of 29 months (range, 1–65), the median event-free survival (EFS) was 6.1 months (95% CI, 5.0–11.5), and the median overall survival (OS) was 12.9 months (95% CI, 8.7–23.4). Patients with a low disease burden (<5% bone marrow blasts) before treatment had markedly enhanced remission duration and survival, with a median EFS of 10.6 months (95% CI, 5.9 to not reached) and a median OS of 20.1 months (95% CI, 8.7 to not reached). Patients with a higher burden of disease (≥5% bone marrow blasts or extramedullary disease) had a greater incidence of the CRS and neurotoxic events and shorter long-term survival than did patients with a low disease burden (Gardner et al. 2017). The latter observation was also made by Maude et al. (2014) (see Chap. 5).

2.3 Non-Hodgkin B-Cell Lymphomas

2.3.1 Phase I, ZUMA-1 Study (Locke et al. 2017a): Primary Results of Axicabtagene Ciloleucel (KTE-C19) with a Focus on Refractory Diffuse Large B-Cell Lymphoma (DLBCL)

In the phase I multicenter ZUMA-1 study, Locke et al. (2017a) evaluated KTE-C19, an autologous CD28-costimulated CAR T-cell therapy, in patients with refractory DLBCL. Patients received concurrent cyclophosphamide (500 mg/m^2) and fludarabine (30 mg/m^2) for 3 days followed by KTE-C19 at a target dose of 2×10^6 CAR T cells/kg of recipient weight. The incidence of dose-limiting toxicity (DLT) was the primary endpoint. Seven patients were treated with KTE-C19, and one patient experienced a DLT of grade IV CRS and neurotoxicity. Grade ≥ III CRS and neurotoxicity were observed in 14% (n = 1 of 7) and 57% (n = 4 of 7) of patients, respectively. All other KTE-C19-related grade ≥III events resolved within 1 month. The overall response rate (ORR) was 71% (n = 5 of 7), and CR rate was 57% (n = 4 of 7). Three patients have ongoing CR (all at 12+ months) at the time of publication. CAR T cells demonstrated peak expansion within 2 weeks and continued to be detectable at 12+ months in patients with ongoing CR. Consistent with the *on-target, off-tumor* effect of KTE-C19, B-cell aplasia and hypogammaglobulinemia were observed in subjects with ongoing CR and persistent CAR T cells at 12 months post-infusion. This multicenter study validated that centralized manufacturing is feasible and established the logistics for transportation of patient-specific product door to door within approximately 2 weeks (Locke et al. 2017a; Lulla and Ramos 2017) (see Chap. 6).

2.3.2 Additional Results of ZUMA-1 Study (Locke et al. 2017b) and US FDA Approval[2] (2017) of Axicabtagene Ciloleucel (KTE-C19)

The safety and efficacy of axicabtagene ciloleucel were established in a multicenter ZUMA-1 clinical trial of 101 adult patients with refractory or relapsed large B-cell lymphoma (Locke et al. 2017a, b). In the subsequent report data from patients enrolled into two cohorts consisting of DLBCL (cohort 1) and primary mediastinal B-cell lymphoma (PMBCL) or transformed follicular lymphoma (TFL) (cohort 2) were reported (Locke et al. 2017b). All patients had chemorefractory disease, with roughly 80% refractory to their last line of chemotherapy, and the remainder relapsing within 12 months of autologous hematopoietic cell transplant (auto-HCT). Patients had received a median of three prior therapies. Prior to infusion of axicabtagene ciloleucel, a conditioning regimen of Flu/Cy was administered. Axicabtagene ciloleucel was administered as a single infusion of modified autologous T cells at a target dose of 2×10^6 CAR^+ T cells/kg of recipient weight. The median follow-up for the primary analysis was 8.7 months, with most patients having data available for 6 months. There were four patients who experienced a CR but did not have assessment data available for 6 months. For the primary analysis, these individuals were classified as nonresponders, suggesting the response rates could be higher. The primary endpoint of the phase II study was ORR, which was significantly satisfied across the full study ($P < 0.0001$). After 6 months, 41% of patients were still in response, with a CR rate of 36% and a partial response (PR) rate of 5%. There was one incidence of a PR improving to a CR after 9 months, suggesting longer follow-up could further alter these numbers. Across the full duration of the study, those with DLBCL ($n = 77$) had an ORR of 82% and a CR rate of 49%. In the PMBCL/TFL group ($n = 24$), the ORR was 83% and the CR rate was 71%. After 6 months of follow-up, the ORR in the DLBCL group was 36%, which included a CR rate of 31%. In the PMBCL/TFL group, the 6-month ORR rate was 54%, with a CR rate of 50%. Median OS was not yet reached. The most common grade ≥ III AEs were anemia (43%), neutropenia (39%), decreased neutrophil count (32%), febrile neutropenia (31%), decreased white blood cell count (29%), thrombocytopenia (24%), encephalopathy (21%), and decreased lymphocyte count (20%). There were three fatal events in the study, two of which were deemed related to axicabtagene ciloleucel: hemophagocytic lymphohistiocytosis (HLH) and cardiac arrest in the setting of CRS. The third death was from pulmonary embolism. Data from 93 patients were available for

[2] https://www.fda.gov/NewsEvents/Newsroom/PressAnnouncements/ucm581216.htm. Accessed July 4, 2018.

the interim analysis from the ZUMA-1 trial (Locke et al. 2017a), whereas the primary assessment contained data for 101 patients (Locke et al. 2017b). With more patients assessed, the rate of CRS declined from 18% at the interim assessment to 13% for the primary analysis. Additionally, neurologic events dropped from 34% in the interim analysis to 28% in the primary assessment. There were no cases of cerebral edema. On the basis of these results, US FDA approved axicabtagene ciloleucel, for use in adult patients with certain types of large B-cell lymphoma after at least two other kinds of treatment have failed, including DLBCL, PMBCL, and DLBCL arising from TFL (see footnote 2). Notably, patients with primary central nervous system lymphoma were excluded from receiving axicabtagene ciloleucel, and the drug is not approved for treatment of patients with this condition.

2.3.3 Phase II Results of ZUMA-1 Study (Neelapu et al. 2017): Axicabtagene Ciloleucel in DLBCL, PMBCL, and Transformed FL

In a multicenter, phase II study, Neelapu et al. (2017) enrolled 111 patients with DLBCL, PMBCL, and TFL who had refractory disease despite undergoing recommended prior therapy. Patients received a target dose of 2×10^6 anti-CD19 CAR T cells/kg of recipient body weight after receiving a conditioning regimen of low-dose Flu/Cy. The primary end point was the rate of objective response (calculated as the combined rates of CR and PR). Secondary end points included OS, safety, and biomarker assessments. Among the 111 patients who were enrolled, axicabtagene ciloleucel was successfully manufactured for 110 (99%) and administered to 101 (91%) patients. The objective response rate was 82%, and the CR rate was 54%. These findings compare favorably with the results of the recent SCHOLAR-1 study (Crump et al. 2017) of conventional therapies for this disease, which showed an objective response rate of 26% and a complete response rate of 7%. With a median follow-up of 15.4 months, 42% of the patients were still in response, with 40% continuing to have a complete response. The overall rate of survival at 18 months was 52%. The most common AEs of grade III or higher during treatment were neutropenia (in 78% of the patients), anemia (in 43%), and thrombocytopenia (in 38%). Grade III or higher CRS and neurologic events occurred in 13% and 28% of the patients, respectively. Three of the patients died during treatment. In this particular study, higher CAR T-cell levels in blood were associated with response. Furthermore, this study (Neelapu et al. 2017) confirmed the feasibility and reliability of centralized manufacturing and coordination of leukapheresis procedures and shipping from multiple centers across the country. The product was manufactured for 99% of the enrolled patients and was administered to 91%. The short 17-day median turnaround time may be important for these patients with refractory large B-cell lymphoma, who generally have rapidly growing disease. The investigators of this multicenter trial (Neelapu et al. 2017) also reported that axicabtagene ciloleucel could be administered safely at medical facilities that perform transplantation, even if such centers had no specific experience in CAR T-cell therapy.

2.3.4 Tisagenlecleucel (CTL019) in Relapsed/Refractory DLBCL and Follicular Lymphoma: Results from University of Pennsylvania (UPenn) (Schuster et al. 2017a)

Patients with DLBCL or FL that is refractory to or which relapses after immunochemotherapy and transplantation have a poor prognosis. High response rates have been reported with the use of T cells modified by CAR that target CD19 in B-cell cancers (Grupp et al. 2013; Porter et al. 2011), although data regarding B-cell lymphomas are limited to small number of patients. Schuster et al. (2017a) used autologous T cells that express a 41BB-costimulated CD19-directed CAR (CTL019) to treat patients with DLBCL or FL that had relapsed or was refractory to previous treatments. Patients were monitored for response to treatment, toxic effects, the expansion and persistence of CTL019 cells in vivo, and immune recovery. A total of 38 patients were enrolled. Twenty-eight patients received tisagenlecleucel, and 18 of 28 had a response (64%; 95% CI, 44–81). CR occurred in 6 of 14 patients with DLBCL (43%; 95% CI, 18–71) and 10 of 14 patients with follicular lymphoma (71%; 95% CI, 42–92). CTL019 cells proliferated in vivo and were detectable in the blood and bone marrow of patients regardless of ultimate response status. Sustained remissions were achieved, and at a median follow-up of 28.6 months, 86% of patients with DLBCL who had a response (95% CI, 33–98) and 89% of patients with FL who had a response (95% CI, 43–98) had maintained the response. In this particular study (Schuster et al. 2017a), the CRS was less frequent and less severe than previously reported for the use of tisagenlecleucel in the treatment of ALL and chronic lymphocytic leukemia (CLL) (Grupp et al. 2013; Porter et al. 2011). The CRS was self-limiting and its severity was not correlated with response to therapy. Severe CRS occurred in five patients (18%). Serious encephalopathy occurred in three patients (11%); two cases were self-limiting and one case was fatal. All patients in CR by 6 months remained in remission at 7.7–37.9 months (median, 29.3 months) after induction, with recovery of normal B cells in 8 of 16 patients and with improvement in levels of IgG in 4 of 10 patients and of IgM in 6 of 10 patients at 6 months or later and in levels of IgA in 3 of 10 patients at 18 months or later. Transient encephalopathy developed in approximately one in three patients and severe CRS developed in one of five patients.

2.3.5 US FDA Approval (2018) of Tisagenlecleucel[3] (CTL019) for Adults with Relapsed/Refractory Large B-Cell Lymphoma: Results of JULIET Study (Schuster et al. 2017b, c)

On May 1, 2018, the US FDA approved tisagenlecleucel, a CD19-directed genetically modified autologous T-cell immunotherapy, for adults with relapsed or refractory large B-cell lymphoma after two or more lines of systemic therapy including

[3] https://www.fda.gov/drugs/informationondrugs/approveddrugs/ucm606540.htm. Accessed July 4, 2018.

DLBCL not otherwise specified (DLBCL-NOS), high-grade B-cell lymphoma, and DLBCL arising from FL (transformed lymphoma) (see footnote 3). Approval was based on a single-arm, open-label, and multicenter, phase II trial (Schuster et al. 2017b) in adults with relapsed or refractory DLBCL and DLBCL after transformation from FL. Eligible patients must have been treated with at least two prior lines of therapy, including an anthracycline and rituximab, or relapsed following auto-HCT. Patients received a single infusion of tisagenlecleucel following completion of lymphodepleting chemotherapy (Flu 25 mg/m^2, Cy 250 mg/m^2/day × 3 days or bendamustine 90 mg/m^2/day × 2 days). The ORR as assessed by an independent review committee for the 68 evaluable patients [presented at multiple national meetings in 2017 (Schuster et al. 2017b, c)] was 50% (95% CI: 37.6, 62.4) with a complete response rate of 32% (95% CI: 21.5, 44.8). With a median follow-up time of 9.4 months, the duration of response was longer in patients with a best overall response of CR, as compared to a best overall response of PR. Among patients achieving CR, the estimated median duration of response was not reached (95% CI: 10.0 months, not estimable). The estimated median response duration among patients in PR was 3.4 months (95% CI: 1.0, not estimable). The most common adverse reactions (incidence >20%) in patients on the trial were CRS, infections-pathogen unspecified, pyrexia, diarrhea, nausea, fatigue, hypotension, edema, and headache. Because of the serious risks of CRS and neurologic toxicities, FDA approved tisagenlecleucel with a Risk Evaluation and Mitigation Strategy (see footnote 3). The recommended dose of tisagenlecleucel for relapsed or refractory adult DLBCL is 0.6–6.0 × 10^8 CAR$^+$ viable T cells (see footnote 3). Like axicabtagene ciloleucel, tisagenlecleucel is also not indicated for the treatment of patients with primary central nervous system lymphoma.

2.3.6 Long Duration of CR in DLBCL After Anti-CD19 CAR T-Cell Therapy: Data from the NCI (Kochenderfer et al. 2017)

Kochenderfer et al. (2017) administered anti-CD19 CAR T cells preceded by Flu/Cy conditioning chemotherapy to patients with relapsed DLBCL. Five of the seven evaluable patients obtained CRs. Four of the five complete remissions had long-term durability with durations of remission of 56, 51, 44, and 38 months; to date (Gardner et al. 2017), none of these four cases of lymphomas have relapsed. Importantly, CRs continued after recovery of nonmalignant polyclonal B cells in three of four patients with long-term CRs. In these three patients, recovery of CD19$^+$ polyclonal B cells took place 28, 38, and 28 months prior to the last follow-up, and each of these three patients remained in CR at the last follow-up. Nonmalignant CD19$^+$ B-cell recovery with continuing complete remissions demonstrated that remissions of DLBCL can continue after the disappearance of functionally effective anti-CD19 CAR T-cell populations. Patients had a low incidence of severe infections despite long periods of B-cell depletion and hypogammaglobulinemia. Only one hospitalization for an infection occurred among the four patients with long-term CRs. Thus, anti-CD19 CAR T cells caused long-term remissions of chemotherapy-refractory DLBCL without substantial chronic toxicities.

2.4 Chronic Lymphocytic Leukemia

2.4.1 CLL and Anti-CD19 CAR T Cells Following Ibrutinib Failure

Turtle et al. (2017) evaluated the safety and feasibility of anti-CD19 CAR T-cell therapy in patients with CLL who had previously received ibrutinib. Twenty-four patients with CLL received lymphodepleting chemotherapy and anti-CD19 CAR T cells at one of three dose levels (2×10^5, 2×10^6, or 2×10^7 CAR T cells/kg). Nineteen patients experienced disease progression while receiving ibrutinib, three were ibrutinib intolerant, and two did not experience progression while receiving ibrutinib. Six patients were venetoclax-refractory, and 23 had a complex karyotype and/or 17p deletion. Four weeks after CAR T-cell infusion, the ORR by International Workshop on Chronic Lymphocytic Leukemia (IWCLL) criteria was 71% (17 of 24). Twenty patients (83%) developed CRS, and eight (33%) developed neurotoxicity, which was reversible in all but one patient with a fatal outcome. Twenty of 24 patients received Flu/Cy lymphodepletion and CD19 CAR T cells at or below the MTD ($\leq 2 \times 10^6$ CAR T cells/kg). In 19 of these patients who were restaged, the ORR by IWCLL imaging criteria 4 weeks after infusion was 74% (CR, 4 of 19, 21%; PR, 10 of 19, 53%), and 15 of 17 patients (88%) with marrow disease before CAR T cells had no disease by FC after CAR T cells. Twelve of these patients underwent deep IGH sequencing, and seven (58%) had no malignant IGH sequences detected in marrow. The absence of the malignant IGH clone in marrow of patients with CLL who responded by IWCLL criteria was associated with 100% PFS and OS (median 6.6 months follow-up) after CAR T-cell immunotherapy. The PFS was similar in patients with lymph node PR or CR by IWCLL criteria. CD19 CAR T cells were highly effective with manageable toxicity in patients with high-risk CLL, including those who were ibrutinib-refractory. Of note, although bone marrow disease was highly responsive to CAR T cells, complete elimination of bulky nodal disease was less common, suggesting the malignant lymph node environment may impair CAR T-cell infiltration and/or function. Thus, CR rates in advanced CLL might be improved if CAR T-cell immunotherapy is delivered when ibrutinib-induced mobilization of lymph node disease into blood and/or marrow is still effective and before the development of bulky lymphadenopathy (Gill et al. 2017). Such a strategy might be used by monitoring patients receiving ibrutinib for development of ibrutinib-resistant mutations or other early evidence of progression (see Chaps. 5 and 6).

2.5 Multiple Myeloma

2.5.1 Results of Anti-BCMA CAR T Cells: Data from NCI (Ali et al. 2016; Brudno et al. 2017)

B-cell maturation antigen (BCMA) is expressed in most cases of MM. Ali et al. (2016) from NCI conducted the first-in-human clinical trial of CAR T cells targeting BCMA. T cells expressing the CAR used in this work (CAR-BCMA) specifically recognized BCMA-expressing cells. The anti-BCMA CAR used in this work incorporated the 11D-5-3 anti-BCMA single-chain variable fragment (scFv), a CD28 costimulatory domain, and the CD3−ζ T-cell activation domain. The cells were transduced with a γ-retroviral vector, and 9 days after the initiation of cultures, CAR-BCMA T cells were infused. Twelve patients received CAR-BCMA T cells in this dose escalation trial. The dose escalation plan called for an initial dose of 0.3×10^6 CAR^+ T cells/kg with threefold increase to each subsequent dose level. Among the six patients treated on the lowest two dose levels, limited antimyeloma activity and mild toxicity occurred. On the third dose level, one patient obtained a very good partial remission (VGPR). Two patients were treated on the fourth dose level of 9×10^6 CAR T cells/kg body weight. Before treatment, the first patient on the fourth dose level had chemotherapy-resistant MM, making up 90% of bone marrow cells. After treatment, plasma cells in the marrow became undetectable by FC, and the patient's MM entered a stringent complete remission (sCR) that lasted for 17 weeks before relapse. The second patient on the fourth dose level had chemotherapy-resistant MM making up 80% of bone marrow cells before treatment. Twenty-eight weeks after this patient received CAR-BCMA T cells, bone marrow plasma cells were undetectable by FC, and the serum monoclonal protein had decreased by >95%. Both patients treated on the fourth dose level had toxicity consistent with CRS including fever, hypotension, and dyspnea. Both patients had prolonged cytopenias. Serum BCMA (sBCMA) served as a tumor marker because substantial decreases in sBCMA occurred in the three patients with the most impressive antimyeloma responses.

Most recently (ASH® annual meeting 2017), the same group presented their updated data of 13 patients treated to date on the highest dose level of 9×10^6 CAR-BCMA T cells/kg (Brudno et al. 2017). The median age of the 13 patients was 54 years (range 43–66). The patients had a median of 11 prior lines of therapy. Five patients (12, 19, 20, 23, and 25) had a chromosome 17p deletion prior to protocol enrollment. Toxicities were consistent with prior reports of CRS after infusions of CAR T cells. Of 13 patients, 4 received the interleukin (IL)-6-receptor antagonist tocilizumab to treat CRS; 2 of these 4 patients also received corticosteroids. While CAR-BCMA T-cell toxicity was severe in some cases, the toxicities were mainly limited to the first 2 weeks after CAR-BCMA T-cell infusion. Because of grade III/IV CRS experienced by some patients with high bone marrow myeloma burdens, investigators of this study modified the clinical protocol to only allow enrollment of patients with lower myeloma burdens defined as MM making up 30% or less of bone marrow cells. Two patients (16 and 18) experienced delayed neutropenia and thrombocytopenia that started approximately 1 month after CAR T-cell infusion when blood counts had recovered from the chemotherapy administered before CAR-BCMA T-cell infusions. These patients were treated with filgrastim, eltrombopag, and prednisone based on the hypothesis that the cytopenias were caused by CAR T cells in the patient's bone marrow. In both cases, cytopenias resolved after approximately 1 month. CAR-BCMA T cells exhibited clear antimyeloma activity. Nine of 11 evaluable patients obtained objective antimyeloma responses with 2 stringent complete responses, 5 very good partial responses, and 2 partial responses; the duration of responses varied. The longest response to date is 66 weeks. Eight of ten evaluable patients obtained MRD-negative status by bone marrow flow cytometry. Consistent with BCMA-specific T-cell activity, plasma cells were reduced on bone marrow core biopsies in all eight evaluated patients and absent in four of these patients 2–3 months after CAR-BCMA T-cell infusion. CAR^+ cell levels have been quantified in the blood of patients. CAR T-cell levels peaked in the first 2 weeks after infusion and persisted at lower levels for many months in some cases. Cytokines were measured in the serum of all patients. In patients with CRS, multiple cytokines including interferon-γ, IL-6, IL-8, and IL-17A were consistently elevated in the serum. Accrual to this trial continues. Toxicity was significant but limited in duration and controllable (Rouce and Heslop 2017).

2.5.2 Anti-BCMA CAR T Cells: Data Presented at ASH® 2017 by UPenn (Cohen et al. 2017)

Cohen and coworkers reported early safety and clinical activity of CART-BCMA without lymphodepleting chemotherapy in highly refractory MM patients during ASH® 2016 (Cohen et al. 2016). Subsequently, they reported extended results from this initial cohort, as well as initial safety and efficacy in additional cohorts at two dose levels in conjunction with Cy at ASH® 2017 (Cohen et al. 2017). Three cohorts are being enrolled: (1) 1–5 × 10^8 CAR T cells alone; (2) Cy 1.5 g/m^2 + 1–5 × 10^7 CAR T cells; and (3) Cy 1.5 g/m^2 + 1–5 × 10^8 CART cells. CART-BCMA cells are given as split-dose infusions (10% on day 0, 30% on day 1, and 60% on day 2), with Cy given on day 3. Participants need serum creatinine (Cr) <2.5 mg/dL or Cr clearance ≥30 mL/min; adequate hepatic, cardiac, and pulmonary function; and absolute CD3 count ≥150/μL. BCMA expression on MM cells is assessed but not required for eligibility. CAR T-BCMA expansion/persistence is assessed by flow cytometry and qPCR. Soluble BCMA levels are measured by ELISA. Responses are assessed by IMWG criteria. As of June 24, 17, 33 patients have consented, with 28 eligible, 21 infused, 4 awaiting infusion, and 3 manufactured but never treated due to rapid progression/clinical deterioration. Of treated patients (n = 21), nine are in cohort 1, five in cohort 2, and seven in cohort 3. Median age is 57 (range 44–73), 71% male, and median 4.3 years from diagnosis. Median lines of therapy is 7 (range 3–11); 100% are proteasome inhibitor and immunomodulatory drugs-refractory, 67% daratumumab-refractory. Ninety-five percent had high-risk cytogenetics, 67% del17p or *TP53* mutation, and 29% extramedullary disease. All expressed BCMA on MM cells and received the minimum target dose of CAR T-BCMA, with 18 patients (86%) receiving full-planned dose and 3 patients receiving 40% of dose (third infusion held due to fevers). Toxicities in cohort 1 ($n = 9$) were previously reported and included CRS in eight patients (three grade III/IV, with four receiving tocilizumab) and neurotoxicity (grade IV encephalopathy) in two patients. In cohorts 2 and 3 ($n = 12$), CRS has occurred in nine patients (three grade III, zero grade IV, none requiring tocilizumab) and neurotoxicity in 1 patient (grade II confusion/aphasia), with no unexpected/DLTs and no TRM. Regarding efficacy, in cohort 1 six of nine patients responded (one stringent CR [sCR], two VGPR, one PR, two MR), with one ongoing sCR at 21 months and other responses lasting 1.5–5 months. In cohort 2, with Cy but tenfold lower CAR T dose, two of five patients responded (one PR, one MR) but progressed at 4 and 2 months, respectively. In cohort 3, median follow-up is currently 1 month, with five of six patients responding (one CR, three PR, one MR) and one not yet evaluable. All patients had detectable CAR T-BCMA expansion by qPCR, and 90% were detectable by FC, with preferential expansion of $CD8^+$ cells and similar degree of expansion in blood and marrow. Median peak expansion (as measured by copies/µg DNA) is 6160, 14,761, and 45,268 in cohorts 1, 2, and 3, respectively, suggesting a benefit with adding Cy, though this was not statistically significant. Achieving PR or better is associated with higher peak CART-BCMA levels and decline in soluble BCMA, but not with baseline soluble BCMA level or intensity of baseline BCMA expression by flow on MM cells. Serial marrow FC demonstrates that five of six patients with ≥PR and detectable residual MM cells have decreased BCMA intensity on MM cells post-infusion compared with baseline. CART-BCMA infusions following Cy lymphodepletion are feasible and have significant clinical activity in highly refractory MM patients with poor-risk genetics and limited treatment options. Efficacy appears lower at the 10^7 dose, compared with 10^8, and remaining patients are now being enrolled in cohort 3. CRS remains a common but manageable toxicity. Decreased BCMA expression on residual MM cells post-infusion may be an escape mechanism reflecting CART-BCMA-induced immune editing. These data also provide further support for exploration of CART-BCMA in relapsed/refractory MM.

2.5.3 CRB-401: A Multicenter Trial Phase I Dose Escalation Trial of bb2121

Berdeja et al. (2017) assessed safety and efficacy of the CAR T-cell modality in relapsed and refractory MM (RRMM), by designing a CAR construct targeting BCMA. They reported the data at ASH® 2017. The bb2121 consists of autologous T cells transduced with a lentiviral vector encoding a novel CAR incorporating an anti-BCMA scFv, a 4-1BB costimulatory motif, and a CD3-zeta T-cell activation domain. CRB-401 (NCT02658929) is a two part, multicenter phase I dose escalation trial of bb2121 in patients with relapsed and refractory MM (RRMM) who have received ≥3 prior regimens, including a proteasome inhibitor and an immunomodulatory agent, or are double-refractory, and have ≥50% BCMA expression on clonal plasma cells. Peripheral blood mononuclear cells are collected via leukapheresis and shipped to a central facility for transduction, expansion, and release testing prior to being returned to the site for infusion. Patients undergo lymphodepletion with Flu (30 mg/m^2) and Cy (300 mg/m^2) daily for 3 days and then receive one infusion of bb2121. The study follows a standard 3 + 3 design with planned dose levels of 50, 150, 450, 800, and 1200 × 10^6 CAR$^+$ T cells. The primary outcome measure is incidence of AEs, including DLTs. Additional outcome measures were quality and duration of clinical response assessed according to the IMWG Uniform Response Criteria for Multiple Myeloma, evaluation of MRD, overall and PFS, quantification of bb2121 in blood, and quantification of circulating soluble BCMA over time. As of May 4, 2017, 21 patients (median age 58 [37–74]) with a median of 5 [1–16] years since MM diagnosis had been infused with bb2121, and 18 patients were evaluable for initial (1-month) clinical response. Patients had a median of 7 prior lines of therapy (range 3–14), all with prior auto-HCT; 67% had high-risk cytogenetics. Fifteen of 21 (71%) had prior exposure to, and 6 of 21 (29%) were refractory to 5 prior therapies (bortezomib/lenalidomide/carfilzomib/pomalidomide/daratumumab). Median follow-up after bb2121 infusion was 15.4 weeks (range 1.4–54.4 weeks). As of data cutoff, no DLTs and no treatment-emergent grade III or higher neurotoxicities similar to those reported in other CAR T clinical studies had been observed. CRS, primarily grade I or II, was reported in 15 of 21 (71%) patients: 2 patients had grade III CRS that resolved in 24 h, and 4 patients received tocilizumab, 1 with steroids, to manage CRS. CRS was more common in the higher-dose groups but did not appear related to tumor burden. One death on study, due to cardiopulmonary arrest more than 4 months after bb2121 infusion in a patient with an extensive cardiac history, was observed while the patient was in sCR and was assessed as unrelated to bb2121. The ORR was 89% and increased to 100% for patients treated with doses of 1.5 × 10^8 CAR$^+$ T cells or higher. No patients treated with doses of 1.50 × 10^8 CAR$^+$ T cells or higher had disease progression, with time since bb2121 between 8 and 54 weeks. MRD-negative results were obtained in all four patients evaluable for analysis. CAR$^+$ T-cell expansion has been demonstrated consistently and three of five patients evaluable for CAR$^+$ cells at 6 months had detectable vector copies. The ORR was 100% at these dose levels with eight ongoing clinical responses at 6 months and one patient demonstrating a sustained response beyond 1 year.

2.5.4 Data from China with Unique Antigen-Binding Domain: Late Breaking Abstract at ASCO® 2017

Fan et al. (2018) reported results using a CAR T designated LCAR-B38M CAR T, which targets two different epitopes on BCMA and induce selective toxicity in BCMA-expressing tumor cells.[4] A single-arm clinical trial was conducted to assess

[4] https://www.cancer.gov/publications/dictionaries/cancer-drug/def/792630. Accessed July 4, 2018.

safety and efficacy of this approach. A total of 19 patients with RRMM were included in the trial. The median number of infused cells was 4.7 (0.6–7.0) × 10^6/kg. The median follow-up was 208 (62–321) days. Among the 19 patients who completed the infusion, 7 patients were monitored for a period of more than 6 months. Six out of the seven achieved CR- and MRD-negative status. The 12 patients who were followed up for less than 6 months met near CR criteria of modified EBMT criteria for various degrees of positive immunofixation. All these effects were observed with a progressive decrease of M-protein and thus may eventually meet CR criteria. In the most recent follow-up examination, all 18 surviving patients were determined to be free of myeloma-related biochemical and hematologic abnormalities. CRS was observed in 14 (74%) patients who received treatment. Among these 14 patients, there were 9 cases of grade I, 2 cases of grade II, 1 case of grade III, and 1 case of grade IV patient who recovered after treatments. A 100% objective response rate (ORR) to LCAR-B38M CAR T cells was observed. Of 18 out of 19 (95%) patients reached CR or near CR status without a single event of relapse in a median follow-up of 6 months. The majority (see footnote 1) of the patients experienced mild or manageable CRS (Gardner et al. 2017).

2.6 Classic Hodgkin and Anaplastic Large-Cell Lymphomas

2.6.1 CD30-Directed CAR T Cell: Phase I Study in Patients with Relapsed/Refractory Classic Hodgkin Lymphoma (cHL) and Anaplastic Large-Cell Lymphoma (ALCL)

In an open-label, phase I study, Wang et al. (2017) reported results of 18 patients including 1 with primary cutaneous ALCL and 17 with cHL. All patients received a conditioning chemotherapy (three regimen options) followed by the CAR T-cell infusion. The level of CAR transgenes in peripheral blood and biopsied tumor tissues was measured periodically according to an assigned protocol by quantitative PCR (qPCR). Eighteen patients were enrolled; most of whom were heavily pretreated or had extensive disease and received a mean of 1.56 × 10^7 CAR-positive T cell/kg (SD, 0.25; range, 1.1–2.1) in total during infusion. CAR T-cell infusion was tolerated, with grade ≥3 toxicities occurring only in 2 of 18 patients. Of 18 patients, 7 achieved partial remission and 6 achieved stable disease. An inconsistent response of lymphoma was observed: lymph nodes presented a better response than extranodal lesions, and the response of lung lesions seemed to be relatively poor. Lymphocyte recovery accompanied by an increase of circulating CAR T cells (peaking between 3 and 9 days after infusion) is a probable indictor of clinical response. Analysis of biopsied tissues by qPCR and immunohistochemistry revealed the trafficking of CAR T cells into the targeted sites and reduction of the expression of CD30 in tumors. The investigators concluded that future clinical trial protocols need to consider the further optimization of conditioning regimens, the trial of multiple-cycle infusions of CAR T cells, and intervention of the CAR T-cell protocol in the early-disease stage.

2.6.2 CD30-Directed CAR T Cell: Another Phase I Study in Patients with Relapsed/Refractory cHL and ALCL

Subsequently, Ramos et al. (2017) conducted a phase I dose escalation study in which nine patients have relapsed/refractory *EBV-negative* cHL ($n = 6$ plus one patient with composite lymphoma [diffuse large B-cell lymphoma evolved to Hodgkin lymphoma]) and ALCL ($n = 2$; one patient had cutaneous anaplastic lymphoma kinase-negative and one patient had anaplastic lymphoma kinase-positive systemic ALCL). The patients were infused with autologous T cells that were gene-modified with a retroviral vector to express the CD30-specific CAR T cell encoding the CD28 costimulatory endodomain. Three dose levels, from 0.2×10^8 to 2×10^8 CAR T cell/m^2, were infused without a conditioning regimen. All other therapy for malignancy was discontinued at least 4 weeks before CAR T-cell infusion. Seven patients had previously experienced disease progression while being treated with brentuximab. No toxicities attributable to CAR T cells were observed. Of seven patients with relapsed cHL, one entered CR lasting more than 2.5 years after the second infusion of CAR T cells, one remained in continued CR for almost 2 years, and three had transient stable disease. Of two patients with ALCL, one had a CR that persisted 9 months after the fourth infusion of CAR T cells. The expansion of CAR T cells in peripheral blood peaked 1 week after infusion, and CAR T cells remained detectable for over 6 weeks. Although CD30 may also be expressed by normal activated T cells, no patients developed impaired virus-specific immunity. The study concluded that appropriate tumor reduction and lymphodepletion before CAR T-cell infusion should enhance their clinical activity without increasing toxicity. Since inhibition of PD1 is an appropriate option in patients with relapsed HL (Ansell et al. 2015), future exploration of the synergy between CAR T cell directed against CD30 and PD1/PD-L1 blockade seems interesting to explore.

2.7 Considerations for Tisagenlecleucel Dosing Rationale

A recent abstract at ASCO® 2018, by Awasthi et al. (2018), analyzed data from pivotal phase II ELIANA [NCT02435849, $n = 75$], ENSIGN [NCT02228096, $n = 29$], and JULIET [NCT02445248, $n = 99$] trials to investigate tisagenlecleucel dose-related impact on efficacy, safety, and exposure. Unlike conventional drugs, the ultimate number of T cells in the patient is a function of in vivo expansion and thus is determined by various factors including patient characteristics (such as disease burden), manufacturing attributes, and indication. Final product attributes (transduction efficiency, percentage T cells, cell viability, total cell count), exposure (maximal in vivo expansion), efficacy, and safety were evaluated against dose. Dose and exposure were independent. Increased probability of any grade or grade III/IV CRS was associated with increase in dose in DLBCL; no impact was observed in B-ALL. Clinically meaningful responses were observed across the dose range. The proposed dose range, as CAR$^+$ viable T cells, were based on totality of these analyses considering the benefit-risk ratio (B-ALL: body weight $\leq$ 50 kg, 0.2–5.0 × 10^6/kg, for weight > 50 kg, 0.1–2.5 × 10^8; DLBCL: 0.6–6.0 × 10^8).

2.8 US FDA Approval of Tocilizumab[5] for Cytokine Release Syndrome

CRS is the most common risk associated with CAR T-cell therapies. On August 30, 2017, the US FDA also (along with tisagenlecleucel [see above]) approved tocilizumab for the treatment of patients 2 years of age or older with CRS that occurs with CAR T-cell therapy. In an analysis of data from clinical trials of CAR T cells, 69% of patients with severe or life-threatening CRS had resolution of CRS within 2 weeks following one or two doses of tocilizumab (see footnote 5).

2.9 Promise of Gene Therapy

After almost 30 years of promise tempered by setbacks, gene therapies are rapidly becoming a critical component of the therapeutic armamentarium for a variety of inherited and acquired human diseases (Dunbar et al. 2018) (see Chaps. 13 and 14). Gene therapy has curative potential, whereby autologous hematopoietic stem cells are genetically modified and transplanted, which would not be limited by a requirement for HLA-matched donors, resulting in onetime, lifelong correction devoid of immune side effects. However, many challenges remain (see Table 2.1). Adeno-associated virus and lentiviral vectors are the basis of several recently approved gene therapies (Dunbar et al. 2018). New gene-editing technologies are in their translational and clinical infancy but are expected to play an increasing role in the field (Dunbar et al. 2018; Antony et al. 2018).

2.9.1 Cerebral Adrenoleukodystrophy

In X-linked adrenoleukodystrophy, mutations in ABCD1 lead to loss of function of the ALD protein. Cerebral adrenoleukodystrophy is characterized by demyelination and neurodegeneration. Disease progression, which leads to loss of neurologic function and death, can be halted only with allo-HCT (Eichler et al. 2017). A single group, open-label phase II/III (STARBEAM) study (Eichler et al. 2017) evaluated the safety and efficacy of autologous $CD34^+$ cells transduced with the elivaldogene tavalentivec (Lenti-D) lentiviral vector for the treatment of early-stage childhood cerebral adrenoleukodystrophy. The inclusion criteria matched widely accepted eligibility criteria for allo-HCT in children with cerebral adrenoleukodystrophy. A total of 17 boys received Lenti-D gene therapy. At the time of the interim analysis, the median follow-up was 29.4 months

[5] https://www.fda.gov/Drugs/InformationOnDrugs/ApprovedDrugs/ucm574154.htm. Accessed July 4, 2018.

Table 2.1 Challenges and future directions in cell-based genetic therapies

• Careful surveillance to assess long-term outcomes is essential
• Large multicenter prospective studies are needed to confirm the clinical efficacy and safety
• Prospective data are needed on the influence of disease biology with CAR T-cell therapies
• Disease- and patient-specific standardization and/or consensus on lymphodepleting conditioning regimens
• Better understanding of therapy associated toxicities
• Identification of pre-therapy biomarkers or models that may allow efficient prediction of clinical response to therapy
• Optimization/standardization of the cell dose and formulation
• Identification of new tumor-specific targets and subsequent development of dual- or even triple-targeting CAR T-cell products
• Expansion of CAR T-cell therapy application to myeloid malignancies and solid tumors
• Exploration of gene therapy earlier in the disease course may be worthwhile in selected group of patients
• Better understanding of in vivo kinetics of gene therapy products with clinical responses and adverse effects is needed
• Exploration of gene-based therapy in mitigating allogeneic hematopoietic cell transplant-associated graft-versus-host disease
• Advancement of third party "allogeneic" CAR T cells clinical trials
• Advancement and selection of best genome editing technologies
• Selected patients might benefit with additional therapeutic modalities pre- or post-CAR T infusion (e.g., epigenetic modulation and PD-1 antibodies)
• Hospital partnerships with biotechnology and pharmaceutical industries with expertise in manufacturing
• Cell and gene therapy product must be delivered in a safe and timely manner
• Standardization of generation and expansion of gene therapy products
• Standardization of quality control is needed

(range, 21.6–42.0). All the patients had gene-marked cells after engraftment, with no evidence of preferential integration near known oncogenes or clonal outgrowth. Measurable ALD protein was observed in all the patients. No TRM or GvHD had been reported; 15 of the 17 patients (88%) were alive and free of major functional disability, with minimal clinical symptoms. One patient, who had had rapid neurologic deterioration, died due to disease progression. Another patient, who had evidence of disease progression on MRI, withdrew from the study to undergo allo-HCT and unfortunately died later from transplantation-related complications. These results suggest that autologous $CD34^+$ cells transduced with Lenti-D are at least as effective as conventional allo-HCT for the treatment of cerebral adrenoleukodystrophy and may be safer.

2.9.2 Transfusion-Dependent β-Thalassemia: Results of HGB-204 and HGB-205 Studies

Donor availability and transplantation-related risks limit the broad use of allo-HCT in patients with transfusion-dependent β-thalassemia. After investigators previously established that lentiviral transfer of a marked β-globin ($\beta^{A\text{-}T87Q}$) gene could substitute for long-term red-cell transfusions in a patient with β-thalassemia, they attempted to evaluate the safety and efficacy of such gene therapy in patients with transfusion-dependent β-thalassemia (Thompson et al. 2018). In the two, phase I/II studies (Thompson et al. 2018), investigators obtained mobilized autologous $CD34^+$ cells from 22 patients (age 12–35 years) with transfusion-dependent β-thalassemia and transduced the cells ex vivo with LentiGlobin BB305 vector, which encodes adult hemoglobin (HbA) with a T87Q amino acid substitution (HbA^{T87Q}). The cells were then reinfused after the patients had undergone myeloablative busulfan conditioning. At a median of 26 months (range, 15–42) after infusion of the gene-modified cells, all but 1 of the 13 patients who had a non-β^0/β^0 genotype no longer required red blood cell transfusions; the levels of HbA^{T87Q} ranged from 3.4 to 10.0 g per deciliter, and the levels of total hemoglobin ranged from 8.2 to 13.7 g per deciliter. Correction of biologic markers of dyserythropoiesis was achieved in evaluated patients with hemoglobin levels near normal ranges. In nine patients with a β^0/β^0 genotype or two copies of the IVS1-110 mutation, the median annualized transfusion volume was decreased by 73%, and red-cell transfusions were discontinued in three patients. Treatment-related AEs were typical of those associated with autologous hematopoietic cell transplantation. No clonal dominance related to vector integration was observed. The study (Thompson et al. 2018) concluded that gene therapy with autologous $CD34^+$ cells transduced with the LentiGlobin BB305 vector reduced or eliminated the need for long-term red-cell transfusions in 22 patients with severe β-thalassemia without serious AEs related to the drug product.

2.10 Challenges

While exciting, it is important to note that most extant clinical data have short-term follow-up. Using CAR T cells for B-ALL as an example, the high response rates at early time-points translate to no higher than 50% disease-free survivals (DFS) beyond 6 months (Park et al. 2018; Maude et al. 2014). Leukemia relapses on these trials occurred either with loss of the CD19 antigen (a form of immunoediting) (Sotillo et al. 2015) or due to inadequate persistence of the CAR T cells (Park et al. 2018; Maude et al. 2014). Responses are lower in lymphomas than in ALL for reasons that remain incompletely elucidated, although complete responses in those lymphoma patients do appear to be durable. Thus, there is clearly room to improve (Table 2.1 and see text below). Widespread clinical deployment of these therapies has only just begun with the recent US FDA approval of tisagenlecleucel (see footnotes 1 and 3) and axicabtagene ciloleucel (see footnote 2) and will highlight logistical challenges associated with centralized manufacturing products from patients located at widely dispersed institutions. As noted above, the registration trials for both tisagenlecleucel (see footnotes 1 and 3) and axicabtagene ciloleucel (see footnote 2) showed that this is feasible, and we now await post-marketing experience. Further challenges to overcome are the frequent and at times severe toxicities that are beginning to seem to be a "class effect" of CAR T cells. CRS appears to be mediated by a cross talk between the infused T cells and the patient's endogenous myeloid cells (Giavridis et al. 2018) yet whether CRS can be dissociated from the antitumor effect remains uncertain. Neurotoxicity, at least in patients with R/R ALL, seems to be related to disruption of the blood-brain barrier and correlates with high tumor burden, peak CAR T-cell expansion, and high levels of serum cytokines (Santomasso et al. 2018). Neurotoxicity is a particular challenge since specific therapy for this complication is lacking. Also noteworthy of reported trials is that patients have received T-cell products comprising often random compositions of $CD4^+$ and $CD8^+$ naive and memory T cells, meaning that each patient received a different therapeutic product. Such variation may have influenced the efficacy of T-cell therapy and complicates comparison of outcomes between different patients and across trials (Sommermeyer et al. 2016). Another barrier to the overall success of CAR T-cell strategies has been the exclusion of research participant enrollment (Singh et al. 2016). In addition, the hurdles for gene therapy for nonmalignant and other non-hematologic disorders remain, including understanding and preventing genotoxicity from integrating vectors or off-target genome editing, improving gene transfer or editing efficiency to levels necessary for treatment of many target diseases, preventing immune responses that limit in vivo administration of vectors or genome editing complexes (Dunbar et al. 2018; Khalil et al. 2016) (Table 2.1).

2.11 Future Directions

More effective and safer genetic engineering approaches have generated great enthusiasm in the field of hematologic malignancies (CAR T cells) and immunodeficiencies or hemoglobinopathies (hematopoietic stem cells gene engineering) (see subsequent chapters in the book). Other than the challenges outlined above and in Table 2.1 for the existing therapies, an enormous challenge remains in translating these therapies beyond the relatively few patients with lymphoid hematologic malignancies. In adults, acute myeloid leukemia is more common than ALL, and myelodysplastic syndromes remain incurable without allo-HCT. Yet due to the lack of a suitable myeloid antigen that is specific to cancer cells, approaches that can bring the power of CAR T-cell therapy to bear on myeloid malignancies remain an area of active investigation (Kim et al. 2018; Buddee et al. 2017) with a paucity of clinical results to date (NCT02159495 (Buddee et al. 2017) and NCT03190278). An even bigger problem and richer prize is the area of solid tumors, where CAR T cells have met with very little success to date. Here the issue is likely to be not only the lack of a suitable antigen but also the presence of a very immunosuppressive tumor microenvironment (TME) that is not conducive to T-cell activity. In the arena of solid tumors, the most convincing (albeit sparse) results have come from the infusion of ex vivo expanded tumor-infiltrating lymphocytes (TILs) into a select few patients with some very impressive results (Zacharakis et al. 2018; Tran et al. 2015, 2016, 2017). It is tempting to speculate that combining antigen-specific T cells with suitable inhibitors of negative signaling in the TME might yield more convincing responses. Finally, further work to streamline, harmonize, and simplify the manufacturing process is underway and could ultimately increase the feasibility and reduce the costs associated with genetically engineered cellular therapy, thereby moving it from a cottage industry into the mainstream.

Conflict of Interest Syed A. Abutalib—None.

Saar I Gill—Research funding (Novartis); Equity (Carisma Therapeutics); Scientific Advisory Board (Carisma Therapeutics, Extellia Therapeutics).

References

Ali SA, Shi V, Maric I et al (2016) T cells expressing an anti-B-cell maturation antigen chimeric antigen receptor cause remissions of multiple myeloma. Blood 128(13):1688–1700

Ansell SM, Lesokhin AM, Borrello I et al (2015) PD-1 blockade with nivolumab in relapsed or refractory Hodgkin's lymphoma. N Engl J Med 372(4):311–319

Antony JS, Haque AKMA, Lamsfus-Calle A et al (2018) CRISPR/Cas9 system: a promising technology for the treatment of inherited and neoplastic hematological diseases. Adv Cell Gene Ther 1:e10. https://onlinelibrary.wiley.com/doi/abs/10.1002/acg2.10

Awasthi R, Mueller KT, Yanik GA et al (2018) Considerations for tisagenlecleucel dosing rationale. J Clin Oncol 36:e15056 (suppl; abstr e15056)

Berdeja JG, Lin Y, Raje N et al (2017) Durable clinical responses in heavily pretreated patients with relapsed/refractory multiple myeloma: updated results from a multicenter study of bb2121 anti-Bcma CAR T cell therapy. Blood 130:740

Brudno J, Lam N, Wang M et al (2017) T cells genetically modified to express an anti-B-cell maturation antigen chimeric antigen receptor with a CD28 costimulatory moiety cause remissions of poor-prognosis relapsed multiple myeloma. Blood 130:524

Buddee LB, Joo Y Song JY, Kim Y et al (2017) Remissions of acute myeloid leukemia and blastic plasmacytoid dendritic cell neoplasm following treatment with CD123-specific CAR T cells: a first-in-human clinical trial. Abstract 811

Buechner J, Grupp SA, Maude SL et al (2017) Global registration trial of efficacy and safety of CTL019 in pediatric and young adults patients with relapsed/refractory (R/R) acute lymphoblastic leukemia (ALL): update of the international interim analysis. In: 2017 European Hematology Association (EHA) annual meeting (Abstract S476)

Cohen AD, Garfall AL, Stadtmauer EA et al (2016) B-cell maturation antigen (BCMA)-specific chimeric antigen receptor T cells (CART-BCMA) for multiple myeloma (MM): initial safety and efficacy from a phase I study. In: 58th American Society of Hematology annual meeting and exposition. Abstract #1147

Cohen AD, Garfall AL, Stadtmauer EA et al (2017) Safety and efficacy of B-cell maturation antigen (BCMA)-specific chimeric antigen receptor T cells (CART-BCMA) with cyclophosphamide conditioning for refractory multiple myeloma (MM). Blood 130:505

Crump M, Neelapu SS, Farooq U et al (2017) Outcomes in refractory diffuse large B-cell lymphoma: results from the international SCHOLAR-1 study. Blood 130:1800–1808

Dunbar CE, High KA, Joung JK et al (2018) Gene therapy comes of age. Science 359:6372

Eichler F, Duncan C, Musolino PL, Orchard PJ, De Oliveira S, Thrasher AJ, Armant M, Dansereau C, Lund TC, Miller WP, Raymond GV, Sankar R, Shah AJ, Sevin C, Gaspar HB, Gissen P, Amartino H, Bratkovic D, NJC S, Paker AM, Shamir E, O'Meara T, Davidson D, Aubourg P, Williams DA (2017) Hematopoietic stem-cell gene therapy for cerebral adrenoleukodystrophy. N Engl J Med 377(17):1630–1638

Fan F, Zhao W, Liu J et al (2018) Durable remissions with BCMA-specific chimeric antigen receptor (CAR)-modified T cells in patients with refractory/relapsed multiple myeloma. J Clin Oncol 35(18_suppl):LBA3001–LBA3001. https://doi.org/10.1200/JCO.2017.35.18_suppl.LBA3001

Gardner RA, Finney O, Annesley C, Brakke H, Summers C, Leger K, Bleakley M, Brown C, Mgebroff S, Kelly-Spratt KS, Hoglund V, Lindgren C, Oron AP, Li D, Riddell SR, Park JR,

Jensen MC (2017) Intent-to-treat leukemia remission by CD19 CAR T cells of defined formulation and dose in children and young adults. Blood 129(25):3322–3331

Giavridis T, van der Stegen SJC, Eyquem J et al (2018) CAR T cell-induced cytokine release syndrome is mediated by macrophages and abated by IL-1 blockade. Nat Med 24(6):731–738

Gill S, Frey NV, Hexner EO et al (2017) CD19 CAR-T cells combined with ibrutinib to induce complete remission in CLL. J Clin Oncol 35:7509 (suppl; abstr 7509)

Grupp SA, Kalos M, Barrett D et al (2013) Chimeric antigen receptor–modified T cells for acute lymphoid leukemia. N Engl J Med 368:1509–1518

Khalil DN, Smith EL, Brentjens RJ et al (2016) The future of cancer treatment: immunomodulation, CARs and combination immunotherapy. Nat Rev Clin Oncol 13:273–290

Kim MY, Yu KR, Kenderian SS et al (2018) Genetic inactivation of CD33 in hematopoietic stem cells to enable CAR T cell immunotherapy for acute myeloid leukemia. Cell 173(6):1439–1453.e19

Kochenderfer JN, Somerville RPT, Lu T et al (2017) Long-duration complete remissions of diffuse large B cell lymphoma after anti-CD19 chimeric antigen receptor T cell therapy. Mol Ther 25(10):2245–2253

Locke FL, Neelapu SS, Bartlett NL et al (2017a) Phase 1 results of ZUMA-1: a multicenter study of KTE-C19 anti-CD19 CAR T cell therapy in refractory aggressive lymphoma. Mol Ther 25(1):285–295

Locke FL, Neelapu SS, Bartlett NL et al (2017b) Primary results from ZUMA-1: a pivotal trial of axicabtagene ciloleucel (Axi-cel; KTE-C19) in patients with refractory aggressive non-Hodgkin lymphoma (NHL). Presented at 2017 AACR annual meeting; April 1–5, 2017; Washington, DC. Abstract CT019

Lulla P, Ramos CA (2017) Expanding accessibility to CD19-CAR T cells: commercializing a “boutique” therapy. Mol Ther 25(1):8–9

Maude SL, Frey N, Shaw PA et al (2014) Chimeric antigen receptor T cells for sustained remissions in leukemia. N Engl J Med 371(16):1507–1517

Neelapu SS, Locke FL, Bartlett NL et al (2017) Axicabtagene ciloleucel CAR T-cell therapy in refractory large B-cell lymphoma. N Engl J Med 377(26):2531–2544

Park JH, Rivière I, Gonen M et al (2018) Long-term follow-up of CD19 CAR therapy in acute lymphoblastic leukemia. N Engl J Med 378(5):449–459

Porter DL, Levine BL, Kalos M, Bagg A, June CH (2011) Chimeric antigen receptor-modified T cells in chronic lymphoid leukemia. N Engl J Med 365:725–733

Ramos CA, Ballard B, Zhang H et al (2017) Clinical and immunological responses after CD30-specific chimeric antigen receptor-redirected lymphocytes. J Clin Invest 127(9):3462–3471

Riddell SR, Sommermeyer D, Berger C, Liu LS, Balakrishnan A, Salter A, Hudecek M, Maloney DG, Turtle CJ (2014) Adoptive therapy with chimeric antigen receptor-modified T cells of defined subset composition. Cancer J 20(2):141–144

Rouce RH, Heslop HE (2017) Equal opportunity CAR T cells. Blood 129(25):3275–3277

Santomasso BD, Park JH, Salloum D et al (2018) Clinical and biologic correlates of neurotoxicity associated with CAR T cell therapy in patients with B-cell acute lymphoblastic leukemia (B-ALL). Cancer Discov 7:811

Schuster SJ, Svoboda J, Chong EA et al (2017a) Chimeric antigen receptor T cells in refractory B-cell lymphomas. N Engl J Med 377(26):2545–2554

Schuster S et al (2017b) Primary analysis of juliet: a global, pivotal, Phase 2 trial of CTL019 in adult patients with relapsed or refractory diffuse large B-cell lymphoma. In: 59th American Society of Hematology annual meeting and exposition. Abstract #577

Schuster SJ, Bishop MR, Tam C et al (2017c) Global pivotal phase 2 trial of the CD19-targeted therapy CTL019 in adult patients with relapsed/refractory (R/R) diffuse large B-cell lymphoma (DLBCL) — an interim analysis. Hematol Oncol 35(Suppl 2):27. Abstract published June 7, 2017

Singh N, Perazzelli J, Grupp SA et al (2016) Early memory phenotypes drive T cell proliferation in patients with pediatric malignancies. Sci Transl Med 8(320):320ra3

Sommermeyer D, Hudecek M, Kosasih PL et al (2016) Chimeric antigen receptor-modified T cells derived from defined CD8+ and CD4+ subsets confer superior antitumor reactivity in vivo. Leukemia 30(2):492–500

Sotillo E, Barrett DM, Black KL et al (2015) Convergence of acquired mutations and alternative splicing of CD19 enables resistance to CART-19 immunotherapy. Cancer Discov 5(12):1282–1295

Thompson AA, Walters MC, Kwiatkowski J et al (2018) Gene therapy in patients with transfusion-dependent β-thalassemia. N Engl J Med 378(16):1479–1493

Tran E, Ahmadzadeh M, Lu YC et al (2015) Immunogenicity of somatic mutations in human gastrointestinal cancers. Science 350(6266):1387–1390

Tran E, Robbins PF, Lu YC et al (2016) T-cell transfer therapy targeting mutant KRAS in cancer. N Engl J Med 375(23):2255–2262

Tran E, Robbins PF, Rosenberg SA (2017) 'Final common pathway' of human cancer immunotherapy: targeting random somatic mutations. Nat Immunol 18(3):255–262

Turtle CJ, Hanafi LA, Berger C, Hudecek M, Pender B, Robinson E, Hawkins R, Chaney C, Cherian S, Chen X, Soma L, Wood B, Li D, Heimfeld S, Riddell SR, Maloney DG (2016) Immunotherapy of non-Hodgkin's lymphoma with a defined ratio of CD8+ and CD4+ CD19-specific chimeric antigen receptor-modified T cells. Sci Transl Med 8(355):355ra116

Turtle CJ, Hay KA, Hanafi LA et al (2017) Durable molecular remissions in chronic lymphocytic leukemia treated with CD19-specific chimeric antigen receptor-modified T cells after failure of ibrutinib. J Clin Oncol 35(26):3010–3020

Wang CM et al (2017) Autologous T cells expressing CD30 chimeric antigen receptors for relapsed or refractory Hodgkin lymphoma: an open-label phase I trial. Clin Cancer Res 23(5):1156–1166

Zacharakis N, Chinnasamy H, Black M et al (2018) Immune recognition of somatic mutations leading to complete durable regression in metastatic breast cancer. Nat Med 24(6):724–730

Part I

Genetically Modified T Cells (Chimeric Antigen Receptors and T Cell Receptors)

Chimeric Antigen Receptor T Cells: Antigen Selection, CAR Development, and Data in Neoplastic Hematology

3

Januario E. Castro and Thomas J. Kipps

3.1 Introduction

The first results of human clinical trials using chimeric antigen receptor T-cell (CAR-T-cell) technology were conducted from 1997 to 2000 in patients infected with the human immune deficiency virus (HIV) (Deeks et al. 2002; Mitsuyasu et al. 2000). These studies provided the proof of concept for this technology and allowed for its application to other diseases, such as cancer. The initial cancer-specific CAR studies were reported in 2006; it used genetically modified T cells in patients with renal cell carcinoma or ovarian cancer (Lamers et al. 2006; Kershaw et al. 2006). Following these initial publications, there have been many basic and clinical research studies that improved the technology, making it more effective and feasible for use in patients with various cancers (Till et al. 2008; Jensen et al. 2010; Porter et al. 2011; Kochenderfer et al. 2012; Brentjens et al. 2011; Davila et al. 2014).

Toxicities are one of the main limiting factors for wide applicability of CAR-T-cell therapy. Those adverse events include neurotoxicity and cytokine release syndrome (CRS). The mechanisms contributing to some of these adverse effects are not fully understood, but significant effort has been devoted to describe the clinical course of these complications and provide strategies to mitigate these toxicities in treated patients (Grupp et al. 2013; Teachey et al. 2016; Lee et al. 2015).

J. E. Castro
Adoptive Cellular Therapy CART-Cell Program, Hematology-Oncology Division, Mayo Clinic Arizona, Phoenix, AZ, USA
e-mail: Castro.Januario@mayo.edu

T. J. Kipps (✉)
Moores UCSD Cancer Center, University of California, San Diego, CA, USA

CLL Research Consortium, San Diego, CA, USA
e-mail: tkipps@ucsd.edu

M.-A. Perales et al. (eds.), *Cell and Gene Therapies*, Advances and Controversies in Hematopoietic Transplantation and Cell Therapy,
https://doi.org/10.1007/978-3-319-54368-0_3

Several questions remain. What are the requirements for antitumor specificity? Can targeted tumor antigens also be expressed by normal tissues, and if so what types of tissues? Can tumor antigens be targeted that are selectively overexpressed by the tumor but still expressed on normal tissues, albeit at low or trace levels? Are all tumors equally sensitive to CAR-T cells? What is the best source of the effector T cells—autologous or allogeneic T cells— or T cells isolated from the blood or from the tumor microenvironment, the so-called tumor-infiltrating lymphocytes (TILs)? Is it better to use TCR or single chain antibodies to redirect CARs? Resolving these questions and other questions will be critical for the full development of an adoptive cellular therapy. Unfortunately, in vitro testing and animal models do not always provide the means to resolve these questions, mandating the use of clinical trials to address these uncertainties.

In spite of these significant obstacles, adoptive cell immunotherapy provides the exciting potential to offer curative treatments to patients with cancers found intractable with current therapies. Moreover, emerging clinical evidence suggests some patients with intractable cancers may have prolonged remissions and a potential cure following treatment with CAR-T cells (Lee et al. 2015; Maude et al. 2015; Scholler et al. 2012; Feldman et al. 2015).

3.2 Generation of Chimeric Antigen Receptors

Conceptually, the CAR design allows the gene-modified cell (T cell, NK cell, or other effector immune cells) to acquire new target specificity. Additional features include built-in stimulation signals such as co-stimulatory molecules, cytokine production, or cell activation/modulatory signals (Gill and June 2015; Rosenberg and Restifo 2015).

Genetically engineered immune receptors used in CARs have minimum five elements:

(1) *A target-binding domain*—this typically is composed of a polypeptide sequence of the light and heavy chains from a single chain antibody (scFV). Other receptor-ligand molecules can replace this domain provided that they have sufficient specificity and affinity. Examples of the latter include protein-protein binding constructs designed using HIV-gp120-binding CD4-CD3ζ (Romeo and Seed 1991), cytokines for cytokine receptors (e.g., IL3-IL-13Rα) (Brown et al. 2012), receptor-ligand constructs (e.g., CD27-CD70) (Shaffer et al. 2011), or pattern recognition receptors, such as Dectin-1 for targeting the β-glycan on *Aspergillus* (Kumaresan et al. 2014).

(2) *A hinge domain*—this provides flexibility to the target-binding domain, allowing it to bind the target antigen without steric hindrance.

(3) *A transmembrane domain*—this allows the chimeric receptor to pass through the plasma membrane and remain tethered to the effector cell.

(4) *A primary signaling domain*—this typically is derived from the T-cell receptor (CD3 ζ chain).

(5) *Co-stimulatory domains*—these stabilize and amplify the activation signal, enhancing proliferation and long-term survival of CAR-expressing T cells. Several examples of such co-stimulatory domains are derived from the cytoplasmic domains of CD27, CD28, CD134 (OX40), CD137 (4-1BB), or CD244 (ICOS). The cytoplasmic domain of CD28 induces expression of IL-2, making the T cell relatively resistant to suppression by regulatory T cells (Maher et al. 2002). CARs constructed with the cytoplasmic domain of CD137 apparently have enhanced in vivo persistence, antitumor activity, and enhanced capacity to traffic to the tumor cells compared to CAR-T cells lacking this domain (Ellebrecht et al. 2016). Contact with tumor cells bearing the target antigen then induces the cytokine production (e.g., IL-2 and others), proliferation, and expansion of CAR-T cells in vivo.

Most CARs have target-binding domains derived from the scFv of antibodies that bind the target antigens. The use of target-binding domain derived from scFv, rather than the standard TCR, confers several advantages, including increased binding affinity and specificity for antigens rather than peptides presented in the context of major histocompatibility complex (MHC) antigens, the typical types of antigens recognized from standard TCRs. Moreover, unlike TCR-based recognition, CAR recognition is not dependent on processing and presentation of antigen by the MHC, which often might be lost on the surface of tumors cells that have escaped host immune surveillance (Spranger 2016). However, CARs generated from antibody scFv may lack the ability to target intracellular molecules that are not expressed on the cell surface. For this reason, some CARs are derived from TCR or engineered receptors that target peptides presented by the MHC. A proof of concept used receptors that exclusively recognized MHC-presented peptides derived from the intracellular protein WT1 (Dao et al. 2013; Houen 2015).

3.3 Different Types of Chimeric Antigen Receptors

The so-called first-generation CARs have one stimulatory cytoplasmic domain (e.g., CD3ζ), whereas the so-called second- or third-generation CARs have a stimulatory cytoplasmic domain and one or two co-stimulatory cytoplasmic domains, respectively (Fig. 3.1). The incorporation of a single co-stimulatory molecule in addition to the CD3 ζ chain (second-generation CAR) enhances persistence, expansion, and other T-cell functions. However, it is not clear whether or not the addition of other co-stimulatory signals provides additional benefit (Rosenberg and Restifo 2015). In addition to signals 1 and 2, T cells typically require a third signal to achieve and sustain full activation. This third signal is mediated through the common γ-chain cytokine receptor, and a coordinated delivery of certain cytokines activates this receptor enhancing CAR-T-cell functions (Brentjens et al. 2011; Davila et al. 2014; Grupp et al. 2013). Particular characteristics and optimization of the CAR depends on the assembly of those domains and their interaction with each other. Intense research is focused now on defining optimal CARs that provide robust clinical responses without collateral toxicities.

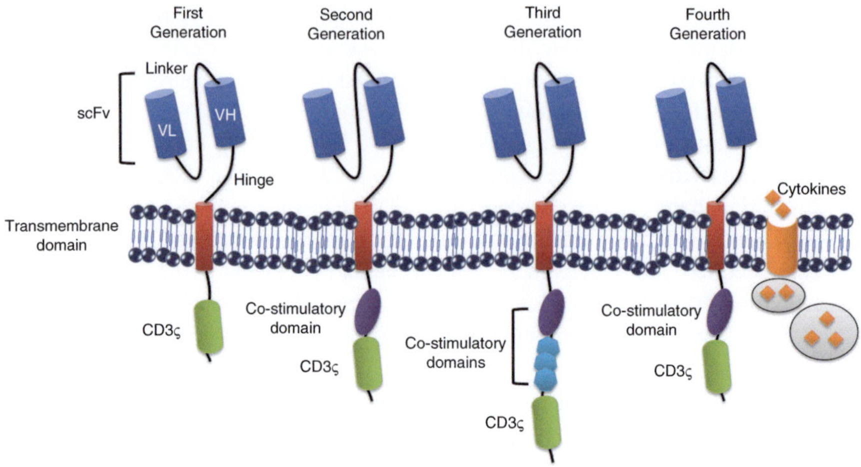

Fig. 3.1 The evolution of CAR-T-cell receptors

In theory, the native TCR complex signaling could participate in the signaling process as well. However, it appears the signaling process through the native TCR complex may be impaired, as implied by the lack of graft-versus-host disease in patients with B-cell acute lymphoblastic leukemia (ALL) who received allogeneic T cells modified to express CARs (Lee et al. 2015; Brudno et al. 2016; Maude et al. 2014). Nonetheless, some investigators have advocated the use of gene-editing techniques to eliminate the expression of native TCR molecules should this turn out to be a problem in future clinical trials using allogeneic T cells as a source of CAR-T cells (Torikai et al. 2012).

3.4 Gene Transfer into T Cells and CAR-T-Cell Expansion

The transfer of the genetic material encoding the CAR into the target cell can be achieved by virus vectors or by physical or mechanical procedures. The most commonly used virus vectors are gamma retrovirus or lentivirus, which each has the capacity to integrate into the host cell genome to potentially allow for long-term transgene expression. Lentivirus vectors have the added advantages of allowing for transgene expression in nondividing cells, being potentially less immunogenic and being able to deliver larger amounts of genetic material (Oldham et al. 2015). Despite concern about potentially disrupting essential genes through the insertion of the virus into the genome, so-called insertional mutagenesis, this has yet to be observed as a problem with the virus vectors used to produce CAR-T cells. Also, virus vectors that do not integrate into the genome, such as adenovirus vectors, allow for only transient gene expression that is not maintained in successive generations of daughter cells (Castro et al. 2012; Chirmule et al. 1999). For this reason, most translational teams use gamma retrovirus vectors or lentivirus vectors, and the selection of the virus-vector platform usually depends on the investigator's expertise with a particular vector system.

Nonetheless, there are examples of nonvector-mediated transfer. These include the transposon/transposase system (*Sleeping Beauty*) (Singh et al. 2015), electroporation of plasmids and in vitro transcribed mRNA among others (Jones et al. 2015). These vectors are much easier to make and to produce, thereby mitigating costs; however, it remains to be seen whether they can provide for the long-term expression of the transgene required for effective CAR-T-cell therapy.

Once gene transfer takes place, the next challenge is to generate large quantities of CAR-T cells using the rigorous Good Manufacturing Practice (GMP) standards that are required for infusion of the vector-modified CAR-T cells into patients. The first step of T-cell activation and expansion is achieved using anti-CD3 (OKT3 clone) plus anti-CD28 antibodies, anti-CD3/CD28 beads, or artificial antigen-presenting cells (Rushworth et al. 2014; Cooper 2015; Levine and June 2013). The final step requires addition of cytokines such as IL-2, IL-7, IL-12, IL-15, and/or IL-21 (Rosenberg and Restifo 2015; Levine and June 2013; Klebanoff et al. 2016). Again, the selected methodology depends greatly on the investigative team's expertise and use of cytokines required to obtain "optimal" expansion, which generally takes 2–6-week time.

Another important aspect is the phenotype of T cells to be amplified. Apheresis products obtained from patients typically contain naïve, central, effector, and possibly memory stem cells. Each subset could differ in their capacity to effect cytotoxicity of the target tumor cell and persist in the patient for sufficient time to be clinically effective. Defining the optimal composition of the "pool" of T cells to be expanded and the phenotype of the final product before infusion to the patient will require evaluation in clinical trials (Feldman et al. 2015).

Overall, one major challenge for CAR technology is the number of variables that needs to be adjusted to generate a product with reproducible characteristics from time to time and facility to facility. Ultimately, rigorous quality controls are required to monitor closely these biological products manufactured under GMP conditions.

3.5 Trafficking Homing and In Vivo Activity of CAR-T Cells

After infusion of CAR-T cells, they must home to the tumor cells and exert cytotoxic activity. As such, these engineered cells need to home to the site of the tumor, overcome immune-suppressive signals elaborated by the cancer cells and/or the tumor microenvironment, and persist and/or multiply to maintain effective immune surveillance against residual cancer cells. The biology involved in most of those steps is not fully known, but some recent findings have helped elucidate critical steps associated with each one of these processes.

Chemotherapy or radiation therapy is used as a conditioning regimen prior to infusion of CAR-T cells. Such conditioning improves CAR-T-cell trafficking, homing, and persistence by reducing the numbers of the patient's own lymphocytes, a process called *lymphodepletion*. Available data suggest that lymphodepletion enables the infused T cells to take advantage of the conditions that facilitate early stages of homing and proliferation. This process is mediated potentially by an inflammatory reaction of lymphoid and cancer tissues, as well as by depleting immune cells that otherwise could complete for resources, such as cytokines/chemokines. The end result is an environment where CAR-T cells find appropriate concentrations of driving cytokines as well as tissue-homing conditions for engraftment and proliferation. The timing of CAR-T-cell infusion after the lymphodepletion regimen also is critical and may determine the functional potential of the infused cells (Gill and June 2015; Oluwole and Davila 2016; Davila et al. 2012; Brentjens et al. 2011).

Another problem is defining the optimal dose of CAR-T cells that are required to mediate an effective antitumor effect. Most clinical trials have based CAR-T-cell dose on body surface area or the patient's weight. However, other factors may be more relevant, such as the extent of the patient's tumor burden, the type of conditioning regimen, the timing of the CAR-T-cell infusion, and the presence of in vivo cytokines or immune-suppressive factors that may enhance or mitigate the function of CAR-T cells (Lee et al. 2015; Chen et al. 2016).

The site of CAR-T-cell distribution and expansion has been studied using tracking techniques. In general, it appears that T cells are distributed throughout highly perfused organs, such as the lung, liver, and spleen (Dobrenkov et al. 2008; Parente-Pereira et al. 2011). After this initial phase of global distribution, CAR-T cells migrate toward tissues that bear the target antigen and/or may be induced to proliferate upon chance encounter with cells bearing the target antigen. Problems with the biodistribution of CAR-T cells and off-target effects can generate significant toxicity (Brudno and Kochenderfer 2016). Recruitment of the infused CAR-T cells and expansion in or near the tumor microenvironment depends on the microcirculation, expression level of the target antigen, and/or the tumor-cell expression of immune-suppressive checkpoint inhibitors of T-cell activation or proliferation (Cherkassky et al. 2016; Beavis et al. 2016).

In addition, the persistence of the CAR-T cells may be impacted by the development of an immune response against the CAR-T cells in the treated patient (Davis et al. 2010), thereby limiting the persistence of the CAR-T cells and limiting the potential for subsequent re-treatment with the same CAR-T cells. The scFv binding sites derived generally are derived from mouse antibodies, which may be more immunogenic than scFv derived from humanized antibodies. Also, the chimeric receptors themselves may make for neo-antigens that could be targeted by the patient's immune system.

After initial expansion of the CAR-T cells, it is important to maintain tumor surveillance and persistence of memory-type CAR-T cells. Certain cytokines, such as IL-7 and IL-15, play important roles in T-cell expansion and persistence of memory T cells without increasing the numbers of regulatory T cell (Barrett et al. 2014). The duration of persistence of CAR-T cells that will provide superior clinical outcome is unknown. However, one can speculate that ongoing CAR-T-cell immune surveillance is required to eradicate minimal residual disease and enhance the chances of achieving curative therapy. It is important to note that memory CAR-T cells can have a life span of many years and long-term follow-up of patients with HIV infections or hematological malignancies has shown that engineered T cells can be detected for more than 10 years after their infusion (Porter et al. 2011; Scholler et al. 2012).

New emerging technologies using cotransduction/transfection of bi-specific target-binding or cytokine domains into the CAR-T cells will allow enhancing these steps of trafficking, homing, and persistence (Magnani et al. 2016; Liu et al. 2016; Riet et al. 2013).

3.6 Cellular Immunotherapy for B-Cell Lymphoma and Leukemia

Our team at the University of California, San Diego (UCSD), conducted the first studies of cellular therapy applied to chronic lymphocytic leukemia (CLL) in the late 1990s, using autologous CLL leukemia cells transduced ex vivo with an adenovirus vector expressing chimeric (mouse/human) CD154 (Ad-CD154) (Castro et al. 2003; Wierda et al. 2000; Kato et al. 1998). The goal of these studies was to generate leukemia cells that express homologs of CD154 so that these cells would stimulate themselves and bystander leukemia cells into becoming proficient antigen-presenting cells capable of inducing antileukemia immune responses.

Transduction of CLL B cells with Ad-CD154 induced the leukemia cells to express immune co-stimulatory molecules, thereby enhancing their capacity to present antigens to autologous T lymphocytes (Kato et al. 1998). Eleven patients received a single infusion of autologous CLL cells transduced ex vivo with Ad-CD154 (Wierda et al. 2000). Nearly all treated patients exhibited increased serum levels of IL-12 and IFN-γ, enhanced expression of immune co-stimulatory molecules on bystander leukemia cells, increased absolute numbers of blood T cells, and reduced blood leukemia cell counts and lymph node size. After additional infusions of Ad-CD154-transduced cells, patients experienced stabilization of disease and/or regression, obviating early additional treatment. Two of the treated patients did not require additional therapy 4 years after treatment (Castro et al. 2003).

On subsequent studies, we tested an adenovirus vector expressing a membrane-stable humanized homolog of CD154 (Ad-ISF35) (Wierda et al. 2010). Patients with CLL (two previously untreated and seven with relapse/refractory disease) received dose-escalation administration of autologous leukemia cells transduced with Ad-ISF35. Similar to what was observed in patients receiving Ad-CD154, the infusions were well-tolerated; clinical benefit was observed in most patients, including patients with high-risk CLL cells that had deletions in the short arm of chromosome 17 (del17p).

We also investigated whether Ad-ISF35 could be directly injected into tumor-infiltrated lymph nodes of patients with CLL. Fifteen patients with CLL received a single ultrasound-guided injection into an enlarged lymph node of 1–30 × 10^{10} Ad-ISF35 viral particles in four different dose cohorts. Injections were well-tolerated with some patients developing local swelling, erythema, and "flu-like" symptoms. Some patients in the highest-dose cohorts had transient and asymptomatic hypophosphatemia and neutropenia. Ad-ISF35 intranodal injection resulted in significant reductions in blood leukemia cell counts, lymphadenopathy, and splenomegaly in the majority of patients. Although there was no evidence for dissemination of Ad-ISF35 beyond the injected lymph node, direct intranodal injection of Ad-ISF35 induced CLL cells circulating in the blood to express death receptors, pro-apoptotic proteins, and immune co-stimulatory molecules, suggesting a "bystander" systemic effect (Castro et al. 2009).

These studies using transduced autologous CLL cells with homologs of CD154 showed the potential to elicit an antileukemia immune response even in patients who have been pretreated with immunosuppressive therapy. Moreover, the antileukemia effect was associated with antibody production against a leukemia-associated surface antigen, which we identified as ROR1 (Fukuda et al. 2008). ROR1 is an oncoembryonic surface antigen and survival-signaling receptor for Wnt5a. We concluded that patients treated with Ad-CD154 transduced CLL cells had significant immune stimulation leading to a break in immune-tolerance to leukemia-associated antigens, such as ROR1.

Our current efforts have focused on development of CAR-T cells that express a svFV specific for ROR1, with the goal of engineering T cells that are cytotoxic for cells bearing this antigen, which is expressed on the neoplastic cells of a variety of human cancers, but not on normal postpartum tissues (Deniger et al. 2015). Using the Sleeping Beauty transposon system, we constructed second-generation ROR1-specific CARs, signaling through CD3ζ and either CD28 (designated ROR1RCD28) or CD137 (designated ROR1RCD137). After transfection, we selected and expanded T cells expressing CARs through co-culture with gamma-irradiated artificial APC cells (AaPC), which co-expressed ROR1 and immune co-stimulatory molecules. Such T cells produced interferon-gamma and had specific cytotoxic activity against $ROR1^+$ tumors. Moreover, such cells could eliminate $ROR1^+$ tumor xenografts, especially T cells expressing ROR1RCD137. We anticipate that current and future clinical trials will help us investigate the ability of ROR1-CAR-T cells to specifically eliminate tumor cells, while maintaining normal B cells, in patients with CLL and other $ROR1^+$ malignancies (NCT02194374).

3.7 CAR-T Cells for B-Cell Lymphoma and Leukemia

The first clinical study using CAR-T cells in hematological malignancies was reported in patients with indolent lymphoma that received T cells that had been electroporated to express an anti-CD20 target-binding domain (Till et al. 2008). Most patients achieved stable disease and toxicities that were manageable; the engineered T cells persisted in treated patients for up to 9 weeks. This proof-of-concept study inspired a rapid development in the field; since 2010 the number of publications has been expanding exponentially (Table 3.1).

Different subtypes of B-cell malignancies have been treated with CAR-T cells to date, including acute and chronic lymphocytic leukemia, as well as low- or high-grade lymphoma. Collectively, these clinical trials have allowed us to evaluate

Table 3.1 Summary of CAR therapy trials for hematologic malignancies

References	No. of patients	Disease	Conditioning regimen	Gene transfer	Target	Cell dose/kg	Response rates CR (%)	Response rates PR (%)	Comments
Brudno et al. (2016)	20	B-cell malignancies	None	Gamma retrovirus	CD19	$1–10 \times 10^6$	30	10	Allogeneic T cells that express an anti-CD19 chimeric antigen receptor
Kalos et al. (2011) Porter et al. (2015)	14	CLL	FLU/CY, PC, Benda	Lentivirus	CD19	$0.14–11 \times 10^8$	29	28	Anti-CD19 CAR-T cells persisted for 14–19 months in some patients
Lee et al. (2015)	21	ALL or NHL	FLU/CY	Retrovirus	CD19	$1–3 \times 10^6$	67	NA	Anti-CD19 CAR-T cells. ALL pediatric or young adults (1–30 years)
Kochenderfer et al. (2015)	14	NHL	FLU/CY	Gamma retrovirus	CD19	$0.3–5.0 \times 10^6$	36	36	Anti-CD19 CAR-T cells. Duration of ongoing CR responses (9–22 months)
Chapuis et al. (2013)	11	Leukemia	Per discretion of treating physician	WT1-specific donor-derived $CD8^+$ cytotoxic T cell	WT1	$3.3 \times 10^9/m^2$–$3.3 \times 10^{10}/m^2$	0	0	HLA A*0201-restricted WT1-specific donor-derived $CD8^+$ cytotoxic T-cell clones were administered post-HCT
Davila et al. (2014) Brentjens et al. (2013)	16	ALL	CY	Retrovirus	CD19	3×10^6	88	NA	Anti-CD19 CAR-T cells. Relapsed/refractory ALL adults. One patient received less than the study dose
Maude et al. (2014) Grupp et al. (2013)	25 5	ALL	Per discretion of treating physician	Lentivirus	CD19	$0.8–21 \times 10^6$	99	NA	Anti-CD19 CAR-T cells. 25 pediatric patients and 5 adult patients

(continued)

Table 3.1 (continued)

References	No. of patients	Disease	Conditioning regimen	Gene transfer	Target	Cell dose/kg	Response rates CR (%)	PR (%)	Comments
Cruz et al. (2013)	4	ALL	None	Retrovirus	CD19	3.2×10^7–1.1×10^8	75	0	Retroviral FMC63 anti-CD19 scFv-CD28-CD3
	4	CLL					0	0	
Kochenderfer et al. (2013)	15	NHL	FLU/CY	Retrovirus	CD19	$1–5 \times 10^6$	53	27	Retroviral FMC63 anti-CD19 scFv-CD28-CD3
Ritchie et al. (2013)	4	AML	FLU/CY	Gamma retrovirus	LeY	$1.4–9.2 \times 10^6$	25	25	Anti-LeY CAR-T cells persisted up to 10 months
Kochenderfer et al. (2012)	7	CLL/NHL	FLU/CY	Gamma retrovirus	CD19	$0.3–4.0 \times 10^6$	43	43	Anti-CD19 CAR-T cells. CAR-T cells persisted <3 months
Till et al. (2012)	3	NHL	CY	Electroporation	CD20	1×10^8/m^2–3.3×10^9/m^2	0	33	Ani-CD20 CAR-T cells. CAR-T cells persisted 9–12 months
Brentjens et al. (2011)	3	CLL	None	Gamma retrovirus	CD19	$1.2–3.0 \times 10^7$	0	0	Anti-CD19 CAR-T cells. This trial included a CAR-T-cell dose escalation and also compared responses in patients treated with or without conditioning chemotherapy before CAR-T-cell infusion
	4		CY	Gamma retrovirus	CD19	$0.4–1.0 \times 10^7$	0	25	Anti-CD19 CAR-T cells. The CY dose (up to 3 g/m^2) is the lowest amount of conditioning treatment among the published trials evaluating CD19-targeted CAR-T cells for NHL
Kalos et al. (2011)	3	CLL	Per discretion of treating physician	Lentivirus	CD19	1.46×10^5–1.6×10^7	100	0	Patients were given a single course of chemotherapy during the week before infusion

Savoldo et al. (2011)	6	NHL	None	Retrovirus	CD19	2×10^7/m^2–2×10^8/m^2	0	0	Retroviral FMC63 anti-CD19 scFv-CD3f and anti-CD19 scFv-CD28-CD3. CAR persistence for 6 weeks
Kochenderfer et al. (2010)	1	Lymphoma	FLU/CY	Retrovirus	CD19	1–3×10^8	100	0	First use of anti-CD19 CAR
Jensen et al. (2010)	2	DLBCL	FLU	Retrovirus	CD19	2×10^9/m^2	100	0	Retroviral FMC63 anti-CD19 scFv-CD3 with thymidine kinase suicide gene
	2	FL					0	0	
Till et al. (2008)	7	NHL	FLU or CY	Electroporation	CD20	1×10^8/m^2–3.3×10^9/m^2	29	14	Anti-CD20 CAR-T cells. CAR-T cells persisted 5–9 weeks

different genetic transfer methods, construct designs, immune co-stimulatory molecules, different T-cell expansion protocols, cell doses, and lymphodepletion regimens (Jensen et al. 2010; Oluwole and Davila 2016; Savoldo et al. 2011; Porter et al. 2011).

The following are important conclusion from those studies: (1) lymphodepletion can promote engraftment and expansion (cyclophosphamide, with or without fludarabine, is most commonly used); (2) second-generation constructs that carry at least one co-stimulatory molecule are more potent; (3) the most responsive disease to date is B-cell ALL; (4) adverse events can be of high grade and include CRS and neurotoxicity; (5) there does not appear to be a clear dose-response relationship between the amount of infused CAR-T cells and the clinical response; (6) CAR-T cells can penetrate the central nervous system, making it possible that CAR-T cells are responsible, at least in part, to the neurotoxicity observed in some treated patients; (7) CRS is mediated in part by the activation of macrophages; and (8) allogeneic donor cells conserve their proliferative and cytotoxic potential and do not appear to induce GvHD (Table 3.2) (Davila et al. 2014; Feldman et al. 2015; Brudno et al. 2016; Cruz et al. 2013).

Despite the excellent initial response observed in patients with B-cell ALL after anti-CD19 CAR-T-cell therapy, it is of concern that some patients relapse with blast cells that are CD19 negative. This appears to result from the selection of variant tumor cells that have lost expression of this B-lineage surface antigen, indicating the potential need for CAR-T cells that target different surface antigens to completely eradicate residual disease; target surface antigens that have been examined in preclinical models for the treatment of B-cell malignancies include CD22, CD23, or ROR1 (Deniger et al. 2015; Haso et al. 2013; Giordano Attianese et al. 2011; Berger et al. 2015). As expected, there are potential advantages and disadvantages of each model, the level of expression of the target molecule in each pathological subtype, variability of expression within the tumor, expression in healthy cells/tissue, and potential for off-target effects are some of the limiting factors that will affect the development of CAR-T cells specific for such target antigens.

3.8 CAR-T-Cell Therapy for Acute Myeloid Leukemia (AML)

Patients with relapsed/refractory AML have a very poor prognosis and high mortality rate. The standard treatment for such patients is allo-HCT, which carries a high risk for complications, such as infection or GvHD, leading to high transplant-related mortality (Schiller 2013). Immune-effector mechanisms may account for the fact that patients with AML appear to have a better outcome following allogeneic stem cell transplantation than autologous stem cell transplantation. However, because AML is a malignancy of the hematopoietic stem cell, it is challenging to find a target antigen that is expressed by AML blast cells that is not expressed on normal hematopoietic stem cells.

For sure, a clinical trial has used CAR-T cells to treat patients with AML. The group at the University of Melbourne treated four patients with a CD28-co-stimulated retrovirus-transduced CAR-T-cell product targeting the Lewis Y

Table 3.2 Ongoing CAR-T-cell trials in hematologic malignancies

Disease	Gene transfer	Target	Center	Comments	Clinicaltrials.gov ID	Clinicaltrials.gov Status
CLL	Retrovirus	CD19	MSKCC	Dose escalation	NCT00466531	Recruiting
B-cell malignancies	Retrovirus	CD19	BCM	With ipilimumab	NCT00586391	Active, not recruiting
				Dose escalation	NCT00608270	Active, not recruiting
				After allo-HCT, viral co-specificity	NCT00840853	Active, not recruiting
B-cell malignancies	Retrovirus	CD19	NCI	With IL-2	NCT00924326	Active, not recruiting
B-cell lymphoma	Retrovirus	CD19	MDACC	With or without IL-2	NCT00968760	Active, not recruiting
B-cell ALL	Retrovirus	CD19	MSKCC		NCT01044069	Recruiting
CLL	Retrovirus	CD19	MSKCC	Upfront therapy	NCT01416974	Active, not recruiting
B-cell ALL	Retrovirus	CD19	MSKCC	After allo-HCT, viral co-specificity	NCT01430390	Recruiting
B-cell malignancies	NA	CD19	MDACC	After allo-HCT	NCT01497184	Active, not recruiting
B-cell malignancies	NA	CD19	NCI		NCT01593696	Active, not recruiting
$CD19^+$ ALL	NA	CD19	Seattle Children's	$EGFR^+$ construct (may allow deletion)	NCT01683279	Active, not recruiting
CLL/SLL	Lentivirus	CD19	ACCUP	2 dose level comparison	NCT01747486	Recruiting

(continued)

Table 3.2 (continued)

Disease	Gene transfer	Target	Center	Comments	Clinicaltrials.gov ID	Clinicaltrials.gov Status
Aggressive B-NHL, relapsed/refractory	Retrovirus	CD19	MSKCC	After autologous SCT	NCT01840566	Active, not recruiting
B-cell ALL	Retrovirus	CD19	MSKCC		NCT01860937	Recruiting
B-cell malignancies	NA	CD19	Beijing		NCT01864889	Recruiting
B-cell malignancies	Lentivirus	CD19	FHCRC		NCT01865617	Recruiting
B-cell NHL	Lentivirus	CD19	Penn		NCT02030834	Recruiting
B-cell ALL	Lentivirus	CD19	Seattle Children's	$EGFR^+$ construct (may allow deletion)	NCT02028455	Recruiting
B-cell ALL	Lentivirus	CD19	ACCUP		NCT02030847	Recruiting
B-cell malignancies	Retrovirus	CD19	BCM	After allo-HCT	NCT02050347	Recruiting
MCL	NA	CD19	Beijing		NCT02081937	Recruiting
B-cell malignancies	Retrovirus	CD19	Sweden		NCT02132624	Recruiting
B-cell NHL	Retrovirus	CD19	Japan		NCT02134262	Recruiting
B-cell malignancies	NA	CD19	China	Sequential CAR-T bridging HCT	NCT02846584	Recruiting
B-cell malignancies	NA	CD19	China		NCT02782351	Recruiting
B-cell malignancies	NA	CD19	NCI		NCT02659943	Recruiting
B-cell lymphoma	NA	CD19	China		NCT02547948	Recruiting
B-cell lymphoma	NA	CD19	Peking University		NCT02247609	Recruiting
B-cell malignancies	NA	CD20	China		NCT02710149	Recruiting
B-cell malignancies	NA	CD22	China		NCT02794961	Recruiting

CD30+ lymphoma (CARCD30)	EBV CTLs	CD30	BCM	EBV CTLs expressing CD30 chimeric receptors	NCT01192464	Active, not recruiting
HL/NHL (CART CD30)	EBV CTLs	CD30	UNCLCCC		NCT01316146	Active, not recruiting
B-cell malignancy or myeloma	Retrovirus	Kappa light chain	BCM		NCT00881920	Recruiting
CLL/SLL	NA	ROR1	MDACC/UCSD		NCT02194374	Active, not recruiting
ALL	Lentivirus	CD19	UCL, Great Ormond Hospital-UK	UCART19-universal donor CAR-T cells	NCT02808442	Recruiting

antigen, a carbohydrate antigen that is expressed by many human tumors (Ritchie et al. 2013). Minimal toxicity was observed and two patients experienced minor responses. Of interest, trafficking studies, using radiolabeled CAR-T cells, showed migration of T cells to sites of the disease. Moreover, one patients with leukemia cutis developed inflammation in a cutaneous lesion, which upon biopsy was found to have CAR-T cells. However, clinical responses were not evident in most patients, despite prolonged persistence of the CAR-T cells, suggesting more work needs to be done to define the target antigen(s) and/or type of CAR-T cell that may be most effective.

Another potential target in AML for development of CAR-T cells is CD123 (IL-3 receptor), expressed both on AML blasts and hematopoietic precursor cells. There is an ongoing clinical study at the City of Hope in Los Angeles, investigating the use of a lentivirus vector to generate CAR-T cells expressing a CD123-binding CAR, which is the CD123-specific, hinge-optimized, CD28-costimulatory construct (NCT02159495).

CD33 also is a potential target, based on the noted clinical activity of the anti-CD33 antibody gemtuzumab ozogamicin in patients with AML (Laszlo et al. 2014). Preclinical studies demonstrated that cytokine-induced killer (CIK) T cells genetically modified to express anti-CD33, or anti-CD123, CARs are cytotoxic for human AML cells engrafted on NOD-SCID IL2Rγnull mice. However, because CD33, like CD123, is expressed by hematopoietic precursor cells, there is a risk that CD33-directed CAR-T cells also may be cytotoxic for hematopoietic stem cells. Early preclinical studies suggest that CD33 CAR-T cells may be more toxic for hematopoietic stem/progenitor cells (HSPCs) than CD123-directed CAR-T cells (Pizzitola et al. 2014).

Other antigens include CD44v6, a CD44 isoform expressed on some AML blasts and myeloma cells. Anti-CD44v6 CAR-T cells mediated potent antitumor effects in mouse models (Casucci et al. 2013). However, this splice variant is expressed on keratinocytes, potentially contributing to the skin inflammation observed in patients treated with anti-CD44v6 mAbs (Casucci et al. 2013). Other antigens that are expressed on HSPCs and could be potential targets for CAR-T cells include CD123, CD47, or CD96, CLL-1, (CLEC12A). However, because expression of these antigens is not restricted to the tumor cells, there is the risk for side effects due to off-target cytotoxicity, constituting perhaps the major obstacle for translation of such CARs to the clinic.

A series of AML-associated antigens were identified using SEREX screening of recombinant cDNA expression libraries from newly diagnosed acute myeloid leukemia (AML) patients. The antigens found included PASD1, SSX2IP, and GRINL1A. RT-PCR analysis showed that these antigens are expressed in AML cells, but not in blood cells of healthy adults. Moreover, antigen presentation assays, using monocyte-derived dendritic cells (mo-DCs), showed that PASD1 could stimulate autologous T cells, suggesting that PASD1 could be a promising target for future immunotherapy clinical trials, including CAR-T-cell-based adoptive immunotherapy (Guinn et al. 2005).

3.9 CAR-T-Cell Therapy for Hodgkin Lymphoma

The hallmarks of Hodgkin lymphoma (HL) are Reed-Sternberg (HRS) cells and a lack of B-cell-associated surface antigens. Instead, HL has intense expression of CD15 and CD30. CD30 can be targeted with brentuximab vedotin, which is an antibody-drug conjugate (ADC) that has produced clinical responses in HL patients who were refractory to chemotherapy. Because of that success, CD30 appears to be a suitable candidate for CAR-T-cell therapy. This has been confirmed through in vitro studies of HL cell lines targeted with anti-CD30 CAR-T cells, as well as in preclinical and clinical studies using an anti-CD30/CD16A bi-specific antibody construct AFM13 (Rothe et al. 2015). There are at least two trials targeting CD30 for treatment of patients with HL (NCT01192464 and NCT01316146).

3.10 CAR-T-Cell Therapy for Myeloma

Multiple myeloma (MM) is still a non-curable disease, despite advances in bone marrow transplantation and biological targeted therapy (Rajkumar 2015). Therefore, there is a need for novel immunotherapy-based strategies. Currently, there are two mAbs approved by the FDA for treatment of patients with refractory MM, daratumumab (anti-CD38 antibody) and elotuzumab (antibody directed against signaling lymphocyte activation molecule family 7—SLAMF7). The clinical activity of these two mAbs makes use of the antigens they find attractive targets for the development of CAR-T cells.

The initial encouraging results from early-phase clinical trials of anti-CD19 CARs for B-cell malignancies prompted interest to test these CAR-T cells in patients with MM. The group from the University of Pennsylvania reported on one patient with refractory MM who received an infusion of anti-CD19 CAR-T cells after myeloablative chemotherapy and autologous stem cell transplantation. One patient achieved a complete response with no evidence of disease progression and no measurable MM protein. What is probably more remarkable is the fact that 99.9% of the malignant plasma cells from this patient did not express CD19, raising the intriguing possibility that the CD19-CAR-T cells targeted a myeloma precursor/stem cell that expresses CD19 and that this was responsible for the observed clinical activity (NCT02135406) (Garfall et al. 2015).

Both CD138 and CD38 are highly expressed by plasma cells but also by epithelial cells and erythrocytes, respectively. This is a potential problem for the development of CAR-T cells that target these antigens. Currently, there is an ongoing phase I/II clinical trial of a CD137-costimulated CAR-T cells against CD138 in Beijing (NCT01886976). Other ongoing preclinical work and CAR-T cell clinical studies are focusing on alternative MM targets, including immunoglobulin kappa light chains, CD138, Lewis Y antigen, B-cell maturation antigen (BCMA), CD38, or the cell surface glycoprotein SLAMF7 (CD319, CS1), which is targeted by elotuzumab, as noted above (Rotolo et al. 2016; Oden et al. 2015; Peinert et al. 2010; Jiang et al.

2014; Drent et al. 2016; Chu et al. 2014). Most of these clinical trials are designed to infuse the CAR-T cells after treating the patients with high-dose chemotherapy and autologous hematopoietic cell transplant; this is to examine whether such CAR-T cells can eradicate minimal-residual disease and/or prolong progression free survival.

3.11 CAR-T-Cell Therapy for T-Cell Malignancies

Patients with T-cell non-Hodgkin lymphoma (NHL) typically have a poor prognosis. Contrary to B-cell lymphomas, standard treatments are not defined, owing to the rarity of T-cell lymphomas relative to B-cell lymphoma and relative dearth of clinical trials. Consequently, there has been only very modest clinical progress in this area.

Targeting T cells with immune-based strategies also is proving to be challenging, mainly because the T cells are cellular vehicles of CAR-T-cell therapy; as such, it is challenging to find T-cell tumor antigens that are expressed by T-cell lymphomas, but not by normal T cells.

Based on previous clinical and preclinical data, T-cell-associated antigens that may be targeted include:

(1) CD30—this is based on the good responses to brentuximab observed in patients with anaplastic large cell lymphoma (Batlevi et al. 2016).
(2) CD52—this is based on the observed activity of alemtuzumab (an anti-CD52 antibody) in T-cell prolymphocytic leukemia and T-cell NHL (Gribben and Hallek 2009).
(3) CD25 (IL-2 receptor)—this is based on the anti-T-NHL activity of CD25-directed denileukin diftitox (Ontak), a fusion protein with interleukin-2 linked to enzymatically active, membrane translocation domains of diphtheria toxin. This chimeric protein is approved by the FDA based on clinical responses in patients with recurrent or persistent cutaneous T-cell lymphoma (CTCL). In addition, the anti-CD25 antibody (basiliximab) is active in GvHD prophylaxis and therapy of active GvHD (Schmidt-Hieber et al. 2005).
(4) EBV-associated proteins—this is based on a recent clinical trial involving patients with NK/T cell lymphomas who were treated with EBV LMP1- and LMP2a-specific cytotoxic T cells.

Even though this trial did not involve the use of CAR-T cells, it showed that specific effector cells against EBV-associated antigens expressed in NK and T cells may be useful in patients with this type of NHL (Cho et al. 2015). However, the problem remains that CAR-T cells engineered to express receptors could be suicidal, making it potentially necessary to consider other effector cells to mediate CAR-directed therapy for T-cell lymphomas, such as natural killer (NK) cells.

3.12 What Are the CARs of the Future

The technological advances in cellular engineering are moving at a fast pace, and more and more CAR models are being tested in vitro and in animal models that are being considered for use in clinical trials. Here are some examples of these platforms:

3.12.1 Combinatorial Antigen-Recognition CARs

Current T-cell engineering approaches redirect patient T cells to tumors by transducing them with one antigen-specific receptor. However, using this strategy, T cells are transduced with two CARs, one that provides suboptimal activation upon binding of one antigen and a second chimeric co-stimulatory receptor (CCR), which recognizes a second antigen. When both CARs are engaged, the activation signal is amplified. This increases the specificity of CAR activation and overcome the need for expression of a solitary tumor-specific antigen on the targeted tumor cell. So far this has been tested using the prostate tumor antigens PSMA and PSCA with good results in vitro (Kloss et al. 2013).

3.12.2 Inhibitory Signaling CARs

This technology takes advantage of the negative feedback loops that regulate cellular signaling, particularly in T cells. Using this design, two CARs are introduced in the T cell. The first one is the activating chimeric receptor, and the second CAR has an inhibitory component, or iCAR, derived from the cytoplasmic domains of immune checkpoint inhibitors, such as CTLA-4- or PD-1. The activation and expansion of these iCARs are modulated by the balance provided by the activation/inhibitory signal, potentially allowing for less toxic antigen recognition, proliferation, and cytotoxic effects. These iCARs provide a dynamic, self-regulating safety switch, which could prevent consequences of inadequate T-cell specificity.

3.12.3 Off-the-Shelf (OTS)–CARs

This is probably one of the most promising strategies that are currently under development. OTS–CARs respond to multiple challenges currently posed by the clinical expansion and application of adoptive cellular therapy using cellular engineering. One of those is the unparalleled logistics involved in the process of production of the patient's product, the rigorous quality controls involved in the process, and, probably the most important, the time that this process takes before the cellular product is delivered to the patient requiring therapy. The delay in generating personalized T-cell products could be highly problematic for patients afflicted with eminently life-threatening malignancies. The ideal OTS-CAR should meet at least some of the following requirements: (1) A cellular product that can be prepared and cryopreserved in advance. (2) The source of the immune cells ideally should be from healthy donors previously screened for certain characteristics. (3) A biological product that already is characterized with lots that are predetermined based on cellular characteristics, activity and other quality control tests. (4) A product that has been generated in a centralized manufacturing facility, meeting standards that allow for reproducibility and comparability, mitigating the risk for batch-to-batch variation in cellular product. (5) A product that is ready to be shipped whenever there is need, minimizing the time required for the patient to wait prior to therapy. (6) A biological product that can be given to nearly all patients, using cells manipulated through gene-editing techniques to remove endogenous TCRs, MHC antigens, and/or minor histocompatibility antigens that potentially could be targeted by the patient's immune system resulting in an anti-CAR-T-cell immune response that rejects the CAR-T cells.

An example of the clinical application of these OTS-CARs was recently reported on a pediatric patient with ALL who was treated on a single-patient protocol under a compassionate-use IND (Qasim et al. 2015). In this report allogeneic HLA-mismatched donor T cells were transduced using a third-generation self-inactivating lentivirus vector encoding a 4g7 CAR19 (CD19 scFv-41BB-CD3ζ) linked to RQR8, an abbreviated sort/suicide gene encoding both CD34 and CD20 epitopes. Alloreactivity and the risk of lethal GvHD were mitigated using *transcription activator-like effector nucleases* (TALENs), which allowed for gene editing of endogenous TCR and CD52 (rendering the cells insensitive to alemtuzumab (anti-CD52 antibody), which was used in vivo as conditioning agent). This universal CAR19 (UCART19) cell bank has been characterized in detail, including sterility, molecular and cytometric analyses, and human/murine functional studies. The patient treated was an infant with refractory B-cell ALL who already had allo-HCT. As part of the cytoreductive chemotherapy regimen, the patient received alemtuzumab prior to infusion of UCART19 cells. The patient tolerated the T-cell infusion well without any observed toxicity or manifestations of CRS. The patient showed a good clinical response with a molecular complete response, reconstitution of donor chimerism, and persistence of detectable UCART19 T cells. This example represents the first-in-man application of TALEN-engineered T cells and provides proof of concept for OTS-CAR-T-cell applications that currently are undergoing testing in early-phase clinical trials (NCT02808442).

3.13 Expert Point of View

The applications of adopted cellular therapy are expanding exponentially, bringing exciting therapeutic alternatives to patients with intractable cancers. Moreover, the expectation is that CAR-T-cell-based immunotherapy will expand beyond oncology into areas such as infectious diseases, autoimmunity, or immune deficiency.

As we see the brisk progress in the field, we also need to realize the importance to address and resolve critical questions before translating these discoveries to the clinic.

The CAR design in itself possesses a big challenge. As described at the beginning of this chapter, there are at least five domains that constitute the basic structure of a CAR, and each one of them could and will be modified and improved in the near future. Evaluation of first-generation and second-generation CARs showed an enhanced persistence and expansion capabilities from the latter (Savoldo et al. 2011). In addition, most CARs are currently derived from murine antibodies, and this increases the risk of human anti-mouse antibodies. Humanization or the target-binding domain will probably abrogate the development of this immunological reaction (Gattenlöhner et al. 2006). How to assemble the most efficient and appropriate CAR for each medical condition will require significant amount of basic research and ultimately evaluation in human subjects. Hence, it is important to conduct clinical trials in a safe and cost-efficient manner.

Optimization of gene transfer methods and large-scale production and expansion of engineered T cells will be required to meet future demands of these new treatments. This will require the development of new equipment and specialized facilities, implementation and optimization of standard operating procedures and the training of expert technicians in the field. Several pharmaceutical companies had established strategic partnerships with academic institutions in an effort to lead this effort (Brewer 2015).

It is likely that the development of adoptive immunotherapy will need to parallel the redundancy that is observed in the normal immune system, which is used to tackle complex problems such as infection and cancer (Casadevall and Pirofski 2003). Most likely, we will need to engineer cells that express more than one CAR to provide that immunological redundancy or infuse a mixture of engineered T cells with different CAR targets/specificities. Furthermore, we might be able to infuse more than one type of effector cell to generate the "perfect immunological cocktail," using redirected engineered T and NK cells, macrophages, dendritic cells, etc. Most likely, "One size will not fit all," and consequently, we will need to develop tailored immune-reconstitution protocols based on adoptive cellular therapy for each specific disease.

Availability of these new immunotherapy treatments is going to be limited and initially accessible only to patients in large specialized centers in the USA, Europe, Australia, Japan, and China (countries that currently have open CAR-T-cell-based protocols). Broadening the coverage of adoptive cellular therapy will require the development of simplified protocols, the use of more effective and safer versions of CARs, and most likely the availability of universal OTS-CARs that can guarantee easier logistics and shorter times for release and shipment of the cellular product.

Once approved by the FDA, the cost of these novel adoptive cellular therapies will become one of an important factor limiting wider use. As we have observed with any new therapy approved in oncology, the cost of the new therapy is always higher than the one of its predecessor. The financial aspects of drug cost and coverage may limit accessibility. In the particular case of CAR-T-cell therapy, we will need to take into consideration not only the cost of manufacturing and administering the engineered T cells but also the cost of management of adverse events and potentially prolonged hospitalizations.

Although the most dramatic results using adoptive immunotherapy have been seen with CAR-T cells, their main problem is that their recognition is limited to cell surface structures. Contrary to that, T-cell receptors (TCRs) can recognize intracellular proteins that could correspond to mutated, misfolded, or overexpressed cancer-associated proteins (Harris and Kranz 2016). Additional studies will be required to define the role of each one of these target-binding platforms and their applicability to cancer therapy.

Another important question is what is the preferred source of cells for adoptive immunotherapy. The majority of studies published to date have used autologous T cells to generate CAR-T cells. This obviates HLA matching and endogenous virus testing. However, it is not certain whether autologous T cells from cancer patients are optimal for generating effective CAR-T cells. Many cancer patients are elderly, and their immune system may be debilitated due to illness, prior therapy, and the inherent biology of their disease (Frumento et al. 2006). On the other hand, healthier allogeneic T cells from younger donors may be better able to proliferate and function, particularly when barriers regarding HLA matching can be minimized by selecting haploidentical or matched unrelated donor cells that are engineered using genetic editing techniques (Qasim et al. 2015). Very likely, those genetic editing tools will make it possible to provide off-the-shelf (OTS) adoptive cellular immunotherapy for immediate administration whenever they are needed. In fact, OTS cellular therapy could solve some of the major obstacles related to immediacy, logistics, and quality consistency required to expand the use of cellular immunotherapy beyond a few academic centers.

CAR-T-cell resistance can be a potential problem due to loss of the target antigen on the surface of the tumor cell (Grupp et al. 2013). The risk for selecting tumors that lack the target antigen may be mitigated using CAR-T cells with two (or more) CARs that react with different target antigens (Roybal et al. 2016; Hegde et al. 2013).

Overall, adoptive immunotherapy using CAR-T cells represents a tremendous advancement toward effective cancer therapy. As seen with other discoveries, now we probably have more questions than answers, and methodical research will help to address those issues. Patients in desperate need for alternative treatments already have benefited from this approach. Definitely, the road ahead looks promising for CARs and other cellular-based therapies. Overcoming the challenges associated with the use of this new technology should optimize the use of these powerful new weapons against cancer.

References

Barrett DM, Singh N, Liu X, Jiang S, June CH, Grupp SA et al (2014) Relation of clinical culture method to T-cell memory status and efficacy in xenograft models of adoptive immunotherapy. Cytotherapy 16(5):619–630

Batlevi CL, Matsuki E, Brentjens RJ, Younes A (2016) Novel immunotherapies in lymphoid malignancies. Nat Rev Clin Oncol 13(1):25–40

Beavis PA, Slaney CY, Kershaw MH, Gyorki D, Neeson PJ, Darcy PK (2016) Reprogramming the tumor microenvironment to enhance adoptive cellular therapy. Semin Immunol 28(1):64–72

Berger C, Sommermeyer D, Hudecek M, Berger M, Balakrishnan A, Paszkiewicz PJ et al (2015) Safety of targeting ROR1 in primates with chimeric antigen receptor-modified T cells. Cancer Immunol Res 3(2):206–216

Brentjens RJ, Riviere I, Park JH, Davila ML, Wang X, Stefanski J et al (2011) Safety and persistence of adoptively transferred autologous CD19-targeted T cells in patients with relapsed or chemotherapy refractory B-cell leukemias. Blood 118(18):4817–4828

Brentjens RJ, Davila ML, Riviere I, Park J, Wang X, Cowell LG et al (2013) CD19-targeted T cells rapidly induce molecular remissions in adults with chemotherapy-refractory acute lymphoblastic leukemia. Sci Transl Med 5(177):177ra38

Brewer V. The CAR-T Cell-Race 2015. Available from: http://www.the-scientist.com/?articles.view/articleNo/42462/title/The-CAR-T-Cell-Race/

Brown CE, Starr R, Aguilar B, Shami AF, Martinez C, D'Apuzzo M et al (2012) Stem-like tumor-initiating cells isolated from IL13Rα2 expressing gliomas are targeted and killed by IL13-zetakine-redirected T cells. Clin Cancer Res 18(8):2199–2209

Brudno JN, Kochenderfer JN (2016) Toxicities of chimeric antigen receptor T cells: recognition and management. Blood 127(26):3321–3330

Brudno JN, Somerville RP, Shi V, Rose JJ, Halverson DC, Fowler DH et al (2016) Allogeneic T cells that express an anti-CD19 chimeric antigen receptor induce remissions of B-cell malignancies that progress after allogeneic hematopoietic stem-cell transplantation without causing graft-versus-host disease. J Clin Oncol 34(10):1112–1121

Casadevall A, Pirofski LA (2003) Exploiting the redundancy in the immune system: vaccines can mediate protection by eliciting 'unnatural' immunity. J Exp Med 197(11):1401–1404

Castro JE, Cantwell MJ, Prussak CE, Bole J, Wierda WG, Kipps TJ (2003) Long-term follow up of chronic lymphocytic leukemia patients treated with CD40-ligand (CD154) gene therapy. Blood 102(11):Abstract 1790

Castro JE, Sandoval-Sus JD, Melo-Cardenas J, Darrah D, Urquiza M, Pakbaz RS et al (2009) Phase I study of intranodal direct injection of adenovirus encoding recombinant CD40-ligand (Ad-ISF35) in patients with chronic lymphocytic leukemia. J Clin Oncol 27(15s):suppl; abstr 3003

Castro JE, Melo-Cardenas J, Urquiza M, Barajas-Gamboa JS, Pakbaz RS, Kipps TJ (2012) Gene immunotherapy of chronic lymphocytic leukemia: a phase I study of intranodally injected adenovirus expressing a chimeric CD154 molecule. Cancer Res 72(12):2937–2948

Casucci M, Nicolis di Robilant B, Falcone L, Camisa B, Norelli M, Genovese P et al (2013) CD44v6-targeted T cells mediate potent antitumor effects against acute myeloid leukemia and multiple myeloma. Blood 122(20):3461–3472

Chapuis AG, Ragnarsson GB, Nguyen HN, Chaney CN, Pufnock JS, Schmitt TM et al (2013) Transferred WT1-reactive CD8+ T cells can mediate antileukemic activity and persist in post-transplant patients. Sci Transl Med 5(174):174ra27

Chen F, Teachey DT, Pequignot E, Frey N, Porter D, Maude SL et al (2016) Measuring IL-6 and sIL-6R in serum from patients treated with tocilizumab and/or siltuximab following CAR T cell therapy. J Immunol Methods 434:1–8

Cherkassky L, Morello A, Villena-Vargas J, Feng Y, Dimitrov DS, Jones DR et al (2016) Human CAR T cells with cell-intrinsic PD-1 checkpoint blockade resist tumor-mediated inhibition. J Clin Invest 126(8):3130–3144

Chirmule N, Propert K, Magosin S, Qian Y, Qian R, Wilson J (1999) Immune responses to adenovirus and adeno-associated virus in humans. Gene Ther 6(9):1574–1583

Cho SG, Kim N, Sohn HJ, Lee SK, Oh ST, Lee HJ et al (2015) Long-term outcome of extranodal NK/T cell lymphoma patients treated with postremission therapy using EBV LMP1 and LMP2a-specific CTLs. Mol Ther 23(8):1401–1409

Chu J, He S, Deng Y, Zhang J, Peng Y, Hughes T et al (2014) Genetic modification of T cells redirected toward CS1 enhances eradication of myeloma cells. Clin Cancer Res 20(15):3989–4000

Cooper LJ (2015) Moving from tinkering in the garage to assembly line production: the manufacture of genetically modified T cells expressing chimeric antigen receptors (CARs) comes on line. Cancer Gene Ther 22(2):64–66

Cruz CR, Micklethwaite KP, Savoldo B, Ramos CA, Lam S, Ku S et al (2013) Infusion of donor-derived CD19-redirected virus-specific T cells for B-cell malignancies relapsed after allogeneic stem cell transplant: a phase 1 study. Blood 122(17):2965–2973

Dao T, Yan S, Veomett N, Pankov D, Zhou L, Korontsvit T et al (2013) Targeting the intracellular WT1 oncogene product with a therapeutic human antibody. Sci Transl Med 5(176):176ra33

Davila ML, Brentjens R, Wang X, Rivière I, Sadelain M (2012) How do CARs work?: Early insights from recent clinical studies targeting CD19. Oncoimmunology 1(9):1577–1583

Davila ML, Riviere I, Wang X, Bartido S, Park J, Curran K et al (2014) Efficacy and toxicity management of 19-28z CAR T cell therapy in B cell acute lymphoblastic leukemia. Sci Transl Med 6(224):224ra25

Davis JL, Theoret MR, Zheng Z, Lamers CH, Rosenberg SA, Morgan RA (2010) Development of human anti-murine T-cell receptor antibodies in both responding and nonresponding patients enrolled in TCR gene therapy trials. Clin Cancer Res 16(23):5852–5861

Deeks SG, Wagner B, Anton PA, Mitsuyasu RT, Scadden DT, Huang C et al (2002) A phase II randomized study of HIV-specific T-cell gene therapy in subjects with undetectable plasma viremia on combination antiretroviral therapy. Mol Ther 5(6):788–797

Deniger DC, Yu J, Huls MH, Figliola MJ, Mi T, Maiti SN et al (2015) Sleeping beauty transposition of chimeric antigen receptors targeting receptor tyrosine kinase-like orphan receptor-1 (ROR1) into diverse memory T-cell populations. PLoS One 10(6):e0128151

Dobrenkov K, Olszewska M, Likar Y, Shenker L, Gunset G, Cai S et al (2008) Monitoring the efficacy of adoptively transferred prostate cancer-targeted human T lymphocytes with PET and bioluminescence imaging. J Nucl Med 49(7):1162–1170

Drent E, Groen RW, Noort WA, Themeli M, Lammerts van Bueren JJ, Parren PW et al (2016) Pre-clinical evaluation of CD38 chimeric antigen receptor engineered T cells for the treatment of multiple myeloma. Haematologica 101(5):616–625

Ellebrecht CT, Bhoj VG, Nace A, Choi EJ, Mao X, Cho MJ et al (2016) Reengineering chimeric antigen receptor T cells for targeted therapy of autoimmune disease. Science 353(6295):179–184

Feldman SA, Assadipour Y, Kriley I, Goff SL, Rosenberg SA (2015) Adoptive cell therapy--tumor-infiltrating lymphocytes, T-cell receptors, and chimeric antigen receptors. Semin Oncol 42(4):626–639

Frumento G, Piazza T, Di Carlo E, Ferrini S (2006) Targeting tumor-related immunosuppression for cancer immunotherapy. Endocr Metab Immune Disord Drug Targets 6(3):233–237

Fukuda T, Chen L, Endo T, Tang L, Lu D, Castro JE et al (2008) Antisera induced by infusions of autologous Ad-CD154-leukemia B cells identify ROR1 as an oncofetal antigen and receptor for Wnt5a. Proc Natl Acad Sci U S A 105(8):3047–3052

Garfall AL, Maus MV, Hwang WT, Lacey SF, Mahnke YD, Melenhorst JJ et al (2015) Chimeric antigen receptor T cells against CD19 for multiple myeloma. N Engl J Med 373(11):1040–1047

Gattenlöhner S, Marx A, Markfort B, Pscherer S, Landmeier S, Juergens H et al (2006) Rhabdomyosarcoma lysis by T cells expressing a human autoantibody-based chimeric receptor targeting the fetal acetylcholine receptor. Cancer Res 66(1):24–28

Gill S, June CH (2015) Going viral: chimeric antigen receptor T-cell therapy for hematological malignancies. Immunol Rev 263(1):68–89

Giordano Attianese GM, Marin V, Hoyos V, Savoldo B, Pizzitola I, Tettamanti S et al (2011) In vitro and in vivo model of a novel immunotherapy approach for chronic lymphocytic leukemia by anti-CD23 chimeric antigen receptor. Blood 117(18):4736–4745

Gribben JG, Hallek M (2009) Rediscovering alemtuzumab: current and emerging therapeutic roles. Br J Haematol 144(6):818–831

Grupp SA, Kalos M, Barrett D, Aplenc R, Porter DL, Rheingold SR et al (2013) Chimeric antigen receptor-modified T cells for acute lymphoid leukemia. N Engl J Med 368(16):1509–1518

Guinn BA, Bland EA, Lodi U, Liggins AP, Tobal K, Petters S et al (2005) Humoral detection of leukaemia-associated antigens in presentation acute myeloid leukaemia. Biochem Biophys Res Commun 335(4):1293–1304

Harris DT, Kranz DM (2016) Adoptive T cell therapies: a comparison of T cell receptors and chimeric antigen receptors. Trends Pharmacol Sci 37(3):220–230

Haso W, Lee DW, Shah NN, Stetler-Stevenson M, Yuan CM, Pastan IH et al (2013) Anti-CD22-chimeric antigen receptors targeting B-cell precursor acute lymphoblastic leukemia. Blood 121(7):1165–1174

Hegde M, Corder A, Chow KK, Mukherjee M, Ashoori A, Kew Y et al (2013) Combinational targeting offsets antigen escape and enhances effector functions of adoptively transferred T cells in glioblastoma. Mol Ther 21(11):2087–2101

Houen G (2015) Peptide antibodies: past, present, and future. Methods Mol Biol 1348:1–6

Jensen MC, Popplewell L, Cooper LJ, DiGiusto D, Kalos M, Ostberg JR et al (2010) Antitransgene rejection responses contribute to attenuated persistence of adoptively transferred CD20/CD19-specific chimeric antigen receptor redirected T cells in humans. Biol Blood Marrow Transplant 16(9):1245–1256

Jiang H, Zhang W, Shang P, Zhang H, Fu W, Ye F et al (2014) Transfection of chimeric anti-CD138 gene enhances natural killer cell activation and killing of multiple myeloma cells. Mol Oncol 8(2):297–310

Jones CH, Hill A, Chen M, Pfeifer BA (2015) Contemporary approaches for nonviral gene therapy. Discov Med 19(107):447–454

Kalos M, Levine BL, Porter DL, Katz S, Grupp SA, Bagg A et al (2011) T cells with chimeric antigen receptors have potent antitumor effects and can establish memory in patients with advanced leukemia. Sci Transl Med 3(95):95ra73

Kato K, Cantwell MJ, Sharma S, Kipps TJ (1998) Gene transfer of CD40-ligand induces autologous immune recognition of chronic lymphocytic leukemia B cells. J Clin Invest 101:1133–1141

Kershaw MH, Westwood JA, Parker LL, Wang G, Eshhar Z, Mavroukakis SA et al (2006) A phase I study on adoptive immunotherapy using gene-modified T cells for ovarian cancer. Clin Cancer Res 12(20 Pt 1):6106–6115

Klebanoff CA, Scott CD, Leonardi AJ, Yamamoto TN, Cruz AC, Ouyang C et al (2016) Memory T cell-driven differentiation of naive cells impairs adoptive immunotherapy. J Clin Invest 126(1):318–334

Kloss CC, Condomines M, Cartellieri M, Bachmann M, Sadelain M (2013) Combinatorial antigen recognition with balanced signaling promotes selective tumor eradication by engineered T cells. Nat Biotechnol 31(1):71–75

Kochenderfer JN, Wilson WH, Janik JE, Dudley ME, Stetler-Stevenson M, Feldman SA et al (2010) Eradication of B-lineage cells and regression of lymphoma in a patient treated with autologous T cells genetically engineered to recognize CD19. Blood 116(20):4099–4102

Kochenderfer JN, Dudley ME, Feldman SA, Wilson WH, Spaner DE, Maric I et al (2012) B-cell depletion and remissions of malignancy along with cytokine-associated toxicity in a clinical trial of anti-CD19 chimeric-antigen-receptor-transduced T cells. Blood 119(12):2709–2720

Kochenderfer JN, Dudley ME, Carpenter RO, Kassim SH, Rose JJ, Telford WG et al (2013) Donor-derived CD19-targeted T cells cause regression of malignancy persisting after allogeneic hematopoietic stem cell transplantation. Blood 122(25):4129–4139

Kochenderfer JN, Dudley ME, Kassim SH, Somerville RP, Carpenter RO, Stetler-Stevenson M et al (2015) Chemotherapy-refractory diffuse large B-cell lymphoma and indolent B-cell malignancies can be effectively treated with autologous T cells expressing an anti-CD19 chimeric antigen receptor. J Clin Oncol 33(6):540–549

Kumaresan PR, Manuri PR, Albert ND, Maiti S, Singh H, Mi T et al (2014) Bioengineering T cells to target carbohydrate to treat opportunistic fungal infection. Proc Natl Acad Sci U S A 111(29):10660–10665

Lamers CH, Sleijfer S, Vulto AG, Kruit WH, Kliffen M, Debets R et al (2006) Treatment of metastatic renal cell carcinoma with autologous T-lymphocytes genetically retargeted against carbonic anhydrase IX: first clinical experience. J Clin Oncol 24(13):e20–e22

Laszlo GS, Estey EH, Walter RB (2014) The past and future of CD33 as therapeutic target in acute myeloid leukemia. Blood Rev 28(4):143–153

Lee DW, Kochenderfer JN, Stetler-Stevenson M, Cui YK, Delbrook C, Feldman SA et al (2015) T cells expressing CD19 chimeric antigen receptors for acute lymphoblastic leukaemia in children and young adults: a phase 1 dose-escalation trial. Lancet 385(9967):517–528

Levine BL, June CH (2013) Perspective: assembly line immunotherapy. Nature 498(7455):S17

Liu X, Barrett DM, Jiang S, Fang C, Kalos M, Grupp SA et al (2016) Improved anti-leukemia activities of adoptively transferred T cells expressing bispecific T-cell engager in mice. Blood Cancer J 6(6):e430

Magnani CF, Turazzi N, Benedicenti F, Calabria A, Tenderini E, Tettamanti S et al (2016) Immunotherapy of acute leukemia by chimeric antigen receptor-modified lymphocytes using an improved Sleeping Beauty transposon platform. Oncotarget 7(32):51581–51597

Maher J, Brentjens RJ, Gunset G, Rivière I, Sadelain M (2002) Human T-lymphocyte cytotoxicity and proliferation directed by a single chimeric TCRzeta/CD28 receptor. Nat Biotechnol 20(1):70–75

Maude SL, Frey N, Shaw PA, Aplenc R, Barrett DM, Bunin NJ et al (2014) Chimeric antigen receptor T cells for sustained remissions in leukemia. N Engl J Med 371(16):1507–1517

Maude SL, Teachey DT, Porter DL, Grupp SA (2015) CD19-targeted chimeric antigen receptor T-cell therapy for acute lymphoblastic leukemia. Blood 125(26):4017–4023

Mitsuyasu RT, Anton PA, Deeks SG, Scadden DT, Connick E, Downs MT et al (2000) Prolonged survival and tissue trafficking following adoptive transfer of CD4zeta gene-modified autologous CD4(+) and CD8(+) T cells in human immunodeficiency virus-infected subjects. Blood 96(3):785–793

Oden F, Marino SF, Brand J, Scheu S, Kriegel C, Olal D et al (2015) Potent anti-tumor response by targeting B cell maturation antigen (BCMA) in a mouse model of multiple myeloma. Mol Oncol 9(7):1348–1358

Oldham RA, Berinstein EM, Medin JA (2015) Lentiviral vectors in cancer immunotherapy. Immunotherapy 7(3):271–284

Oluwole OO, Davila ML (2016) At the bedside: clinical review of chimeric antigen receptor (CAR) T cell therapy for B cell malignancies. J Leukoc Biol 100(6):1265–1272

Parente-Pereira AC, Burnet J, Ellison D, Foster J, Davies DM, van der Stegen S et al (2011) Trafficking of CAR-engineered human T cells following regional or systemic adoptive transfer in SCID beige mice. J Clin Immunol 31(4):710–718

Peinert S, Prince HM, Guru PM, Kershaw MH, Smyth MJ, Trapani JA et al (2010) Gene-modified T cells as immunotherapy for multiple myeloma and acute myeloid leukemia expressing the Lewis Y antigen. Gene Ther 17(5):678–686

Pizzitola I, Anjos-Afonso F, Rouault-Pierre K, Lassailly F, Tettamanti S, Spinelli O et al (2014) Chimeric antigen receptors against CD33/CD123 antigens efficiently target primary acute myeloid leukemia cells in vivo. Leukemia 28(8):1596–1605

Porter DL, Levine BL, Kalos M, Bagg A, June CH (2011) Chimeric antigen receptor-modified T cells in chronic lymphoid leukemia. N Engl J Med 365(8):725–733

Porter DL, Hwang WT, Frey NV, Lacey SF, Shaw PA, Loren AW et al (2015) Chimeric antigen receptor T cells persist and induce sustained remissions in relapsed refractory chronic lymphocytic leukemia. Sci Transl Med 7(303):303ra139

Qasim W, Amrolia PJ, Samarasinghe S, Pule M (2015) First clinical application of Talen engineered universal CAR19 T cells in B-ALL. Blood 126:2046 (S)

Rajkumar SV (2015) Myeloma today: disease definitions and treatment advances. Am J Hematol 91(1):90–100

Riet T, Holzinger A, Dörrie J, Schaft N, Schuler G, Abken H (2013) Nonviral RNA transfection to transiently modify T cells with chimeric antigen receptors for adoptive therapy. Methods Mol Biol 969:187–201

Ritchie DS, Neeson PJ, Khot A, Peinert S, Tai T, Tainton K et al (2013) Persistence and efficacy of second generation CAR T cell against the LeY antigen in acute myeloid leukemia. Mol Ther 21(11):2122–2129

Romeo C, Seed B (1991) Cellular immunity to HIV activated by CD4 fused to T cell or Fc receptor polypeptides. Cell 64(5):1037–1046

Rosenberg SA, Restifo NP (2015) Adoptive cell transfer as personalized immunotherapy for human cancer. Science 348(6230):62–68

Rothe A, Sasse S, Topp MS, Eichenauer DA, Hummel H, Reiners KS et al (2015) A phase 1 study of the bispecific anti-CD30/CD16A antibody construct AFM13 in patients with relapsed or refractory Hodgkin lymphoma. Blood 125(26):4024–4031

Rotolo A, Caputo V, Karadimitris A (2016) The prospects and promise of chimeric antigen receptor immunotherapy in multiple myeloma. Br J Haematol 173(3):350–364

Roybal KT, Rupp LJ, Morsut L, Walker WJ, McNally KA, Park JS et al (2016) Precision tumor recognition by T cells with combinatorial antigen-sensing circuits. Cell 164(4):770–779

Rushworth D, Jena B, Olivares S, Maiti S, Briggs N, Somanchi S et al (2014) Universal artificial antigen presenting cells to selectively propagate T cells expressing chimeric antigen receptor independent of specificity. J Immunother 37(4):204–213

Savoldo B, Ramos CA, Liu E, Mims MP, Keating MJ, Carrum G et al (2011) CD28 costimulation improves expansion and persistence of chimeric antigen receptor-modified T cells in lymphoma patients. J Clin Invest 121(5):1822–1826

Schiller GJ (2013) High-risk acute myelogenous leukemia: treatment today … and tomorrow. Hematology Am Soc Hematol Educ Program 2013:201–208

Schmidt-Hieber M, Fietz T, Knauf W, Uharek L, Hopfenmüller W, Thiel E et al (2005) Efficacy of the interleukin-2 receptor antagonist basiliximab in steroid-refractory acute graft-versus-host disease. Br J Haematol 130(4):568–574

Scholler J, Brady TL, Binder-Scholl G, Hwang WT, Plesa G, Hege KM et al (2012) Decade-long safety and function of retroviral-modified chimeric antigen receptor T cells. Sci Transl Med 4(132):132ra53

Shaffer DR, Savoldo B, Yi Z, Chow KK, Kakarla S, Spencer DM et al (2011) T cells redirected against CD70 for the immunotherapy of CD70-positive malignancies. Blood 117(16):4304–4314

Singh H, Moyes JS, Huls MH, Cooper LJ (2015) Manufacture of T cells using the Sleeping Beauty system to enforce expression of a CD19-specific chimeric antigen receptor. Cancer Gene Ther 22(2):95–100

Spranger S (2016) Mechanisms of tumor escape in the context of the T-cell-inflamed and the non-T-cell-inflamed tumor microenvironment. Int Immunol 28(8):383–391

Teachey DT, Lacey SF, Shaw PA, Melenhorst JJ, Maude SL, Frey N et al (2016) Identification of predictive biomarkers for cytokine release syndrome after chimeric antigen receptor T-cell therapy for acute lymphoblastic leukemia. Cancer Discov 6(6):664–679

Till BG, Jensen MC, Wang J, Chen EY, Wood BL, Greisman HA et al (2008) Adoptive immunotherapy for indolent non-Hodgkin lymphoma and mantle cell lymphoma using genetically modified autologous CD20-specific T cells. Blood 112(6):2261–2271

Till BG, Jensen MC, Wang J, Qian X, Gopal AK, Maloney DG et al (2012) CD20-specific adoptive immunotherapy for lymphoma using a chimeric antigen receptor with both CD28 and 4-1BB domains: pilot clinical trial results. Blood 119(17):3940–3950

Torikai H, Reik A, Liu PQ, Zhou Y, Zhang L, Maiti S et al (2012) A foundation for universal T-cell based immunotherapy: T cells engineered to express a CD19-specific chimeric-antigen-receptor and eliminate expression of endogenous TCR. Blood 119(24):5697–5705

Wierda WG, Cantwell MJ, Woods SJ, Rassenti LZ, Prussak CE, Kipps TJ (2000) CD40-ligand (CD154) gene therapy for chronic lymphocytic leukemia. Blood 96(9):2917–2924

Wierda WG, Castro JE, Aguillon R, Sampath D, Jalayer A, McMannis J et al (2010) A phase I study of immune gene therapy for patients with CLL using a membrane-stable, humanized CD154. Leukemia 24(11):1893–1900

Chimeric Antigen Receptor T Cells for Leukemias in Children: Methods, Data, and Challenges

4

Mala K. Talekar and Stephan A. Grupp

4.1 Introduction: "The Race"

The past few decades have brought enormous improvements in the cure rates of childhood acute leukemia; about 85% of all children with newly diagnosed acute lymphoblastic leukemia (ALL) and 50–60% with acute myeloid leukemia (AML) experience long-term disease control after multimodal treatments that often include intensified chemotherapy (Hunger et al. 2012; Sander et al. 2010). However, despite improved supportive care resources, intensifying chemotherapeutic regimens and harnessing the graft-versus-leukemia effect by allogeneic hematopoietic cell transplantation (HCT) for relapsed and very high-risk leukemic patients, leukemia still remains the leading cause of cancer death in children (Jeha et al. 2006). Relapsed and refractory leukemia patients pose a challenging subset of the pediatric leukemic population due to highly resistant disease and, very often, underlying organ dysfunction, calling for development of novel therapeutic approaches and innovative strategies with the power to kill refractory leukemic cells. Although combinations of unconventional chemotherapies with non-overlapping toxicities are being tested, each subsequent relapse makes achieving and maintaining remission more difficult, resulting in poor long-term survival. Advanced laboratory technologies have provided new insights into mechanisms of relapse and leukemic cell evolution. Newer

M. K. Talekar (✉)
Division of Oncology, Children's Hospital of Philadelphia, Philadelphia, PA, USA

Oncology Clinical Development, GlaxoSmithKline, Collegeville, PA, USA
e-mail: talekarm@email.chop.edu

S. A. Grupp
Division of Oncology, Children's Hospital of Philadelphia, Philadelphia, PA, USA

Department of Pediatrics, Perelman School of Medicine, University of Pennsylvania, Philadelphia, PA, USA

M.-A. Perales et al. (eds.), *Cell and Gene Therapies*, Advances and Controversies in Hematopoietic Transplantation and Cell Therapy,
https://doi.org/10.1007/978-3-319-54368-0_4

formulations of older drugs, antibody-based therapies, and molecularly targeted agents are some of the current strategies under investigation for treatment of relapsed ALL. Whole-genome sequencing has allowed characterization of the transcriptional profile of the leukemic cell, facilitating targeted therapy and leading us one step closer to precision medicine (Bhojwani and Pui 2013). One successful example of this is the efficacy of imatinib for BCR-ABL1-positive ALL; however, driver lesions have been identified in only a small proportion of ALL (Maude et al. 2012; Roberts et al. 2012; Schultz et al. 2014). In this rapidly evolving "race" for better and non-toxic treatments, we find ourselves in an era of the new "CARs"—chimeric antigen receptor(s)—that are defining a role for immunotherapy in childhood leukemia.

4.2 "The CAR"

Surveillance by the immune system may play a role in preventing malignancy, and there is no question that there are multiple steps in carcinogenesis directed at immune evasion. This process of evading immune surveillance is termed cancer immunoediting (Swann and Smyth 2007) and may involve at various levels the activites of tumor-infiltrating lymphocytes (TILs)—T cells, NK cells, or NKT cells—of which the best known example is the strong correlation between improved survival and presence of TILs in patients with melanoma (Mihm et al. 1996). Immunotherapy, which is the elimination of tumor cells via harnessing the immune system, has long been a goal and is the basis for the development of cancer vaccines and cellular therapies including allogeneic HCT and the rationale for donor lymphocyte infusion (DLI) after allogeneic HCT (Loren and Porter 2008; Maude et al. 2015). These approaches have evolved into the concept of adoptive transfer of autologous CAR-T cells, which have been genetically reprogrammed to express a chimeric tumor-specific antigen receptor enabling identification and elimination of neoplastic cells (Maude et al. 2015).

4.2.1 "Blueprint of CAR"

CARs are synthetic polypeptides (Fig. 4.1): they are composed of an extracellular domain, a spacer or transmembrane domain, and intracellular signaling moieties (Kenderian et al. 2015). The extracellular domain provides the antigen recognition that enables the interaction between the T cell and the target cell. In currently used CARs, these are single-chain variable fragments (scFv) derived from monoclonal antibody, although other approaches to target recognition and binding are possible. A key point is that CAR molecules only recognize antigens which are on the cell surface. The intracellular signaling domains provide both signals required for full T-cell activation. Signal 1, the initial activation signal, is provided by CD3ζ (zeta) component. Signal 2, the co-stimulatory signal, can be provided by signaling domains from CD28 or 4-1BB. These designs result in T cells bearing CAR

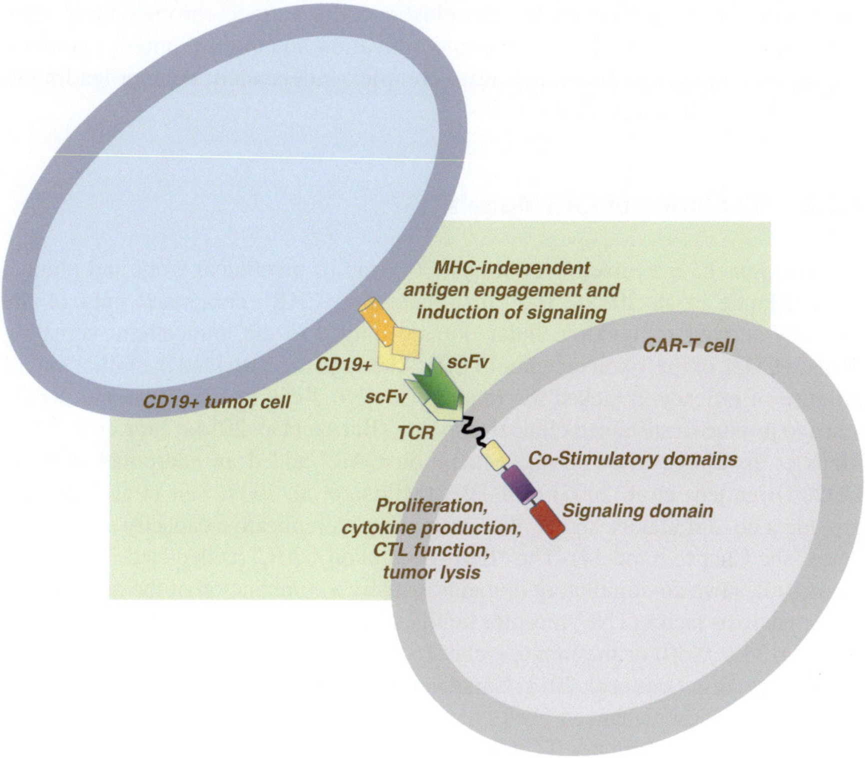

Fig. 4.1 Construct of a CD19-directed CAR-T cell. *TCR* T-cell receptor, *CD* cluster of differentiation, *CTL* cytolytic, *scFv* single-chain variable fragment, *MHC* major histocompatibility complex

molecules (CAR-T cells), which combine the antigen specificity of a monoclonal antibody with the potent cytolytic effector functions of T lymphocytes.

4.2.2 "Manufacturing a CAR"

Modalities utilized to engineer T cells to express the CARs employ gene transfer technologies which can range from messenger RNA-based vectors that confer transient gene expression (hindering persistence and requiring multiple infusions in a clinical setting) to retro- or lentiviral-based approaches that cause permanent modification in the T-cell genome, leading to the potential for persistent on-target toxicity (see Chap. 2). From a regulatory perspective, these permanent genetic modifications come with a theoretical risk of potential T-cell transformation as a result of gene dysregulation. Fortunately, this has not been observed in hundreds of patient-years of follow-up after lentivirally transduced CAR-T therapies (June et al. 2014). The CAR-T cells recognize and bind to the target antigen expressed on the neoplastic cell's surface through their scFv domain; once engaged, T cells undergo activation and elicit a potent cytotoxic response in a major histocompatibility complex-independent manner leading to elimination of the target tumor cell.

4.2.3 "Evolution of CAR Models"

CAR designs have evolved over almost 30 years of preclinical work and clinical trials (Maude et al. 2015). The "first-generation CAR" comprised only of the antibody-derived *scFv* extracellular domain hinged to the intracellular signaling domain CD3ζ of the T-cell receptor (TCR). Although this provided the initial hint of promise of efficacy, it lacked the required in vivo T-cell proliferation and persistence to produce a sustained clinical response (Barrett et al. 2014a; June et al. 2014; Maus et al. 2014). The "second-generation CAR" added an additional domain, CD28 (Brentjens et al. 2007) or 4-1BB (Milone et al. 2009; Seif et al. 2009), to provide a co-stimulatory signal, thus increasing its replicative capacity and persistence (see Chaps. 2 and 14). The "third-generation CAR," as depicted in Fig. 4.1, incorporates two co-stimulatory domains, usually a combination of the members of tumor necrosis factor (TNF) receptor family such as CD27, CD28, CD137 (4-1BB), and CD134 (OX40) or the immune checkpoint protein ICOS (inducible T-cell co-stimulator) (Brentjens et al. 2011; Campana et al. 2014; Barrett et al. 2014b; Pegram et al. 2014). These enhanced CARs have been modeled to mimic normal physiology, where both a primary TCR signal and a second co-stimulatory signal are required for full activation of T cells (Till et al. 2012). All of the CAR-T-cell products showing a high activity in current clinical trials are second-generation CARs (Table 4.1). Third-generation CARs, with alternate or multiple co-stimulatory domains, have been proposed but are in early clinical testing only (e.g., third-generation GD2-CAR-T cells for neuroblastoma NCT01822652) and not in setting of ALL. Researchers at different institutions have used different vectors/components in the CAR construct targeting ALL (Fig. 4.2). The differences in the CAR construct result in variations in persistence and efficacy and are under investigation in ongoing clinical trials.

4.2.4 "The CAR Destination"

An ideal target antigen for CARs with high specificity would have the following characteristics: an antigen that (1) is expressed homogeneously on all cells of the target malignancy; (2) is expressed on the cell surface, as CARs do not "see" intracellular antigens; (3) should not be expressed on normal cells or only on an expendable cell type; (4) is not shed into circulation; and (5) is essential to the growth or survival of the cancer cell and thus not easily lost under selective pressure (Maude and Barrett 2016). A true, tumor-specific antigen would require a

Table 4.1 A representative listing of clinical trials evaluating CAR-T-cell therapy for pediatric B-ALL

	ClinicalTrials.gov identifier	Study title	Ages eligible for study	Center(s)
1	NCT01626495	Phase I/IIA Study of CART19 Cells for Patients With Chemotherapy Resistant or Refractory CD19$^+$ Leukemia and Lymphoma (Pedi CART19)	1–24 years	University of Pennsylvania, PA, USA
2	NCT02650414	CD22 Redirected Autologous T Cells for ALL	1–24 years	University of Pennsylvania, PA, USA
3	NCT02228096	Study of Efficacy and Safety of CTL019 in Pediatric ALL Patients (ENSIGN)	2–21 years	Multicenter
4	NCT02374333	Pilot Study of Redirected Autologous T Cells Engineered to Contain Humanized Anti-CD19 in Patients With Relapsed or Refractory CD19$^+$ Leukemia and Lymphoma Previously Treated With Cell Therapy NCT02374333	1–24 years	University of Pennsylvania, PA, USA
5	NCT02435849	Determine Efficacy and Safety of CTL019 in Pediatric Patients with Relapsed and Refractory B-cell ALL (ELIANA)	3–21 years	Global, phase II, multicenter (26 locations), registration trial
6	NCT02445222	CD19 CART Long Term Follow Up (LTFU) Study	All	Multicenter (21 locations)
7	NCT02588456	Pilot Study of Autologous Anti-CD22 Chimeric Antigen Receptor Redirected T Cells In Patients With Chemotherapy Resistant Or Refractory Acute Lymphoblastic Leukemia	18 years and older	University of Pennsylvania, PA, USA
8	NCT01551043	Allo CART-19 Protocol	18 years and older	University of Pennsylvania, PA, USA
9	NCT02030847	Phase II Study of Redirected Autologous T Cells Engineered to Contain Anti-CD19 Attached to TCR and 4-1BB Signaling Domains in Patients With Chemotherapy Resistant or Refractory Acute Lymphoblastic Leukemia	18 years and older	University of Pennsylvania, PA, USA
10	NCT01747486	CD19 Redirected Autologous T Cells	18 years and older	University of Pennsylvania, PA, USA

(continued)

Table 4.1 (continued)

	ClinicalTrials.gov identifier	Study title	Ages eligible for study	Center(s)
11	NCT02623582	CD123 Redirected Autologous T Cells for AML	18 years and older	University of Pennsylvania, PA, USA
12	NCT01044069	Precursor B Cell Acute Lymphoblastic Leukemia (B-ALL) Treated With Autologous T Cells Genetically Targeted to the B Cell Specific Antigen CD19	18 years or older	Memorial Sloan Kettering Cancer Center, New York, USA
13	NCT01029366	Pilot Study of Redirected Autologous T-cells Engineered to Contain Anti-CD19 Attached to TCR and 4-1BB Signaling Domains in Patient With Chemotherapy Resistant or Refractory $CD19^+$ Leukemia and Lymphoma	18 years and older	University of Pennsylvania, PA, USA
14	NCT01860937	A Phase I Trial of T-Lymphocytes Genetically Targeted to the B-Cell Specific Antigen CD19 in Pediatric and Young Adult Patients With Relapsed B-Cell Acute Lymphoblastic Leukemia	Up to 26 years	Dana-Farber Cancer Institute, MD and Memorial Sloan Kettering Cancer Center, NY, USA
15	NCT01430390	A Phase I Dose Escalation Trial Using In Vitro Expanded Allogeneic Epstein-Barr Virus Specific Cytotoxic T-Lymphocytes (EBV-CTLs) Genetically Targeted to the CD19 Antigen in B-cell Malignancies	Up to 18 years	Memorial Sloan Kettering Cancer Center, NY, USA
16	NCT01044069	A Phase I Trial of Precursor B Cell Acute Lymphoblastic Leukemia (B-ALL) Treated With Autologous T Cells Genetically Targeted to the B Cell Specific Antigen CD19	18 years and older	Memorial Sloan Kettering Cancer Center, NY, USA
17	NCT02028455	Pediatric and Young Adult Leukemia Adoptive Therapy (PLAT)-02: A Phase 1/2 Feasibility and Safety Study of CD19-CAR T Cell Immunotherapy for $CD19^+$ Leukemia	1–26 years	Seattle Children's Hospital, Washington, USA
18	NCT01853631	Phase I Study of Activated T-Cells Expressing Second or Third Generation CD19-Specific Chimeric Antigen Receptors for Advanced B-Cell Non-Hodgkin's Lymphoma, Acute Lymphocytic Leukemia and Chronic Lymphocytic Leukemia (SAGAN)	Up to 75 years	Baylor College of Medicine, Texas, USA

Table 4.1 (continued)

	ClinicalTrials.gov identifier	Study title	Ages eligible for study	Center(s)
19	NCT01683279	Pediatric Leukemia Adoptive Therapy (PLAT)-01: A Phase 1 Feasibility and Safety Study of Cellular Immunotherapy for Relapsed Pediatric $CD19^+$ Acute Lymphoblastic Leukemia Using Autologous T-cells Lentivirally Transduced To Express a CD19-Specific Chimeric Antigen Receptor	1–26 years	Seattle Children's Hospital, Washington, USA
20	NCT02529813	$CD19^+$ Chimeric Antigen Receptor T Cells for Patients With Advanced Lymphoid Malignancies	1–80 years	University of Texas, MD Anderson Cancer Center, Texas, USA
21	NCT01362452	Donor-Derived, CD19-Specific *T Cell* Infusion in Patients With B-Lineage Lymphoid Malignancies After Umbilical Cord Blood Transplantation	1–75 years	University of Texas, MD Anderson Cancer Center, Texas, USA
22	NCT01497184	CD19-Specific T Cell Infusion in Patients With B-Lineage Lymphoid Malignancies After Allogeneic Hematopoietic Stem Cell Transplantation	1–65 years	University of Texas, MD Anderson Cancer Center, Texas, USA
23	NCT02028455	A Pediatric and Young Adult Trial of Genetically Modified T Cells Directed Against CD19 for Relapsed/Refractory $CD19^+$ Leukemia	1–26 years	Seattle Children's Hospital, Washington, USA
24	NCT02315612	Anti-CD22 Chimeric Receptor T Cells in Pediatric and Young Adults With Recurrent or Refractory CD22-expressing B Cell Malignancies	1–30 years	National Cancer Institute
25	NCT02625480	A Multi-Center Study Evaluating KTE-C19 in Pediatric and Adolescent Subjects With Relapsed/Refractory B-precursor Acute Lymphoblastic Leukemia (ZUMA-4)	2–21 years	Multisite

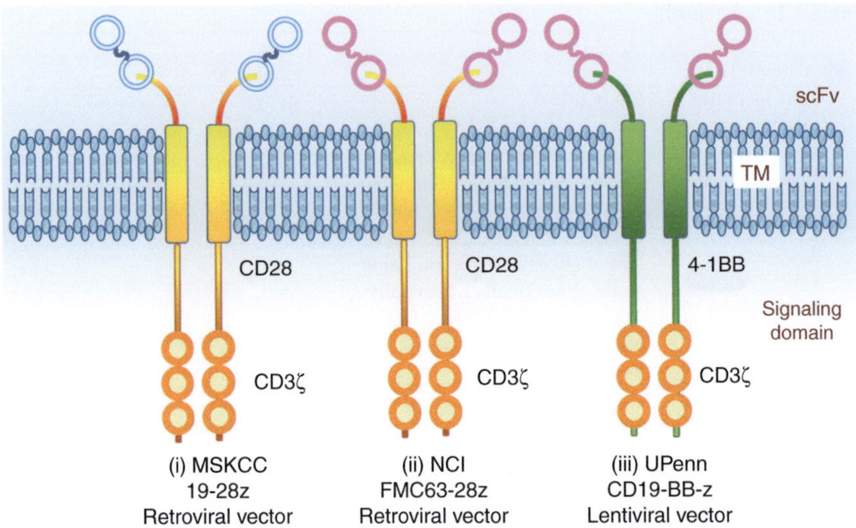

Fig. 4.2 Schematic diagram of different models of chimeric antigen receptors (CARs) used to treat patients with ALL at (i) MSKCC, (ii) NCI, and (iii) UPenn. (i) 19–28ζ (MSKCC). (ii) FMC63–28ζ (NCI). (iii) 19-BB-ζ (UPenn). Groups at MSKCC and NCI have reported use of a CD28ζ second-generation CAR design introduced by a retroviral vector. The UPenn and CHOP group have used a 4–1BBζ design and a lentiviral vector. The MSKCC group used the SJ single-chain variable fragment (scFv), while researchers at NCI and UPenn have used the FMC63 scFv. TM, transmembrane. Adapted from Davila et al. (2012)

cell surface molecule that is unique to the malignancy, either by mutation leading to altered configuration, a fusion protein, or altered expression (Maude et al. 2015). In the realm of B-cell malignancies, CD19 is a tumor-associated antigen that is not cancer-specific but only expressed on normal B cells, which are not required for survival. It is expressed throughout B-cell development until the plasma cell stage and is uniformly expressed on nearly all B-cell malignancies. Expression on a single-cell lineage (B lymphocytes) whose function is replaceable (i.e., by immunoglobulin administration) and given that patients can tolerate prolonged B-cell aplasia, CD19 represents an excellent target for the CAR-modified T cell. Additionally, CD22, another B-cell-specific surface molecule, is also currently being investigated (Haso et al. 2013). In contrast, T-cell ALL and myeloid leukemias pose a significant challenge. In regard to T-cell ALL, the neoplastic cells express the same antigens as do the normal T cells, and unlike B cells, T-cell aplasia is not tolerated and is not as easily treatable. Similarly, in case of myeloid leukemias, currently the known repertoire of cell surface antigens that are unique to neoplastic myeloid clone but which spare normal hematopoietic cells is very limited. In that context, CAR therapy directed against the AML blasts would potentially be myelotoxic and therefore require time-limited expression (allowing hematopoietic recovery) or replacement of hematopoiesis with allogeneic HCT (Gill et al. 2014).

4.3 Methods to Administration: "Prepping the Raceway"

4.3.1 Recipient Lymphodepletion

Induction of lymphopenia in the recipient of adoptive cell therapy has been shown to promote in vivo T-cell expansion (Cui et al. 2009). Through this "homeostatic proliferation," the T cells assume an antigen-experienced or memory phenotype, which in turn is associated with enhanced effector functions (Wu et al. 2004; Goldrath et al. 2000; Cho et al. 2000). In a patient with cancer, lymphodepletion before adoptive transfer of tumor-reactive T cells has been shown to provide a platform for augmented in vivo function of the transferred cells and improved therapeutic outcome (Klebanoff et al. 2005). In a cohort of patients with metastatic melanoma, Dudley et al. showed that by eliminating competition for endogenous serum cytokines, lymphodepletion may directly affect the survival, persistence, and proliferation of adoptively transferred TIL cells (Dudley et al. 2008).

In the setting of CAR therapy, host lymphodepletion is typically accomplished by chemotherapy or targeted monoclonal antibodies. Most groups use cyclophosphamide and fludarabine in the week prior to planned CAR-T-cell infusion (Maude et al. 2014a). In vivo T-cell expansion can then be further enhanced by application of supportive cytokines such as interleukin (IL)-7 and IL-15 as shown by Klebanoff et al. (2005).

4.4 The Efficacy of CAR-T Cells in Pediatric Leukemias: The "Speedway"

4.4.1 Acute Lymphoblastic Leukemia

The advent of CAR-T therapy for leukemias has dramatically changed the outlook of children with relapsed/refractory disease. The unprecedented early success of CD19-directed CAR-modified T-cell clinical trials has given rise to new optimism and laid the foundation for further exploration of therapeutic potential of CAR-T cells in ALL and of targeted immunotherapy. Initial studies by various groups showed remarkable responses in a small series of patients with disease that was chemotherapy refractory and considered incurable and provided compelling proof of principle (Brentjens et al. 2013; Grupp et al. 2013). Subsequently, larger studies by other groups substantiated early results and reported complete remission (CR) rates of 70–90% (Maude et al. 2014a; Davila et al. 2014; Lee et al. 2015).

Our group reported a CR rate of 90% in 30 pediatric and adult patients with relapsed/refractory ALL treated with CD19-directed CAR-modified T cells (Maude et al. 2014a). This phase I/IIa trial conducted at the Children's Hospital of Philadelphia (CHOP) and University of Pennsylvania (UPenn) utilized a lentiviral engineered autologous T-cell construct expressing a second-generation CAR composed of anti-CD19 scFv, CD3ζ as a signaling domain, and 4-1BB as co-stimulatory domain. The cohort included two patients with blinatumomab-refractory disease and 15 who had undergone allogeneic HCT. Sustained remission was achieved with a 6-month event-free survival (EFS) rate of about 70% and an overall survival (OS) rate of about 80%, and durable remission up to 24 months was observed (Maude et al. 2014a).

The group at Memorial Sloan Kettering Cancer Center (MSKCC) reported a complete remission (CR) of 88% in a cohort of 16 adult patients with relapsed/refractory B-ALL; their group utilized a 19-28z CAR-T construct (Davila et al. 2014). Lee et al. reported a CR of 70% in an intention-to-treat phase I dose escalation trial with the TCR ζ (zeta)/CD28 CAR-T construct in a cohort of 20 children and young adults with relapsed/refractory B-ALL conducted at the National Cancer Institute (NCI) (Lee et al. 2015). In an expanded cohort of 59 pediatric patients with ALL reported initially at the European Hematology Association meeting in 2015 and later at ASCO annual meeting in 2016, our group reported a 93% CR and a 12-month overall survival (OS) of 79% (95% CI, 69–91%) (Maude and Barrett 2016; Maude et al. 2016). Table 4.1 lists the clinical trials evaluating CAR-T therapy for pediatric B-ALL that are currently active/recruiting at various centers across the USA.

Some initial reports demonstrating high CR rates with a CD19 CAR focused on providing a bridge to definitive curative therapy with allogeneic HCT. However, given that persistence out to 5 years has been observed with a 4-1BB second-generation CAR (Porter et al. 2015), it has become evident that T-cell persistence can sustain durable remissions. This in turn suggests that patients with refractory disease could have a better quality of life (QoL) without the need for further chemotherapy and may be able to avoid allogeneic HCT. The CAR-T cells have additionally been observed in the cerebrospinal fluid (CSF) of the recipients, where they have been shown to persist at high levels for at least 12 months (Grupp et al. 2013; Rheingold et al. 2015). The highly efficient migration of CAR-directed T cells to the CSF potentially provides a mechanism for surveillance to prevent and perhaps treat even isolated CNS relapses in leukemias and is being investigated in current clinical trials. Although longer follow-up is needed to establish the most efficacious CAR designs, including elucidating differences in the co-stimulatory domains, persistent B-cell aplasia at the longest follow-up of 4–5 years with the 4-1BB CARs provides an indirect but compelling evidence for continued effector functions of infused CAR-T cells in the CHOP/Penn cohort (Maude and Barrett 2016). An update to the interim analysis of the global registration trial of efficacy and safety of CD19 directed CAR-T cells (CTL019) in pediatric and young adult patients with RR ALL was recently presented at EHA 2017. Of the 63 patients who were evaluable for efficacy, the confirmed overall remission rate as assessed by independent central review was 82.5% (95% CI 70.9%–91%), consisting of 63% of patients with CR and 19% with complete remission with incomplete hematological recovery

(CRi). All patients with a confirmed CR or CRi were minimal residual disease negative by flow cytometry. Median remission duration was not reached (range: 1.2 to 14.1+ months). The most common adverse reactions (incidence greater than 20%) were cytokine release syndrome (CRS), hypogammaglobulinemia, infections-pathogen unspecified, pyrexia, decreased appetite, headache, encephalopathy, hypotension, bleeding episodes, tachycardia, nausea, diarrhea, vomiting, viral infectious disorders, hypoxia, fatigue, acute kidney injury, and delirium. Grade 3 or 4 adverse events were noted in 84% of patients. It was these and other supporting compelling data that led to the approval of first CAR-T-cell therapy in B-ALL in 2017 (discussed later in the chapter).

4.4.2 Acute Myeloid Leukemia

Although the leukemic blasts of AML express a host of cell surface molecules that could potentially be attractive targets for CAR-directed therapy, the hindrance has been the ubiquitous expression of those antigens on normal hematopoietic progenitors and stem cells (Rambaldi et al. 2015). Unlike CAR-directed therapy for B-ALL, wherein the consequences of long-term B-cell aplasia can be managed by immunoglobulin administration, CAR-T therapy for currently known targets in AML is likely to cause persistent suppression of marrow progenitors, which would result in bone marrow aplasia unless the active T cells can be eliminated. Targets under scrutiny include CD33, CD34, CD38, CD116, and CD123 (Kenderian et al. 2015; Gill et al. 2014; Nakazawa et al. 2016). Preclinical studies of CD123 CAR in xenograft mouse models of AML by our group demonstrated eradication of normal myelopoiesis—however, this on-target/off-tumor toxicity could be recognized as the potential novel application for CART123 as a chemotherapy-free myeloablative conditioning (MAC) regimen for HCT (Gill et al. 2014). This also calls for consideration of CARs with in-built mechanisms for limiting expression, suicide genes or using combinations of CARs with Boolean properties to modulate T-cell receptor signaling that could improve specificity, thereby restricting toxicity (Maude and Barrett 2016; Saez-Rodriguez et al. 2007; Wang et al. 2015). Table 4.1 lists a number of clinical trials evaluating CAR-T therapy for pediatric leukemias that are active/recruiting at various centers across the USA.

4.5 Toxicities and Challenges: The "Bumps in the Road"

4.5.1 Cytokine Release Syndrome

Although in vivo proliferation (and persistence) of CAR-T cells is the desired intent of engineered cell therapy infusions, the potent inflammatory response associated with an exponential multiplication (100 to 100,000×) of activated cells incites marked elevations in cytokine levels. CRS, the clinical syndrome resulting from this phenomenon, is not unique to CAR-T cells and has been seen in other T-cell engaging therapies such as bispecific T-cell engaging (BiTE) antibodies like blinatumomab and can also be associated with many of the characteristics of macrophage activation syndrome (MAS) (Teachey et al. 2013, 2016).

CRS is the most common and severe toxicity associated with CD19 directed CAR-T cells. Although data from our group and others suggests a correlation between *development* of CRS and efficacy, the *degree* of CRS has not been found to be predictive of response to therapy (Maude et al. 2014a; Davila et al. 2014; Lee et al. 2015). The severity of CRS has rather been found to correlate with disease burden at the time of CAR-T-cell infusion (Maude et al. 2014a, 2015; Teachey et al. 2016).

Clinical symptoms of CRS can range from mild and flu-like (headaches, myalgias, fevers) to a severe inflammatory syndrome including vascular leak, hypotension, shock, pulmonary edema, and coagulopathy leading to multi-organ failure (MOF); and recently, Gore et al. reported a CRS-related death after blinatumomab (Maude et al. 2014b; Gore et al. 2013). Various groups have attempted to establish criteria for grading CRS (Porter et al. 2015; Lee et al. 2014; Brudno and Kochenderfer 2016), and these systems have yet to be systematized across CAR trials, although efforts are underway to do so. This has come out of an appreciation that the Common Terminology Criteria for Adverse Events (CTCAE) grading for CRS is more relevant to treatment with monoclonal antibodies rather than T-cell-based immunotherapies (Health UDo 2012). Published criteria grade CRS on basis of presence of fevers, key clinical events such as hypotension and hypoxia, and other organ dysfunctions, which may be seen in setting of elevation of characteristic cytokines (Davila et al. 2014; Porter et al. 2015). As more is appreciated about neurologic toxicities such as mental status changes, aphasia, and seizures, these events may need to be graded separately or merged into CRS grading scale. Our group has used the grading system described in Table 4.2. This approach focuses on events of greatest clinical concern, identifying as grade 4 events that almost universally require treatment with tocilizumab which was also recently approved by US Food and Drug Administration (FDA). Serum cytokine measurements are not used in the grading scale, as rapid turnaround for such tests is not feasible at most centers. CRS has been graded as ranging from grade 1 to grade 5. Grade 1 (mild) refers to CRS requiring only symptomatic management; grade 2 (moderate) refers to CRS requiring moderate intervention such as low oxygen requirement or hypotension responsive to intravenous (IV) fluids; grade 3 (severe) refers to CRS that would manifest with clinical symptomatology that requires medical and pharmacologic intervention such as high oxygen requirement, vasopressors, and organ toxicity; and grade 4 (life threatening) refers to CRS requiring ventilator support or grade 4 organ toxicity (Table 4.2).

Cytokine elevations are measurable in most patients, although some patients manifest symptoms without marked increase in cytokine levels, whereas others have laboratory findings out of proportion to clinical symptoms (Klinger et al. 2012). Several groups have consistently demonstrated elevations in levels of acute phase reactants such as C-reactive protein (CRP), ferritin, lactate dehydrogenase (LDH), and transaminases and additionally in biomarkers such as interleukins

Table 4.2 UPenn grading system for CAR-T-cell-associated cytokine release syndrome

Grade 1	*Mild reaction*: Treated with supportive care such as antipyretics and antiemetics
Grade 2	*Moderate*: Requiring intravenous therapies or parenteral nutrition; some signs of organ dysfunction (i.e., grade 2 renal toxicity rise or grade 3 liver toxicity) related to CRS and not attributable to any other condition. Hospitalization for management of CRS-related symptoms including fevers with associated neutropenia
Grade 3	*More severe reaction*: Hospitalization required for management of symptoms related to organ dysfunction including grade 4 liver toxicity or grade 3 renal toxicity related to CRS and not attributable to any other conditions; excludes management of fever or myalgias. Includes hypotension treated with intravenous fluids[a] or low-dose pressors, coagulopathy requiring fresh frozen plasma or cryoprecipitate, and hypoxia requiring supplemental O2 (nasal cannula oxygen, high-flow O2, CPAP, or BiPAP). Patients admitted for management of suspected infection due to fevers and/or neutropenia may have grade 2 CRS
Grade 4	*Life-threatening* complications such as hypotension requiring multiple, escalating or high-dose vasopressors[b], hypoxia requiring mechanical ventilation, requirement for dialysis
Grade 5	*Death*

CRS cytokine release syndrome, *O2* oxygen, *CPAP* continuous positive pressure airway, *BiPAP* bilevel positive airway pressure
[a]Defined as multiple fluid boluses for blood pressure support
[b]Modified from Porter et al. (2015). Please refer to this reference for definition of high-dose vasopressors

(IL-2R, IL-6, IL-10, IL-13), IFNγ, sgp130, MIP1α, and MIP1β (Teachey et al. 2016; Chen et al. 2016). Generally, these elevations (including CRP and IL-6) correlate well with the degree of CRS, but they do not predict CRS. Predictive models are being developed by the CHOP group and others, and elevations in cytokines such as IFNγ and sgp130 can predict severe CRS when measured within the first 72 h after engineered T-cell infusion (Teachey et al. 2016). Cytokine-directed approaches to manage CRS could be limited by the potential to inhibit T-cell activity and thereby clinical efficacy.

The interventions to limit CRS have to weigh the benefit of accelerated T-cell proliferation against the risk of loss of efficacy/persistence of activated T cells making the management of CRS challenging. The obvious choice is suppression of immune activation; however, blunting the intended cytotoxic response of CAR-T cells is undesirable. Although corticosteroids have been employed in both treatment and prophylaxis of CRS arising secondary to BiTE therapy (see text above), the known negative impact of steroids on therapeutic T-cell proliferation suggests the need to avoid steroid therapy in treating CRS after CAR-T-cell therapy. This led to the proposal that it might be worth targeting the elevated cytokines directly as a potential management tool. IL-10, IL-6, and IFNγ have been found to be the most significantly elevated cytokines during CRS. With IL-10 being a negative regulator while IFNγ being an effector cytokine released by activated T cells and potentially required for efficacy, they are probably not the ideal and perhaps unsavory targets for toxicity management. IL-6, in contrast, was not thought to be required for T-cell efficacy. For this reason, combined with the striking elevations of IL-6, we have observed in CAR-T patients, IL-6 signaling was first targeted by our group (Grupp et al. 2013). IL-6 blockade with tocilizumab was found to be effective in reversing life-threatening CRS without compromising efficacy of T-cell engaging therapies (Grupp et al. 2013; Teachey et al. 2013).

Although early observations indicated the potential for abnormalities in standard laboratory tests such as CRP, ferritin, LDH, etc., in predicting CRS severity, a large comprehensive analysis of clinical and biologic manifestations of CRS after CAR-T-cell therapy by our group gave more credence to the elevations of IFNγ, IL10, spg130, and MIP1α using multiple predictive models (Teachey et al. 2016) with sensitivities and specificities exceeding 85–90%. Despite the frequency and improved recognition of CRS after CAR-T-cell infusion, the underlying biology of the interplay between the components of the inflammatory cytokines and the homeostatic milieu in CRS is not well understood. In the future, improved understanding of cytokine activation in CRS could perhaps enhance the ability to prevent the serious complications of CRS.

4.5.2 Neurotoxicity

Neurologic toxicities have been reported after T-cell engaging therapies, both with BiTE (blinatumomab) and CD19 and CD22 directed CAR-T therapies (Davila et al. 2014; Schlegel et al. 2014; Topp et al. 2011). Neurologic symptoms ranging from headaches to delirium to global encephalopathy and even seizures have been reported. The CHOP/Penn group reported a distinct encephalopathy-like syndrome in 6 of 30 ALL patients treated with CD19 directed CAR-T cells (CTL019), that occurred after resolution of CRS. The post-CAR-T-cell encephalopathy has been brief and self-limited, resolving over several days without apparent sequelae. Although CAR-T cells have been identified in the CSF of the affected patients, imaging and lumbar punctures did not provide insight into the etiology (Maude et al. 2015). Larger studies with longer follow-ups are needed to better characterize the pathophysiology and spectrum of neurotoxicity associated with CAR-T cells.

4.5.3 B-Cell Aplasia

Successful CD19-directed CAR-T-cell therapy entails elimination of normal B cells as an on-target/off-tumor toxicity. Hypogammaglobulinemia as a result of chronic B-cell aplasia is an anticipated outcome and is manageable with immunoglobulin replacement; however, longer follow-up will be needed to help determine any late effects of continued B-cell aplasia.

4.5.4 Challenges

CAR-T-cell therapy is changing the landscape of refractory/relapsed leukemias in children, but it also brings forth several clinical challenges. Increasing access to improve delivery to more patients requires a comprehensive clinical care team setup with experience in managing the toxicities of this novel therapy (Fig. 4.3). Consistency across institutions and parallel advancements in techniques need coordinated efforts and incur financial burdens.

Although striking responses have been seen with this therapy, unfortunately relapse after CAR-T-cell therapy remains a challenge. Relapses have been seen in two forms—reappearance of disease that remains CD19-positive and emergence of a CD19-negative clone. Disease relapse with CD19-positive disease most likely reflects poor persistence of CAR-T cells or suboptimal CAR-T function for another reason. Both of these can be potentially prevented with future optimization of CAR designs and improvements in the current manufacturing processes, including assessment of most efficacious co-stimulatory domains. The MSKCC group has proposed fourth-generation "armored" CARs with co-stimulatory ligands or incorporation of additional genes encoding pro-proliferative cytokines (Brentjens and Curran 2012). Using serial CAR-T-cell infusions directed against a second antigen (such as CAR-T against CD22) or using a combination or tandem of CAR joining 2 antigen moieties may prevent escape clones and needs investigation and validation with future studies.

4.5.5 Expert Point of View and Future Directions

The field of highly active engineered T-cell therapy has been launched with observations from several groups of high CR rates and long-term disease control in patients with CD19^{+} malignancies. This advance has been the result of GMP cell manufacturing approaches which produce "younger" and more proliferative T cells for adoptive transfer (particularly using CD3/CD28 beads to stimulate the

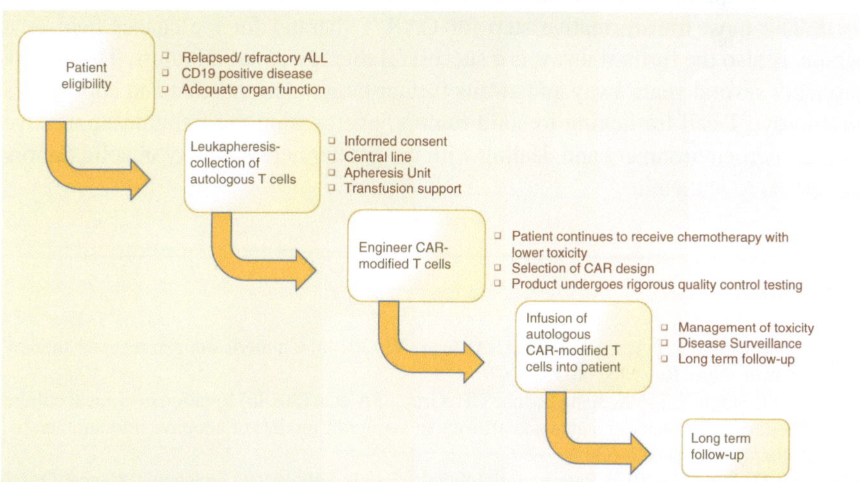

Fig. 4.3 Algorithm for CD19-directed CAR-T-cell therapy

manufactured T cells) and the addition of co-stimulatory domains to CAR constructs that provide signal 2 in addition to the activating signal 1 to the T cells (refer to the text above). Even within the B-cell malignancy space, responses and toxicity differ, with ALL studies showing very high response rates as well as higher rates of severe CRS, while CAR therapy in CLL and NHLs has resulted in striking and durable responses in highly resistant disease but lower rates of both CR and CRS. The next few years will bring results from trials carried out in multicenter settings, demonstrating the ability of groups to translate single-center results to larger groups, while hopefully maintaining efficacy with acceptable safety. Each of the large centers has developed industry partnerships, and we will see data addressing the ability of groups to take cell manufacturing processes developed under academic GMP conditions to centralized cell manufacturing facilities run by pharmaceutical industries. Recently, on August 30, 2017, the US Food and Drug Administration granted regular approval to tisagenlecleucel (CD19 CAR-T cells) for the treatment of patients up to age 25 years with B-cell precursor ALL that is refractory or in second or later relapse. Tisagenlecleucel consists of autologous T cells collected in a leukapheresis procedure that are genetically modified with a new gene containing a CAR protein allowing the T cells to identify and eliminate CD19-expressing normal and malignant cells. Approval of tisagenlecleucel was based on a phase II single-arm trial (Funded by Novartis Pharmaceuticals; ClinicalTrials.gov number, NCT02435849) of 63 patients with relapsed or refractory pediatric precursor B-cell ALL, including 35 patients who had a prior hematopoietic cell transplantation. Patients received a single dose of tisagenlecleucel intravenously within 2–14 days following the completion of lymphodepleting chemotherapy. In this global study, a single infusion of tisagenlecleucel produced high remission rates, had manageable toxic effects and demonstrated durable remissions without any additional therapy in high-risk pediatric and young adult patients with relapsed or refractory B-cell ALL. In the near future, we hope to see results from trials extending CAR-T therapy successfully to diseases like multiple myeloma and AML as well. The most transformative step for CAR-T therapy for the cancer field as a whole, is also the furthest away, is a successful therapy of solid tumors. This step is probably several years away and awaits further target identification and approaches to improve T-cell trafficking to solid tumors, overcoming the immunosuppressive tumor microenvironment and dealing with the greater heterogeneity of solid tumors compared to leukemia.

References

Barrett DM, Singh N, Porter DL, Grupp SA, June CH (2014a) Chimeric antigen receptor therapy for cancer. Annu Rev Med 65:333–347

Barrett DM, Singh N, Liu X, Jiang S, June CH, Grupp SA et al (2014b) Relation of clinical culture method to T-cell memory status and efficacy in xenograft models of adoptive immunotherapy. Cytotherapy 16(5):619–630

Bhojwani D, Pui CH (2013) Relapsed childhood acute lymphoblastic leukaemia. Lancet Oncol 14(6):e205–e217

Brentjens RJ, Curran KJ (2012) Novel cellular therapies for leukemia: CAR-modified T cells targeted to the CD19 antigen. Hematology Am Soc Hematol Educ Program 2012:143–151
Brentjens RJ, Santos E, Nikhamin Y, Yeh R, Matsushita M, La Perle K et al (2007) Genetically targeted T cells eradicate systemic acute lymphoblastic leukemia xenografts. Clin Cancer Res 13(18 Pt 1):5426–5435
Brentjens RJ, Riviere I, Park JH, Davila ML, Wang X, Stefanski J et al (2011) Safety and persistence of adoptively transferred autologous CD19-targeted T cells in patients with relapsed or chemotherapy refractory B-cell leukemias. Blood 118(18):4817–4828
Brentjens RJ, Davila ML, Riviere I, Park J, Wang X, Cowell LG et al (2013) CD19-targeted T cells rapidly induce molecular remissions in adults with chemotherapy-refractory acute lymphoblastic leukemia. Sci Transl Med 5(177):177ra38
Brudno JN, Kochenderfer JN (2016) Toxicities of chimeric antigen receptor T cells: recognition and management. Blood 127(26):3321–3330
Campana D, Schwarz H, Imai C (2014) 4-1BB chimeric antigen receptors. Cancer J 20(2):134–140
Chen F, Teachey DT, Pequignot E, Frey N, Porter D, Maude SL et al (2016) Measuring IL-6 and sIL-6R in serum from patients treated with tocilizumab and/or siltuximab following CAR T cell therapy. J Immunol Methods 434:1–8
Cho BK, Rao VP, Ge Q, Eisen HN, Chen J (2000) Homeostasis-stimulated proliferation drives naive T cells to differentiate directly into memory T cells. J Exp Med 192(4):549–556
Cui Y, Zhang H, Meadors J, Poon R, Guimond M, Mackall CL (2009) Harnessing the physiology of lymphopenia to support adoptive immunotherapy in lymphoreplete hosts. Blood 114(18):3831–3840
Davila ML, Brentjens R, Wang X, Riviere I, Sadelain M (2012) How do CARs work?: Early insights from recent clinical studies targeting CD19. Oncoimmunology 1(9):1577–1583
Davila ML, Riviere I, Wang X, Bartido S, Park J, Curran K et al (2014) Efficacy and toxicity management of 19-28z CAR T cell therapy in B cell acute lymphoblastic leukemia. Sci Transl Med 6(224):224ra25
Dudley ME, Yang JC, Sherry R, Hughes MS, Royal R, Kammula U et al (2008) Adoptive cell therapy for patients with metastatic melanoma: evaluation of intensive myeloablative chemoradiation preparative regimens. J Clin Oncol 26(32):5233–5239
Gill S, Tasian SK, Ruella M, Shestova O, Li Y, Porter DL et al (2014) Preclinical targeting of human acute myeloid leukemia and myeloablation using chimeric antigen receptor-modified T cells. Blood 123(15):2343–2354
Goldrath AW, Bogatzki LY, Bevan MJ (2000) Naive T cells transiently acquire a memory-like phenotype during homeostasis-driven proliferation. J Exp Med 192(4):557–564
Gore L, Zugmaier G, Handgretinger R, Locatelli F, Trippett TM, Rheingold SR, et al (eds) (2013) Cytological and molecular remissions with blinatumomab treatment in second or later bone marrow relapse in pediatric acute lymphoblastic leukemia (ALL). ASCO Annual Meeting Proceedings
Grupp SA, Kalos M, Barrett D, Aplenc R, Porter DL, Rheingold SR et al (2013) Chimeric antigen receptor-modified T cells for acute lymphoid leukemia. N Engl J Med 368(16):1509–1518
Haso W, Lee DW, Shah NN, Stetler-Stevenson M, Yuan CM, Pastan IH et al (2013) Anti-CD22-chimeric antigen receptors targeting B-cell precursor acute lymphoblastic leukemia. Blood 121(7):1165–1174
Health UDo, Services H. National Cancer Institute. Common terminology criteria for adverse events (CTCAE). Version v4. 03. 2012
Hunger SP, Lu X, Devidas M, Camitta BM, Gaynon PS, Winick NJ et al (2012) Improved survival for children and adolescents with acute lymphoblastic leukemia between 1990 and 2005: a report from the Children's Oncology Group. J Clin Oncol 30(14):1663–1669
Jeha S, Gaynon PS, Razzouk BI, Franklin J, Kadota R, Shen V et al (2006) Phase II study of clofarabine in pediatric patients with refractory or relapsed acute lymphoblastic leukemia. J Clin Oncol 24(12):1917–1923
June CH, Maus MV, Plesa G, Johnson LA, Zhao Y, Levine BL et al (2014) Engineered T cells for cancer therapy. Cancer Immunol Immunother 63(9):969–975

Kenderian SS, Ruella M, Shestova O, Klichinsky M, Aikawa V, Morrissette JJ et al (2015) CD33-specific chimeric antigen receptor T cells exhibit potent preclinical activity against human acute myeloid leukemia. Leukemia 29(8):1637–1647

Klebanoff CA, Khong HT, Antony PA, Palmer DC, Restifo NP (2005) Sinks, suppressors and antigen presenters: how lymphodepletion enhances T cell-mediated tumor immunotherapy. Trends Immunol 26(2):111–117

Klinger M, Brandl C, Zugmaier G, Hijazi Y, Bargou RC, Topp MS et al (2012) Immunopharmacologic response of patients with B-lineage acute lymphoblastic leukemia to continuous infusion of T cell-engaging CD19/CD3-bispecific BiTE antibody blinatumomab. Blood 119(26):6226–6233

Lee DW, Gardner R, Porter DL, Louis CU, Ahmed N, Jensen M et al (2014) Current concepts in the diagnosis and management of cytokine release syndrome. Blood 124(2):188–195

Lee DW, Kochenderfer JN, Stetler-Stevenson M, Cui YK, Delbrook C, Feldman SA et al (2015) T cells expressing CD19 chimeric antigen receptors for acute lymphoblastic leukaemia in children and young adults: a phase 1 dose-escalation trial. Lancet 385(9967):517–528

Loren AW, Porter DL (2008) Donor leukocyte infusions for the treatment of relapsed acute leukemia after allogeneic stem cell transplantation. Bone Marrow Transplant 41(5):483–493

Maude S, Barrett DM (2016) Current status of chimeric antigen receptor therapy for haematological malignancies. Br J Haematol 172(1):11–22

Maude SL, Tasian SK, Vincent T, Hall JW, Sheen C, Roberts KG et al (2012) Targeting JAK1/2 and mTOR in murine xenograft models of Ph-like acute lymphoblastic leukemia. Blood 120(17):3510–3518

Maude SL, Frey N, Shaw PA, Aplenc R, Barrett DM, Bunin NJ et al (2014a) Chimeric antigen receptor T cells for sustained remissions in leukemia. N Engl J Med 371(16):1507–1517

Maude SL, Barrett D, Teachey DT, Grupp SA (2014b) Managing cytokine release syndrome associated with novel T cell-engaging therapies. Cancer J 20(2):119–122

Maude SL, Teachey DT, Porter DL, Grupp SA (2015) CD19-targeted chimeric antigen receptor T-cell therapy for acute lymphoblastic leukemia. Blood 125(26):4017–4023

Maude SL, Teachey DT, Rheingold SR, Shaw PA, Aplenc R, Barrett DM et al (2016) Sustained remissions with CD19-specific chimeric antigen receptor (CAR)-modified T cells in children with relapsed/refractory ALL. Am Soc Clin Oncol 34(15_suppl):3011

Maus MV, Grupp SA, Porter DL, June CH (2014) Antibody-modified T cells: CARs take the front seat for hematologic malignancies. Blood 123(17):2625–2635

Mihm MC Jr, Clemente CG, Cascinelli N (1996) Tumor infiltrating lymphocytes in lymph node melanoma metastases: a histopathologic prognostic indicator and an expression of local immune response. Lab Investig 74(1):43–47

Milone MC, Fish JD, Carpenito C, Carroll RG, Binder GK, Teachey D et al (2009) Chimeric receptors containing CD137 signal transduction domains mediate enhanced survival of T cells and increased antileukemic efficacy in vivo. Mol Ther 17(8):1453–1464

Nakazawa Y, Matsuda K, Kurata T, Sueki A, Tanaka M, Sakashita K et al (2016) Anti-proliferative effects of T cells expressing a ligand-based chimeric antigen receptor against CD116 on CD34(+) cells of juvenile myelomonocytic leukemia. J Hematol Oncol 9:27

Pegram HJ, Park JH, Brentjens RJ (2014) CD28z CARs and armored CARs. Cancer J 20(2):127–133

Porter DL, Hwang WT, Frey NV, Lacey SF, Shaw PA, Loren AW et al (2015) Chimeric antigen receptor T cells persist and induce sustained remissions in relapsed refractory chronic lymphocytic leukemia. Sci Transl Med 7(303):303ra139

Rambaldi A, Biagi E, Bonini C, Biondi A, Introna M (2015) Cell-based strategies to manage leukemia relapse: efficacy and feasibility of immunotherapy approaches. Leukemia 29(1):1–10

Rheingold SR, Chen LN, Maude SL, Aplenc R, Barker C, Barrett DM et al (2015) Efficient trafficking of Chimeric Antigen Receptor (CAR)-modified T cells to CSF and induction of durable CNS remissions in children with CNS/combined relapsed/refractory ALL. Blood 126(23):3769

Roberts KG, Morin RD, Zhang J, Hirst M, Zhao Y, Su X et al (2012) Genetic alterations activating kinase and cytokine receptor signaling in high-risk acute lymphoblastic leukemia. Cancer Cell 22(2):153–166

Saez-Rodriguez J, Simeoni L, Lindquist JA, Hemenway R, Bommhardt U, Arndt B et al (2007) A logical model provides insights into T cell receptor signaling. PLoS Comput Biol 3(8):e163
Sander A, Zimmermann M, Dworzak M, Fleischhack G, von Neuhoff C, Reinhardt D et al (2010) Consequent and intensified relapse therapy improved survival in pediatric AML: results of relapse treatment in 379 patients of three consecutive AML-BFM trials. Leukemia 24(8):1422–1428
Schlegel P, Lang P, Zugmaier G, Ebinger M, Kreyenberg H, Witte KE et al (2014) Pediatric post-transplant relapsed/refractory B-precursor acute lymphoblastic leukemia shows durable remission by therapy with the T-cell engaging bispecific antibody blinatumomab. Haematologica 99(7):1212–1219
Schultz KR, Carroll A, Heerema NA, Bowman WP, Aledo A, Slayton WB et al (2014) Long-term follow-up of imatinib in pediatric Philadelphia chromosome-positive acute lymphoblastic leukemia: Children's Oncology Group study AALL0031. Leukemia 28(7):1467–1471
Seif AE, Barrett DM, Milone M, Brown VI, Grupp SA, Reid GS (2009) Long-term protection from syngeneic acute lymphoblastic leukemia by CpG ODN-mediated stimulation of innate and adaptive immune responses. Blood 114(12):2459–2466
Swann JB, Smyth MJ (2007) Immune surveillance of tumors. J Clin Investig 117(5):1137–1146
Teachey DT, Rheingold SR, Maude SL, Zugmaier G, Barrett DM, Seif AE et al (2013) Cytokine release syndrome after blinatumomab treatment related to abnormal macrophage activation and ameliorated with cytokine-directed therapy. Blood 121(26):5154–5157
Teachey DT, Lacey SF, Shaw PA, Melenhorst JJ, Maude SL, Frey N et al (2016) Identification of predictive biomarkers for cytokine release syndrome after chimeric antigen receptor T cell therapy for acute lymphoblastic leukemia. Cancer Discov 6(6):664–679
Till BG, Jensen MC, Wang J, Qian X, Gopal AK, Maloney DG et al (2012) CD20-specific adoptive immunotherapy for lymphoma using a chimeric antigen receptor with both CD28 and 4-1BB domains: pilot clinical trial results. Blood 119(17):3940–3950
Topp MS, Kufer P, Gokbuget N, Goebeler M, Klinger M, Neumann S et al (2011) Targeted therapy with the T-cell-engaging antibody blinatumomab of chemotherapy-refractory minimal residual disease in B-lineage acute lymphoblastic leukemia patients results in high response rate and prolonged leukemia-free survival. J Clin Oncol 29(18):2493–2498
Wang E, Wang LC, Tsai CY, Bhoj V, Gershenson Z, Moon E et al (2015) Generation of potent T-cell immunotherapy for cancer using DAP12-based, multichain, chimeric immunoreceptors. Cancer Immunol Res 3(7):815–826
Wu Z, Bensinger SJ, Zhang J, Chen C, Yuan X, Huang X et al (2004) Homeostatic proliferation is a barrier to transplantation tolerance. Nat Med 10(1):87–92

Chimeric Antigen Receptor-T Cells for Leukemias in Adults: Methods, Data and Challenges

5

Mark B. Geyer, Jae H. Park, and Renier J. Brentjens

5.1 CAR T-Cell Therapeutics in Adult Leukemias: A General Introduction

Within the past several years, renewed interest in immunotherapy has been observed in multiple fields of oncology, including antibody-based therapeutics (e.g., checkpoint blockade) and adoptive cellular therapies. In the field of adult leukemia, such

M. B. Geyer · J. H. Park
Department of Medicine, Memorial Sloan Kettering Cancer Center, New York, NY, USA

Leukemia Service and Cellular Therapeutics Center, Division of Hematologic Oncology, Department of Medicine, Memorial Sloan-Kettering Cancer Center, New York, NY, USA

Joan and Sanford I. Weill Department of Medicine, Weill Cornell Medical College, New York, NY, USA

Center for Cell Engineering, Memorial Sloan Kettering Cancer Center, New York, NY, USA
e-mail: geyerm@mskcc.org; parkj6@mskcc.org

R. J. Brentjens (✉)
Department of Medicine, Memorial Sloan Kettering Cancer Center, New York, NY, USA

Leukemia Service and Cellular Therapeutics Center, Division of Hematologic Oncology, Department of Medicine, Memorial Sloan-Kettering Cancer Center, New York, NY, USA

Joan and Sanford I. Weill Department of Medicine, Weill Cornell Medical College, New York, NY, USA

Center for Cell Engineering, Memorial Sloan Kettering Cancer Center, New York, NY, USA

Molecular Pharmacology and Chemistry Program, Memorial Sloan Kettering Cancer Center, New York, NY, USA
e-mail: brentjer@mskcc.org

M.-A. Perales et al. (eds.), *Cell and Gene Therapies*, Advances and Controversies in Hematopoietic Transplantation and Cell Therapy,
https://doi.org/10.1007/978-3-319-54368-0_5

interest has been driven by the limitations of presently available therapies to induce durable remissions reliably in patients with relapsed or refractory leukemia. For instance, while an increasing proportion of children and young adults with B-cell acute lymphoblastic leukemia (B-ALL) have achieved long-term overall survival in recent decades, most adults diagnosed with B-ALL continue to experience relapse, and adults with relapsed or refractory B-ALL continue to have a poor prognosis when treated with standard salvage chemotherapy (Kantarjian et al. 2010; Gokbuget et al. 2012). The natural history of chronic lymphocytic leukemia (CLL) is considerably more heterogeneous, and a subset of patients will never require therapy. However, patients with unfavorable cytogenetic or molecular features, or with persistent or recurrent disease following initial purine analog-based therapy, continue to have a guarded prognosis when treated with standard therapy regimens (Tam et al. 2008; Kay et al. 2007). The development of oral molecularly targeted therapies such as ibrutinib has now brought a highly efficacious line of therapy to patients with newly diagnosed or relapsed CLL (Byrd et al. 2013, 2015). However, such therapies require an indefinite duration of treatment, are associated with few complete (vs. partial) responses, and are limited by toxicity or development of resistance in a subset of patients.

The adoptive transfer of genetically modified autologous T-cells aims to rapidly establish specific antitumor activity. This strategy requires targeting of autologous T-cells by means of a transgene-encoded antigen receptor, consisting of a chimeric antigen receptor (CAR), as will be discussed herein, or T-cell receptor (TCR) chains. The rationale for targeting CD19 specifically in B-cell malignancies is discussed in a previous chapter. To summarize, CD19 is a surface-exposed 95 kDa glycoprotein present on B-cells from early development until differentiation into plasma cells and represents an integral component of a cell surface signal transduction complex positively regulating signal transduction through the B-cell receptor (Stamenkovic and Seed 1988; Bradbury et al. 1993; Matsumoto et al. 1993; Fearon and Carter 1995). CD19 is nearly universally expressed by B-ALL, CLL, and hairy cell leukemia, while not expressed on normal tissues other than B-cells, including multipotent hematopoietic progenitor cells (De Rossi et al. 1993; Uckun et al. 1988; Schwonzen et al. 1993; Robbins et al. 1993). A CAR is a recombinant receptor construct composed of an extracellular antibody-derived single-chain variable fragment (scFv), linked to intracellular T-cell signaling domains of the T-cell receptor, thereby redirecting T-cell specificity in an HLA-independent manner (Park and Brentjens 2010). As discussed in a previous chapter, multiple generations of CARs have been developed and investigated in clinical studies. First-generation CARs consist of a target-specific scFv fused to the CD3ζ endodomain of the T-cell receptor/CD3 complex. As first-generation CAR T-cells exhibited limited persistence, expansion, and antitumor efficacy in preclinical and clinical studies, second-generation CARs incorporated cytoplasmic signaling domains of T-cell costimulatory receptors (e.g., CD28, 4-1BB) to provide a costimulatory "signal 2" to the T-cell. Third-generation CARs place multiple costimulatory domains in tandem (Fig. 5.1). Several groups have presented early data demonstrating that CAR-modified T-cells targeting CD19 can induce meaningful responses in patients with relapsed or chemotherapy-refractory

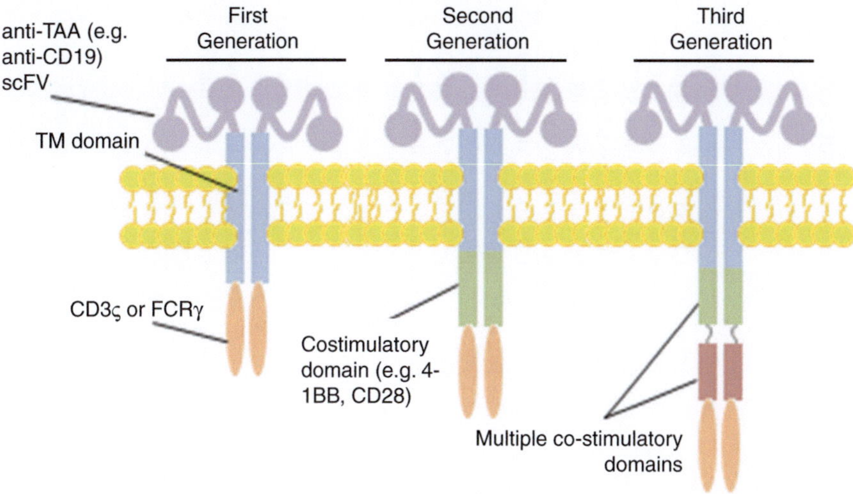

Fig. 5.1 Schematic depicting structure of chimeric antigen receptors in largest published series to date. *scFv* single-chain variable region fragment, *TM* transmembrane

B-cell leukemias (Park et al. 2016). In 2017, tisagenlecleucel, a CD19-targeted CAR T-cell product bearing a 4-1BB costimulatory domain, was approved by the US Food and Drug Administration for children and young adults <26 years old with refractory B-ALL or in second or greater relapse and became the first commercially available CAR T-cell product (U.S. Food and Drug Administration 2017). The largest clinical series described herein, reflecting treatment of adults with B-ALL and CLL, have employed second-generation CD19-targeted CAR T-cells. In this chapter, we review clinical outcomes of adults with leukemia treated with CAR T-cells, toxicities associated with CAR T-cell administration, present challenges limiting therapeutic efficacy, and future directions, including novel targets and enhancements to improve antileukemic activity.

5.2 CD19-Targeted CAR T-Cells in B-ALL

The largest series to date treating adults with relapsed or refractory B-ALL with CD19-targeted CAR T-cells are summarized in Table 5.1. Important differences between these studies include the use of autologous vs. allogeneic T-cells for genetic modification, as well as different transduction methods, costimulatory domains, regimens of lymphodepleting chemotherapy, CAR T-cell doses, and CAR T-cell product composition. Investigators from Memorial Sloan Kettering Cancer Center (MSKCC) were the first to report the efficacy of CD19-targeted CAR T-cells incorporating a CD28 costimulatory domain (19-28z) in generating durable molecular remissions in five adults with relapsed ALL (Brentjens et al. 2013; Davila et al. 2014) and have since reported the largest series of adults with ALL treated with

Table 5.1 CAR T-cell design and production and clinical aspects of largest reported clinical series to date investigating CD19-targeted CAR T-cells in the treatment of B-ALL

Institution/Reference	# of patients reported	Gene transfer method	scFv	Costimulatory domain	Lymphodepleting chemotherapy	CAR T-cell doses	Disease-related outcomes
Memorial Sloan Kettering Cancer Center (Brentjens et al. 2013; Davila et al. 2014; Park et al. 2018)	53	*Gammaretrovirus*	SJ25C1	CD28	Cy or Cy/Flu	1×10^6 vs. 3×10^6 CAR⁺ T-cells/kg	CR: 83% (MRD-negative in 67%); 17 of 44 in CR underwent allo-HSCT Median EFS: 6.1 months (all) and 12.5 months (pts in MRD-negative CR)
Fred Hutchinson Cancer Research Center (Turtle et al. 2016)	30	*Lentivirus*	FMC63	4-1BB	Cy 2–4 g/m^2 (± etoposide 100 mg/m^2 × 3 days) or Cy 30–60 mg/kg + Flu 25 mg/m^2 × 3–5 days	2×10^5, 2×10^6, and 2×10^7 CAR^+ T-cells/kg	CR: 10/12 (MRD-negative by flow cytometry) among pts receiving Cy or Cy/etoposide; 16/17 (MRD-negative by flow cytometry and FISH/karyotype) among pts receiving Flu/Cy Median DFS: not yet reached in Flu/Cy arm
University of Pennsylvania (Frey et al. 2014)	12	*Lentivirus*	FMC63	4-1BB	Investigator's choice	6.5–8.45×10^6 CAR^+ T-cells/kg	CR: 89% (8/9) of evaluable pts, all MRD-negative; 3 non-evaluable patients died in the setting of refractory CRS
National Cancer Institute (Brudno et al. 2016)	5	*Gammaretrovirus*	FMC63	CD28	None (administered following allo-HCT)	4.2–7.1×10^6 CAR^+ T-cells/kg	CR: 80% (4/5, all MRD-negative)

Cy cyclophosphamide, *Flu* fludarabine, *EFS* event-free survival, *DFS* disease-free survival, *CR* complete response, *MRD* minimal residual disease, *Allo-HCT* allogeneic hematopoietic cell transplantation

CD19-targeted CAR T-cells (Park et al. 2018). Patients' high-risk characteristics include ≥3 prior lines of treatment (n = 32), prior allogeneic hematopoietic cell transplantation (allo-HCT, n = 19), and Philadelphia (Ph) chromosome positivity (n = 16). Subsequent to salvage therapy or allo-HCT but prior to CAR T-cell infusion, 27 patients had morphologic disease (≥5% blasts in the bone marrow [BM] or measurable extramedullary disease) and 26 patients had minimal disease (<5% blasts in BM). Patients received cyclophosphamide (Cy) alone or Cy in combination with fludarabine (Flu) as lymphodepleting chemotherapy 2 days prior to 19-28z CAR T-cell infusion. Initially, all patients received 3×10^6 19-28z CAR T-cells/kg regardless of pretreatment disease burden. However, after observing a higher incidence of treatment-related toxicities at this dose in patients with morphologic disease (see section on "Toxicities"), the CAR T-cell dose was adjusted based on the disease burden, such that patients with morphologic disease received 1×10^6 19-28z CAR T-cells/kg and patients with minimal disease continued to receive 3×10^6 19-28z CAR T-cells/kg. In the entire cohort (i.e., at all CAR T-cell doses), 44 of 53 evaluable patients achieved or remained in complete response (CR) following 19-28z CAR T-cell infusion; 32 of 44 patients in CR evaluated for minimal residual disease (MRD) by multiparameter flow cytometry or deep sequencing achieved MRD-negative CR. Similar rates of CR were observed regardless of age, disease burden prior to CAR T-cell infusion, number of prior therapies, and prior allo-HCT. Seventeen of 44 patients in CR following CAR T-cell infusion underwent allo-HCT. However, as of most updated analysis, 6-month overall survival (OS) appeared similar between those who did and did not undergo post-CAR T-cell allo-HCT. Twenty-five patients achieving CR experienced morphologic relapse during follow-up; four of these patients relapsed with CD19-negative blasts by flow cytometry. Median event-free survival among all patients and among those who achieved MRD-negative CR was 6.1 months and 12.5 months, respectively (Brentjens et al. 2013; Davila et al. 2014; Park et al. 2015, 2018). 19-28z CAR T-cells were generally detectable by flow cytometry and quantitative PCR (qPCR) for 1–6 months post-infusion (Park et al. 2018).

Investigators from the Fred Hutchinson Cancer Research Center (FHCRC) also reported mature results of their phase I trial of CD19-targeted CAR T-cells in 30 adults with relapsed/refractory B-ALL (Turtle et al. 2016). In contrast to MSKCC's approach, the FHCRC's treatment protocol uses lentiviral transduction and a CD19-targeted CAR bearing a 4-1BB costimulatory domain (rather than the CD28 costimulatory domain). In addition, $CD4^+$ and $CD8^+$ T-cells are expanded separately in vitro prior to infusion at a defined ratio of 1:1 $CD4^+$:$CD8^+$ CAR T-cells, at total infused doses of 2×10^5, 2×10^6, and 2×10^7 CAR T-cells/kg. In support of this methodology, investigators from FHCRC have reported preclinical data demonstrating that transduced CAR T-cell subsets exhibit different effector functions, noting weak lytic activity from isolated $CD4^+$ CAR T-cells, but greater IFN-γ, TNF-α, and IL-2 cytokine production from naïve $CD4^+$ CAR T-cells after stimulation with $CD19^+$ tumor cells, and greatest direct antitumor potency from $CD8^+$ CAR T-cells with a central memory phenotype. In NOD/SCID/$\gamma c^{-/-}$ (NSG) mice engrafted with the Raji/ffluc ($CD19^+$) tumor cell lines, treatment with patient-derived CAR T-cells products with defined subset composition resulted in enhanced survival (Sommermeyer et al. 2016). As such, this strategy may allow for a lower requisite overall CAR T-cell dose and more uniform product composition between patients. In the FHCRC trial, the 30 treated patients had received a median of 3 prior intensive chemotherapy regimens (range, 1–11), and 11 had experienced relapse following prior allo-HCT. Most had morphologic B-ALL at the time of infusion (median BM blast burden 21%, range, 0.014–97%), and seven had extramedullary disease. Thirteen patients received lymphodepleting chemotherapy consisting of Cy-based regimens without Flu; 10 of 12 evaluable patients achieved BM CR without evidence of disease by flow cytometry, though 7 of 10 experienced relapse at a median of 66 days following CAR T-cell infusion (Turtle et al. 2015, 2016). While five of these patients were retreated, no response was observed; an endogenous $CD8^+$ T-cell response directed against the murine scFv component of the transgene was observed and hypothesized to contribute to CAR T-cell rejection and in vivo expansion failure. Of note, investigators from the National Cancer Institute (NCI) reported T-cell mediated anti-CAR responses in several pediatric patients with relapsed or refractory B-ALL treated with CD19-targeted CAR T-cells (Lee et al. 2015). As the FHCRC investigators hypothesized that greater lymphodepletion would reduce the risk of CAR T-cell rejection, they added Flu 25 $mg/m^2/day$ for 3–5 days to Cy 60 mg/kg prior to CAR T-cell infusion in 17 subsequent patients, observed BM CR by flow cytometry and cytogenetic studies in 16 of 17 patients, and noted significantly improved disease-free survival compared with patients in the prior cohort who had not received Flu (Turtle et al. 2016). Additionally, greater $CD4^+$ and $CD8^+$ CAR T-cell levels were observed 28 days following infusion of 2×10^6 CAR T-cells in patients receiving Flu/Cy vs. Cy-based lymphodepleting chemotherapy (Turtle et al. 2016). Of note, due to greater toxicity observed in patients with >20% BM blasts treated with $\geq 2 \times 10^6$ CAR T-cells, the investigators ultimately adopted a risk-adapted strategy in which these patients received a lower dose of 2×10^5 CAR T-cells, similar to MSKCC's approach as above (Turtle et al. 2016).

As discussed in a separate chapter, investigators from the University of Pennsylvania (UPenn) and Children's Hospital of Philadelphia (CHOP) have reported on the use of CTL019, a CD19-targeted CAR T-cell product containing a 4-1BB costimulatory domain, in children and adolescents with relapsed or refractory B-ALL (Maude et al. 2014, 2018). This group has additionally reported on 12 adults with relapsed or refractory B-ALL treated with CTL019 following investigator's choice of lymphodepleting chemotherapy. Eight of nine evaluable patients achieved MRD-negative CR at 1 month. However, substantial toxicity was observed as noted in a subsequent section (Frey et al. 2014). While mature data reflecting CTL019 persistence in adults with B-ALL has not yet been reported, this group has noted CTL019 persistence by qPCR and B-cell aplasia for ≥2 years following infusion in pediatric patients with B-ALL who achieved MRD-negative CR (Grupp et al. 2015).

While most studies of CD19-targeted CAR T-cell therapeutics to date have employed autologous T-cells, investigators from the NCI have additionally investigated the use of donor-derived (i.e., allogeneic) CAR T-cell products in patients with progressive B-ALL or other B-cell malignancies post-allo-HCT. Eligible patients had ≤grade I acute graft-versus-host disease (GvHD) and ≤mild chronic GvHD; DLI was not required for recipients with B-ALL. The investigators modified T-cells derived from the related or unrelated donor used for the patient's allo-HCT to express a CD19-targeted CAR incorporating a CD28 costimulatory domain. The five reported patients with progressive or relapsed B-ALL at infusion received a single dose of 4.2–7.1 × 10^6 CAR T-cells/kg (median 5.6 × 10^6/kg) without antecedent lymphodepleting chemotherapy. Four of these patients achieved MRD-negative CR, with recovery of normal hematopoiesis, including normal polyclonal B-cells; remission was durable (16+ months) in one patient with B-ALL treated with this approach, and another patient underwent second allo-HCT while in MRD-negative CR (Brudno et al. 2016).

5.3 CD19-Targeted CAR T-Cells in CLL

Following several early clinical reports of CD20- and CD19-targeted CAR T-cells in patients with relapsed or refractory B-cell non-Hodgkin lymphoma, several groups reported their early experience treating patients with relapsed or refractory CLL with CD19-targeted CAR T-cells (see Table 5.2 for largest/most mature series). MSKCC initially reported on eight patients with purine analog-refractory CLL and bulky lymphadenopathy treated with 19-28z CAR T-cells. Seven of eight patients had additional adverse cytogenetic or molecular features (del17p, del11q, and/or unmutated IgHV). No objective responses were observed in three patients who received 1.2–3.0 × 10^7 19-28z CAR T-cells/kg without any prior lymphodepleting chemotherapy. A fourth patient developed fevers, hypotension, and renal failure following 19-28z CAR T-cell therapy and died within 48 h of a suspected sepsis syndrome, possibly related to subacute infection prior to CAR T-cell therapy (Brentjens et al. 2010). Four subsequent patients received Cy 1.5–3.0 g/m^2 followed by 0.4–1.0 × 10^7 CAR T-cells/kg, infused in split doses over 2 days. One patient demonstrated marked reduction of peripheral adenopathy after an initial period of stable to progressed disease, two others demonstrated stable disease, and another demonstrated progression (Brentjens et al. 2011). Updated clinical results have noted objective responses in a subset of patients with CLL receiving conditioning chemotherapy prior to 19-28z CAR T-cell therapy, however (Geyer et al. 2016a). In a subsequent phase I trial at MSKCC, we enrolled patients with untreated CLL and administered 19-28z CAR T-cells to patients with residual disease following initial chemoimmunotherapy consisting of pentostatin, Cy, and rituximab (PCR). Eight such patients attained PR and then subsequently received Cy 600 mg/m^2 followed 2 days later by escalating doses of 19-28z CAR T-cells (3 × 10^6, $n = 3$; 1 × 10^7, $n = 3$; 3 × 10^7, $n = 2$, in 19-28z CAR T-cells/kg), administered outpatient. Most treated patients had unfavorable cytogenetic or molecular features (unmutated IgHV, $n = 7$; del11q, $n = 1$). Two patients achieved CR as best response, three achieved stable disease (with BM PR in one), and three had progression of disease, one of whom had a rising ALC by the time of 19-28z CAR T-cell infusion and two

Table 5.2 CAR T-cell design and production and clinical aspects of selected clinical series to date investigating CD19-targeted CAR T-cells in the treatment of CLL

Institution	# of patients reported	Gene transfer method	scFv	Costimulatory domain	Lymphodepleting chemotherapy	Infused cell doses	Responses observed
National Cancer Institute (Kochenderfer et al. 2012)	4	*Gammaretrovirus*	FMC63	CD28	Cy 60 mg/kg × 2 days + Flu 25 mg/m^2 × 5 days	0.3–2.8 × 10^7 CAR$^+$ T-cells/kg	ORR: 3/4 (CR, $n = 1$; PR, $n = 2$)
National Cancer Institute (Kochenderfer et al. 2015)	4	*Gammaretrovirus*	FMC63	CD28	Cy 60 mg/kg × 1–2 days + Flu 25 mg/m^2 × 5 days	1–4 × 10^6 CAR$^+$ T-cells/kg	ORR: 4/4 (CR, $n = 3$; PR, $n = 1$)
National Cancer Institute (Brudno et al. 2016)	5	*Gammaretrovirus*	FMC63	CD28	None (administered following Allo-HCT)	0.4–3.1 × 10^6 CAR$^+$ T-cells/kg	ORR: 2/5 (CR, $n = 1$; PR, $n = 1$; SD, $n = 1$)
Fred Hutchinson Cancer Research Center (Turtle et al. 2017)	19	*Lentivirus*	FMC63	4-1BB	Cy 30–60 mg/kg × 1 + Flu 25 mg/m^2 × 3 days	2 × 10^5, 2 × 10^6, or 2 × 10^7 CAR$^+$ T-cells/kg; 1:1 CD4$^+$:CD8$^+$	ORR: 14/19 (CR, $n = 4$; PR, $n = 10$)
University of Pennsylvania (Porter et al. 2015)	14	*Lentivirus*	FMC63	4-1BB	Investigator's choice	0.14–11 × 10^8 CAR$^+$ T-cells (median, 1.6 × 10^8 cells)	ORR: 8/14 (MRD-negative CR, $n = 4$; PR, $n = 4$) Median PFS: 7 months Median OS: 29 months
University of Pennsylvania (Porter et al. 2016)	35	*Lentivirus*	FMC63	4-1BB	Investigator's choice	5 × 10^7 vs. 5 × 10^8 CAR$^+$ T-cells	ORR: 9/17 (CR, $n = 6$; PR, $n = 3$) among pts receiving 5 × 10^8 CAR$^+$ T-cells

Cy cyclophosphamide, *Flu* fludarabine, *OS* overall survival, *PFS* progression-free survival, *CR* complete response, *PR* partial response, *MRD* minimal residual disease, *Allo-HCT* allogeneic hematopoietic cell transplantation

of whom achieved BM response (MRD-positive CR in one, PR in the other) with progression noted in lymph node; median PFS was 13.6 months (Geyer et al. 2016b; Park et al. 2014). CAR T-cells were detectable for a maximum of 48 days post-infusion by flow cytometry and/or qPCR.

Investigators from UPenn have treated >40 patients with relapsed or refractory CLL with CTL019 (Frey et al. 2014). This group published an initial report describing durable CR in a patient with refractory, p53-deficient CLL following pentostatin + Cy followed by 1.5 × 10^5 CTL019/kg (Porter et al. 2011). The investigators subsequently published detailed follow-up on 14 patients with relapsed or refractory CLL treated on their pilot study with CTL019. Treated patients had several high-risk features, including a median of five prior therapies, loss of TP53 or chromosome 17p ($n = 6$), and unmutated IgHV ($n = 9$). Patients received one of several lymphodepleting regimens, including bendamustine ($n = 6$), Cy/Flu ($n = 3$), or Cy/pentostatin, followed by infusion of CTL019 (median dose, 1.6 × 10^8 CTL019) over 1–3 days. Eight of 14 patients completed the full 3-day regimen, with others receiving only one ($n = 3$) or two fractions ($n = 3$) due to fevers within 24 h of infusion. Eight of 14 patients attained objective response at median follow-up of 19 months, including 4 patients who achieved MRD-negative CR, of whom 3 have experienced durable responses (28–53 months), while 1 died of unrelated causes 21 months post-CTL019 infusion with no evidence of disease. Four patients achieved PR within the first month of infusion, lasting 5–13 months, and two patients with PR completely cleared detectable CLL from the blood and BM. Six patients had no objective response and experienced progressive disease within 9 months of CTL019 infusion. Median OS for all patients was 29 months, 18-month OS was 71%, and 18-month PFS was 28.6%. Though subgroup analysis is limited considerably by the small number of patients, number of previous therapies, abnormalities of chromosome 17p, IgHV mutation status, and CTL019 dose did not appear to be correlated with response (Porter et al. 2015). CTL019 expansion peaked within 1 month of infusion, and patients achieving CR exhibited greater peak expansion than those who did not achieve CR. Persistence of CTL019 by qPCR or flow cytometry and B-cell aplasia were noted through last follow-up (as long as ≥4 years) in patients achieving MRD-negative CR (Porter et al. 2015). UPenn additionally presented a phase II dose optimization study in which 28 patients with relapsed or refractory CLL were randomly assigned to receive either 5 × 10^7 or 5 × 10^8 CTL019 (stage 1) and subsequent patients received 5 × 10^8 CTL019 (stage 2) following conditioning chemotherapy. Among 17 patients who received the higher CTL019 dose, 9 achieved objective response (CR, $n = 6$, and PR, $n = 3$) (Porter et al. 2014, 2016).

Several other groups have reported results in patients with CLL treated with CD19-targeted CAR T-cells on prospective studies enrolling patients with different B-cell malignancies. Investigators from the NCI have included several patients with CLL in their prospective trials of CD19-targeted CAR T-cell therapies in B-cell NHL. In their initial series, they treated eight patients with indolent B-NHL, including CLL, with Flu/Cy followed by CD19-targeted CAR T-cell, and IL-2 post-infusion. Three of four patients with CLL experienced objective response, including one patient who achieved a durable CR (Kochenderfer et al. 2012). In a subsequent study that omitted IL-2 following CAR T-cell infusion, they again observed responses in all four enrolled patients with relapsed CLL; three of these patients achieved CR, ongoing as of the time of publication (Kochenderfer et al. 2015). Investigators from the FHCHC also reported on 19 patients with relapsed and refractory CLL treated with CD19-targeted CAR T-cells, with 4 patients achieving CR (Turtle et al. 2017). Finally, as above, investigators from the NCI have additionally investigated the use of CD19-targeted allogeneic CAR T-cell infusion post-allo-HCT, including in patients with progression of CLL post-allo-HCT who had ≤grade I acute GvHD (aGvHD), including following at least ≥1 donor lymphocyte infusion (DLI). Patients received no antecedent lymphodepleting chemotherapy. Best responses were CR ($n = 1$), PR ($n = 1$), and stable disease ($n = 1$) among the five enrolled patients with CLL (Brudno et al. 2016).

5.4 Toxicities Associated with CD19-Targeted CAR T-Cells

The principal toxicities of CD19-targeted CAR T-cells observed to date include cytokine release syndrome (CRS), a spectrum of neurologic toxicities, and the on-target/off-tumor effect of B-cell aplasia. CRS may be defined broadly as a systemic inflammatory response in the hours to days following CAR T-cell infusion characterized by fevers, myalgias, malaise, and, in more severe cases, capillary leak syndrome with hypotension, hypoxia, and, more rarely, acute kidney injury and coagulopathy. CRS appears to arise in the setting of brisk CAR T-cell activation and expansion and marked elevations in pro-inflammatory cytokines (Davila et al. 2014). Severe CRS may be treated initially using the IL-6 receptor inhibitor tocilizumab, with the addition of lymphotoxic corticosteroids if symptoms persist. Intravenous immune globulin (IVIG) may be used to manage hypogammaglobulinemia in the setting of B-cell aplasia.

Among adults with B-ALL treated with CAR T-cells, the incidence and severity of severe CRS appears to be associated with underlying disease burden and with CAR T-cell dose (Davila et al. 2014; Park et al. 2018; Turtle et al. 2016; Frey et al. 2014). Classification systems for CRS severity vary between reported studies to date, complicating cross-trial comparisons (Lee et al. 2015; Porter et al. 2015). At MSKCC, severe CRS (i.e., requiring vasopressors or mechanical ventilation) has been observed almost exclusively among adults with morphologic B-ALL (vs. MRD alone) at the time of CAR T-cell infusion. After 3 of 11 patients at MSKCC with morphologic B-ALL experienced fatal treatment-related toxicity following infusion of 3×10^6 19-28z CAR T-cells/kg, CAR T-cell dose was lowered to 1×10^6 19-28z CAR T-cells/kg for patients with morphologic B-ALL and maintained at 3×10^6/kg for those patients with MRD only. Subsequently, no grade 5 toxicity was observed in patients treated according to this risk-adapted approach (Park et al. 2015, 2018). The FHCRC reported 25 of 30 adults with B-ALL treated with CD19-targeted CAR T-cells developed any CRS between 6 h and 9 days following CAR T-cell infusion, most commonly characterized by fevers and/or hypotension and elevated levels of IL-6 and IFN-γ; 7 patients had severe CRS requiring ICU care, and 2 patients died of treatment-related toxicity (severe CRS in one, irreversible neurologic toxicity in the other). Pretreatment disease burden and CAR T-cell dose were correlated with the incidence of CRS. After the first two patients were treated with 2×10^7 CAR T-cells/kg developed severe treatment-related toxicities, this dose level was determined to be too toxic. Moreover, as all six patients with >20% BM blasts treated with $\geq 2 \times 10^6$ CAR T-cells/kg required ICU care for CRS and developed severe neurologic toxicity, they implemented a risk-adapted approach in which patients with >20% BM blasts received 2×10^5 CAR T-cells/kg and those with ≤20% BM blasts received 2×10^6 CAR T-cells/kg. Thereafter, only one of ten patients with >20% BM blasts required ICU care (Turtle et al. 2016). Investigators from UPenn noted severe CRS in 11 of 12 adults with B-ALL treated with CTL019 on a phase I trial, including 3 patients with CRS refractory to tocilizumab and corticosteroids who died within 3–15 days of infusion; all treated patients had high pretreatment disease burden, and patients with fatal CRS had received a higher dose of CTL019 compared to the others (Frey et al. 2014). While data describing CRS in patients with CLL treated with CD19-targeted CAR T-cells are more limited, a preliminary report describing MSKCC's initial phase I trial utilizing 19-28z CAR T-cells in patients with CLL noted that all patients became febrile following 19-28z CAR T-cell infusion and two developed hypotension (Brentjens et al. 2011). In their subsequent trial of CAR T-cell therapy as consolidation following PCR chemoimmunotherapy in patients with CLL, four of five patients receiving $\geq 1 \times 10^7$ 19-28z CAR T-cells/kg were readmitted with fevers and mild, self-limited CRS not requiring ICU transfer, anti-cytokine therapy, or corticosteroids (Geyer et al. 2016b; Park et al. 2014). UPenn reported 9 of 14 CLL patients treated with CTL019 on their phase I trial developed ≥grade 1 CRS, 5 of whom required tocilizumab and/or corticosteroids and 4 of whom required ICU admission; in abstract form, they reported 19 of 35 patients with CLL treated with CTL019 on their phase II study developed any CRS, of whom 4 required tocilizumab ± corticosteroids (Porter et al. 2014, 2015, 2016). A similar proportion of patients with CLL or other B-NHL treated by the NCI with CD19-targeted CAR T-cells experienced fever (12 of 15) or hypotension (4 of 15) consistent with CRS (Kochenderfer et al. 2015).

A range of generally reversible neurologic toxicity has been observed following CAR T-cell infusion in children and adults, including delirium, seizure-like activity, confusion, word-finding difficulty, aphasia, and frank obtundation (Davila et al. 2014; Turtle et al. 2016; Porter et al. 2015; Kochenderfer et al. 2015). These neurologic toxicities may occur independently of CRS. Twenty-two of 53 adults with B-ALL treated with 19-28z CAR T-cells at MSKCC have experienced ≥grade 3 neurologic toxicity, including 14% of patients with MRD only at the time of CAR T-cell infusion, suggesting a less intimate correlation between the development of such toxicity and tumor burden (Park et al. 2015, 2018). FHCRC reported ≥grade 3 neurologic toxicity in 15 of 30 adults with B-ALL treated with CD19-targeted CAR T-cells, either concurrent with or after resolution of CRS, including generalized seizures in 3 patients (Turtle et al. 2016). Investigators from UPenn reported neurologic toxicity including hallucinations, confusion, and delirium in 6 of 14 adults (≤grade 2, $n = 5$) with relapsed/refractory CLL treated with CTL019 (Porter et al.

2015). The NCI has reported a similar incidence and spectrum of neurologic toxicity in patients with CLL and other B-NHL treated with CD19-targeted CAR T-cells (Kochenderfer et al. 2015). A correlation between CAR T-cell concentrations in the CSF has been postulated, but not consistently observed, and the pathogenesis of such toxicity remains uncertain (Davila et al. 2014; Lee et al. 2015).

5.4.1 Expert Point of View

CD19-targeted CAR-modified T-cells have emerged as one of the most effective available therapies in treating adults with relapsed or refractory B-ALL, including those with relapse following allo-HSCT, with high rates of MRD-negative CR now observed in multiple reported series, despite differences in therapeutic strategies, including differences in CAR design (e.g., scFv, costimulatory domain), lymphodepleting chemotherapy, and CAR T-cell dose, source (e.g., autologous vs. allogeneic), and product composition. A more modest proportion of patients with refractory CLL treated with second-generation CAR T-cells achieve durable clinical benefit, though long-term CRs have been observed in several reports. Potential strategies for extending this technology to non-B-cell leukemias are noted in the following section.

CAR T-cell therapies remain a new and evolving approach in the treatment of refractory adult leukemia, and further review of mature data will be required to draw firm conclusions regarding optimal therapeutic strategy. The broad, clinically relevant themes of studies to date have suggested the importance of costimulation and adequate lymphodepletion in promoting CAR T-cell persistence and expansion. Limited data suggests a trend toward longer persistence of CAR T-cells containing a 4-1BB (vs. CD28) costimulatory domain, such as CTL019. However, treatment with this 4-1BB-containing CAR T-cell product additionally appears associated with a greater incidence of CD19^{-} B-ALL escape variants when relapse occurs post-CR following CAR T-cell therapy. Additionally, differences in clinical trial design and patient selection make it extremely difficult to conclude whether costimulatory domain selection affects the incidence of relapse after achieving CR or long-term EFS/OS (Park et al. 2018; Turtle et al. 2016; Maude et al. 2014; Grupp et al. 2015).

Several lines of evidence support the need for adequate lymphodepletion prior to CAR T-cell therapy; while the exact mechanisms remain unclear, lymphodepleting chemotherapy may enhance antigen-presenting cell activation and eradicate immune-suppressive regulatory T-cells and homeostatic cytokine "sinks." The absence of significant rise in pro-inflammatory cytokine levels, poor CAR T-cell expansion, and limited clinical efficacy have been observed in adults with B-cell malignancies treated with CAR T-cell products without antecedent lymphodepleting chemotherapy (Brentjens et al. 2011; Cruz et al. 2013). Additionally, investigators from the FHCRC noted that the addition of Flu to Cy appeared to enhance CAR T-cell persistence and expansion, decrease the incidence of transgene-directed immune responses, and possibly improve EFS in adults with relapsed B-ALL treated with CAR T-cells (Turtle et al. 2016). Potential strategies for enhancing the persistence, expansion, and clinical efficacy of CAR T-cells in patients with CLL are discussed in a subsequent section.

Optimizing CAR T-cell therapeutics in adult leukemias additionally warrants consideration of management following CAR T-cell therapy. Challenges proximal to therapy include acquiring greater understanding of the pathogenesis and optimal management of treatment-related neurologic toxicity and in prevention and management of refractory CRS. Challenges more distal to therapy include defining an optimal consolidation strategy for patients with B-ALL achieving MRD-negative CR and management of escape variants (i.e., loss of target tumor-associated antigen) at relapse. In MSKCC's experience to date treating refractory B-ALL with 19-28z CAR T-cells, we have identified no significant difference in OS among patients achieving MRD-negative CR, regardless of whether the patient underwent subsequent allo-HCT (Park et al. 2015, 2018). However, in other series utilizing this approach, including the NCI's experience in treating pediatric patients with relapsed B-ALL, most patients achieving MRD-negative CR have undergone allo-HCT (Lee et al. 2015); whether consolidative allo-HCT or >1 cycle of CAR T-cell therapy will improve long-term EFS in this setting remains uncertain. We and others have additionally described loss of detectable CD19 by flow cytometry in relapsing B-ALL blasts in a subset of patients with B-ALL treated with CD19-targeted CAR T-cell therapy, a finding that parallels reports of CD19-negative relapse following therapy with the bispecific T-cell engager blinatumomab (Park et al. 2018; Turtle et al. 2016; Lee et al. 2015; Maude et al. 2014; Frey et al. 2014; Grupp et al. 2015; Topp et al. 2014). One of several potential mechanisms underlying this phenomenon appears to be alternative splicing of CD19 mRNA compromising the target epitope, and in turn, CAR T-cell efficacy, while preserving cytoplasmic domains required for kinase recruitment and signaling to permit leukemic maintenance (Sotillo et al. 2015). Antigen escape might be treated by the use of CAR T-cells targeting other immature B-cell antigens (e.g., CD22), as is being investigated in several ongoing studies (NCT02650414, NCT02315612), and might be prevented by use of CAR T-cells targeting multiple tumor-associated antigens at once or by therapies designed to enhance early T-cell expansion and overcome inhibitory effects of the tumor microenvironment as described in the next section.

5.4.2 Future Directions

The dramatic responses observed in many patients with refractory B-ALL treated with CD19-targeted CAR T-cells have led several groups of investigators to consider potential strategies for extending CAR T-cell therapy to acute myeloid leukemia (AML) and T-cell leukemias. While CD19 is in many ways an ideal target surface antigen for B-cell malignancies, as previously discussed, selection of a target for AML is far more challenging given the lack of known surface antigens unique to malignant myeloid blasts and not expressed on normal hematopoietic cells or myeloid precursors. Using a lentiviral anti-CD123 vector costimulated via

4-1BB, investigators from UPenn noted that CD123-targeted CAR T-cells (CART123) exhibited potent antileukemic activity in NSG mice bearing human AML cell lines (e.g., MOLM14) as well as NSG mice transgenic for IL-3, stem cell factor, and GM-CSF (NSGS mice) bearing patient-derived AML samples. However, CART123 administration appeared to ablate normal hematopoiesis in NSG mice engrafted with human $CD34^{+}$ hematopoietic progenitor cells, even at 1 month post-infusion (Gill et al. 2014). Administration of T-cells transduced with an anti-CD33 lentiviral vector (encoding an scFv derived from the anti-CD33 monoclonal antibody-drug conjugate gemtuzumab ozogamicin and a 4-1BB costimulatory domain) leads to severe hematopoietic toxicity in similar humanized xenograft models (Kenderian et al. 2015). As such, this group subsequently investigated a transiently expressed mRNA CD33-targeted CAR as a potential means to circumvent the myeloablation observed with CART123 and CART33 and thereby expand the therapeutic index of CAR T-cell therapy for AML. The mRNA construct is electroporated into human T-cells to generate the RNA-CART33 product, resulting in high-level CAR expression that diminished over 7 days, with cytotoxicity decreasing over time post-electroporation. MOLM14-engrafted NSG mice exhibited enhanced survival following Cy + RNA-CART33 vs. Cy + untransduced T-cells (Kenderian et al. 2015). Further development of "biodegradable" CAR T-cells and other strategies to modulate the therapeutic effect of CAR T-cells with potent antileukemic activity may permit safer application of CAR T-cell therapeutics in AML. Alternatively, CAR T-cells with greater hematologic toxicity might be used in patients with AML as a bridge to allo-HCT, as is being investigated in ongoing clinical trials utilizing CD33-targeted and CD123-targeted CAR T-cells (NCT02623582, NCT01864902). There also remains an unmet need for effective therapies for patients with relapsed or refractory T-cell malignancies, including T-ALL. However, the potential use of CAR T-cells targeted to T-cell antigens raises immediate concerns of on-target/off-tumor toxicity against endogenous T-cells and infused CAR T-cells (i.e., fratricide). Investigators from the Baylor College of Medicine/Texas Children's Hospital have conducted preclinical studies of CD5-targeted CAR T-cells, as CD5 is expressed on the surface of most T-ALL and T-NHL. Specifically, human T-cells transduced with a retrovirus encoding a CD5-targeted CAR costimulated via CD28 eliminate malignant T-cell lines in vitro and in xenograft NSG mouse models in vivo while exhibiting only limited fratricide, with sparing of native central and effector memory T-cells as well as virus-specific T-cells (Mamonkin et al. 2015).

The more modest observed clinical efficacy of CD19-targeted CAR T-cells in CLL, compared with B-ALL, may be related in part to a hostile tumor microenvironment. CLL cells exploit a variety of mechanisms to escape elimination from the endogenous immune system, including upregulation of inhibitory ligands inducing impairment of T-cell immunologic synapses (e.g., CD200, PD-L1), production of soluble plasma factors leading to suppression of NK cytotoxicity (e.g., BAG6), release of exosomes promoting a cancer-associated fibroblast phenotype in stromal cells and supporting leukemic maintenance, and induction of $CD8^{+}$ T-cell exhaustion (as marked by decreased proliferative and cytotoxic capacity and increased expression of exhaustion markers PD-1, CD160, and CD244) (Reiners et al. 2013; Ramsay et al. 2012; Gorgun et al. 2005; McClanahan et al. 2015; Riches et al. 2013; Paggetti et al. 2015). Several strategies to overcome this inhibitory microenvironment have been described and are being investigated in forthcoming clinical studies, including further genetic modification of CD19-targeted CAR T-cells with an additional costimulatory ligand, such as 4-1BB ligand (4-1BBL) or CD40 ligand (CD40L), or incorporation of the pro-inflammatory cytokine IL-12 (Pegram et al. 2012, 2015; Stephan et al. 2007). Several investigators have hypothesized that coadministration of checkpoint inhibitors targeting the programmed death-1 (PD-1)/PD-L1 pathway may abrogate CAR T-cell exhaustion, deplete myeloid-derived suppressor cells at disease sites, and thereby enhance antitumor response (John et al. 2013). Additionally, ibrutinib appears to have immunomodulatory effects independent of inhibition of Bruton's tyrosine kinase (BTK), including inhibition of interleukin-2-inducible T-cell kinase (ITK), which may in turn enhance Th1 responses (Sagiv-Barfi et al. 2015). Investigators from the University of Pennsylvania have observed decreased levels of PD-1 expression on endogenous $CD8^+$ T-cells in patients with CLL treated with ibrutinib, as well as superior CTL019 expansion ex vivo in patients treated with ibrutinib for ≥5 months, and enhanced proliferation and engraftment in vivo in patients with CLL treated with ibrutinib prior to CTL019 infusion (Fraietta et al. 2016). Early clinical data from MSKCC supports the potential efficacy of ibrutinib in promoting ex vivo T-cell expansion and enhancing clinical response (Geyer et al. 2016a). These findings suggest a potential role for combination therapy with ibrutinib and CD19-targeted CAR T-cells in future clinical studies in CLL.

References

Bradbury LE, Goldmacher VS, Tedder TF (1993) The CD19 signal transduction complex of B lymphocytes. Deletion of the CD19 cytoplasmic domain alters signal transduction but not complex formation with TAPA-1 and Leu 13. J Immunol 151:2915–2927

Brentjens R, Yeh R, Bernal Y, Riviere I, Sadelain M (2010) Treatment of chronic lymphocytic leukemia with genetically targeted autologous T cells: case report of an unforeseen adverse event in a phase I clinical trial. Mol Ther 18:666–668

Brentjens RJ et al (2011) Safety and persistence of adoptively transferred autologous CD19-targeted T cells in patients with relapsed or chemotherapy refractory B-cell leukemias. Blood 118:4817–4828

Brentjens RJ et al (2013) CD19-targeted T cells rapidly induce molecular remissions in adults with chemotherapy-refractory acute lymphoblastic leukemia. Sci Transl Med 5:177ra138

Brudno JN et al (2016) Allogeneic T cells that express an anti-CD19 chimeric antigen receptor induce remissions of B-cell malignancies that progress after allogeneic hematopoietic stem-cell transplantation without causing graft-versus-host disease. J Clin Oncol 34:1112–1121

Byrd JC et al (2013) Targeting BTK with ibrutinib in relapsed chronic lymphocytic leukemia. N Engl J Med 369:32–42

Byrd JC et al (2015) Three-year follow-up of treatment-naive and previously treated patients with CLL and SLL receiving single-agent ibrutinib. Blood 125:2497–2506

Cruz CR et al (2013) Infusion of donor-derived CD19-redirected virus-specific T cells for B-cell malignancies relapsed after allogeneic stem cell transplant: a phase 1 study. Blood 122:2965–2973

Davila ML et al (2014) Efficacy and toxicity management of 19-28z CAR T cell therapy in B cell acute lymphoblastic leukemia. Sci Transl Med 6:224ra225
De Rossi G et al (1993) Immunophenotype of acute lymphoblastic leukemia cells: the experience of the Italian Cooperative Group (Gimema). Leuk Lymphoma 9:221–228
Fearon DT, Carter RH (1995) The CD19/CR2/TAPA-1 complex of B lymphocytes: linking natural to acquired immunity. Annu Rev Immunol 13:127–149
Fraietta JA et al (2016) Ibrutinib enhances chimeric antigen receptor T-cell engraftment and efficacy in leukemia. Blood 127:1117–1127
Frey NV et al (2014) Refractory cytokine release syndrome in recipients of chimeric antigen receptor (CAR) T cells. Blood 124:2296–2296
Geyer MB et al (2016a) Implications of concurrent ibrutinib therapy on CAR T-cell manufacturing and phenotype and on clinical outcomes following CD19-targeted CAR T-cell administration in adults with relapsed/refractory CLL. Blood 128:58–58
Geyer MB et al (2016b) Updated results: phase I trial of autologous CD19-targeted CAR T cells in patients with residual CLL following initial purine analog-based therapy. J Clin Oncol 34:7526
Gill S et al (2014) Preclinical targeting of human acute myeloid leukemia and myeloablation using chimeric antigen receptor-modified T cells. Blood 123:2343–2354
Gokbuget N et al (2012) Outcome of relapsed adult lymphoblastic leukemia depends on response to salvage chemotherapy, prognostic factors, and performance of stem cell transplantation. Blood 120:2032–2041
Gorgun G, Holderried TA, Zahrieh D, Neuberg D, Gribben JG (2005) Chronic lymphocytic leukemia cells induce changes in gene expression of CD4 and CD8 T cells. J Clin Investig 115:1797–1805
Grupp SA et al (2015) Durable remissions in children with relapsed/refractory ALL treated with T cells engineered with a CD19-targeted chimeric antigen receptor (CTL019). Blood 126:681
John LB et al (2013) Anti-PD-1 antibody therapy potently enhances the eradication of established tumors by gene-modified T cells. Clin Cancer Res 19:5636–5646
Kantarjian HM et al (2010) Defining the course and prognosis of adults with acute lymphocytic leukemia in first salvage after induction failure or short first remission duration. Cancer 116:5568–5574
Kay NE et al (2007) Combination chemoimmunotherapy with pentostatin, cyclophosphamide, and rituximab shows significant clinical activity with low accompanying toxicity in previously untreated B chronic lymphocytic leukemia. Blood 109:405–411
Kenderian SS et al (2015) CD33-specific chimeric antigen receptor T cells exhibit potent preclinical activity against human acute myeloid leukemia. Leukemia 29:1637–1647
Kochenderfer JN et al (2012) B-cell depletion and remissions of malignancy along with cytokine-associated toxicity in a clinical trial of anti-CD19 chimeric-antigen-receptor-transduced T cells. Blood 119:2709–2720
Kochenderfer JN et al (2015) Chemotherapy-refractory diffuse large B-cell lymphoma and indolent B-cell malignancies can be effectively treated with autologous T cells expressing an anti-CD19 chimeric antigen receptor. J Clin Oncol 33:540–549
Lee DW et al (2015) T cells expressing CD19 chimeric antigen receptors for acute lymphoblastic leukaemia in children and young adults: a phase 1 dose-escalation trial. Lancet 385:517–528
Mamonkin M, Rouce RH, Tashiro H, Brenner MK (2015) A T-cell-directed chimeric antigen receptor for the selective treatment of T-cell malignancies. Blood 126:983–992
Matsumoto AK et al (1993) Functional dissection of the CD21/CD19/TAPA-1/Leu-13 complex of B lymphocytes. J Exp Med 178:1407–1417
Maude SL et al (2014) Chimeric antigen receptor T cells for sustained remissions in leukemia. N Engl J Med 371:1507–1517
Maude SL et al (2018) Tisagenlecleucel in children and young adults with B-cell lymphoblastic leukemia. N Engl J Med 378:439–448
McClanahan F et al (2015) PD-L1 checkpoint blockade prevents immune dysfunction and leukemia development in a mouse model of chronic lymphocytic leukemia. Blood 126:203–211

Paggetti J et al (2015) Exosomes released by chronic lymphocytic leukemia cells induce the transition of stromal cells into cancer-associated fibroblasts. Blood 126:1106–1117

Park JH, Brentjens RJ (2010) Adoptive immunotherapy for B-cell malignancies with autologous chimeric antigen receptor modified tumor targeted T cells. Discov Med 9:277–288

Park JH et al (2014) Phase I trial of autologous CD19-targeted CAR-modified t cells as consolidation after purine analog-based first-line therapy in patients with previously untreated CLL. J Clin Oncol 32:7020

Park JH et al (2015) Implications of minimal residual disease negative complete remission (MRD-CR) and allogeneic stem cell transplant on safety and clinical outcome of CD19-targeted 19-28z CAR modified T cells in adult patients with relapsed, refractory B-cell ALL. Blood 126:682–682

Park JH, Geyer MB, Brentjens RJ (2016) CD19-targeted CAR T-cell therapeutics for hematologic malignancies: interpreting clinical outcomes to date. Blood 127:3312–3320

Park JH et al (2018) Long-term follow-up of CD19 CAR therapy in acute lymphoblastic leukemia. N Engl J Med 378:449–459

Pegram HJ et al (2012) Tumor-targeted T cells modified to secrete IL-12 eradicate systemic tumors without need for prior conditioning. Blood 119:4133–4141

Pegram HJ et al (2015) IL-12-secreting CD19-targeted cord blood-derived T cells for the immunotherapy of B-cell acute lymphoblastic leukemia. Leukemia 29:415–422

Porter DL, Levine BL, Kalos M, Bagg A, June CH (2011) Chimeric antigen receptor-modified T cells in chronic lymphoid leukemia. N Engl J Med 365:725–733

Porter DL et al (2014) Randomized, phase II dose optimization study of chimeric antigen receptor modified T cells directed against CD19 (CTL019) in patients with relapsed, refractory CLL. Blood 124:1982

Porter DL et al (2015) Chimeric antigen receptor T cells persist and induce sustained remissions in relapsed refractory chronic lymphocytic leukemia. Sci Transl Med 7:303ra139

Porter DL et al (2016) Randomized, phase II dose optimization study of chimeric antigen receptor (CAR) modified T cells directed against CD19 in patients (pts) with relapsed, refractory (R/R) CLL. J Clin Oncol 34:3009

Ramsay AG, Clear AJ, Fatah R, Gribben JG (2012) Multiple inhibitory ligands induce impaired T-cell immunologic synapse function in chronic lymphocytic leukemia that can be blocked with lenalidomide: establishing a reversible immune evasion mechanism in human cancer. Blood 120:1412–1421

Reiners KS et al (2013) Soluble ligands for NK cell receptors promote evasion of chronic lymphocytic leukemia cells from NK cell anti-tumor activity. Blood 121:3658–3665

Riches JC et al (2013) T cells from CLL patients exhibit features of T-cell exhaustion but retain capacity for cytokine production. Blood 121:1612–1621

Robbins BA et al (1993) Diagnostic application of two-color flow cytometry in 161 cases of hairy cell leukemia. Blood 82:1277–1287

Sagiv-Barfi I et al (2015) Therapeutic antitumor immunity by checkpoint blockade is enhanced by ibrutinib, an inhibitor of both BTK and ITK. Proc Natl Acad Sci U S A 112:E966–E972

Schwonzen M et al (1993) Immunophenotyping of low-grade B-cell lymphoma in blood and bone marrow: poor correlation between immunophenotype and cytological/histological classification. Br J Haematol 83:232–239

Sommermeyer D et al (2016) Chimeric antigen receptor-modified T cells derived from defined CD8(+) and CD4(+) subsets confer superior antitumor reactivity in vivo. Leukemia 30:492–500

Sotillo E et al (2015) Convergence of acquired mutations and alternative splicing of CD19 enables resistance to CART-19 immunotherapy. Cancer Discov 5:1282–1295

Stamenkovic I, Seed B (1988) CD19, the earliest differentiation antigen of the B cell lineage, bears three extracellular immunoglobulin-like domains and an Epstein-Barr virus-related cytoplasmic tail. J Exp Med 168:1205–1210

Stephan MT et al (2007) T cell-encoded CD80 and 4-1BBL induce auto- and transcostimulation, resulting in potent tumor rejection. Nat Med 13:1440–1449

Tam CS et al (2008) Long-term results of the fludarabine, cyclophosphamide, and rituximab regimen as initial therapy of chronic lymphocytic leukemia. Blood 112:975–980
Topp MS et al (2014) Phase II trial of the anti-CD19 bispecific T cell-engager blinatumomab shows hematologic and molecular remissions in patients with relapsed or refractory B-precursor acute lymphoblastic leukemia. J Clin Oncol 32:4134–4140
Turtle CJ et al (2015) Addition of fludarabine to cyclophosphamide lymphodepletion improves in vivo expansion of CD19 chimeric antigen receptor-modified T cells and clinical outcome in adults with B cell acute lymphoblastic leukemia. Blood 126:3773–3773
Turtle CJ et al (2016) CD19 CAR-T cells of defined CD4+:CD8+ composition in adult B cell ALL patients. J Clin Investig 126:2123–2138
Turtle CJ et al (2017) Durable molecular remissions in chronic lymphocytic leukemia treated with CD19-specific chimeric antigen receptor-modified T cells after failure of ibrutinib. J Clin Oncol 35:3010–3020
U.S. Food and Drug Administration (2017) FDA approves tisagenlecleucel for B-cell ALL and tocilizumab for cytokine release syndrome. FDA, Silver Spring
Uckun FM et al (1988) Detailed studies on expression and function of CD19 surface determinant by using B43 monoclonal antibody and the clinical potential of anti- CD19 immunotoxins. Blood 71:13–29

Chimeric Antigen Receptor T Cells for Lymphomas: Methods, Data, and Challenges

6

Yakup Batlevi and Craig S. Sauter

6.1 Introduction

The cluster of differentiation antigen 19 (CD19) is a 95 kD transmembrane glycoprotein ubiquitously expressed on B cells from pro-B to mature B-cell phenotypes, thus making it an optimal target for targeted cellular therapy against all B-cell non-Hodgkin lymphomas (B-NHL)/chronic lymphocytic leukemia/small lymphocytic lymphoma (CLL/SLL) and B-cell acute lymphoblastic leukemia (B-ALL). CD19 is not expressed on other hematopoietic, or organ, cell populations. Targeting CD19 can hypothetically result in prolonged B-cell aplasia. Given the clinical experience with the anti-CD20 monoclonal antibody rituximab with temporary B-cell aplasia, severe clinical consequence has not been observed. Intravenous gamma globulin has proven to effectively supplement humoral immunity in hypogammaglobulinemic patients. Thus, CD19 continues to serve as an acceptable tumor antigen to target with cellular therapy. Genetically engineered recombinant T-cell receptors directed against a specific tumor antigen (chimeric antigen receptors, CARs) can

Y. Batlevi
Adult Bone Marrow Transplant Service, Memorial Sloan Kettering Cancer Center, New York, NY, USA
e-mail: batleviy@mskcc.org

C. S. Sauter (✉)
Adult Bone Marrow Transplant Service, Memorial Sloan Kettering Cancer Center, New York, NY, USA

Cellular Therapeutics Center, Department of Medicine, Memorial Sloan Kettering Cancer Center, New York, NY, USA

Department of Medicine, Weill Cornell Medical College, New York, NY, USA
e-mail: sauterc@mskcc.org

M.-A. Perales et al. (eds.), *Cell and Gene Therapies*, Advances and Controversies in Hematopoietic Transplantation and Cell Therapy,
https://doi.org/10.1007/978-3-319-54368-0_6

recognize and kill tumor cell targets. This review will focus on the clinical experience of targeting CD19 with CAR-modified T cells (19-CAR-T) for B-cell lymphomas, excluding CLL/SLL and multiple myeloma.

The initial CAR constructs consisted of a single-chain antigen recognizing variable fragment (scFv) extracellular domain from an antibody in conjunction with a transmembrane link to a functional CD3ζ intracellular signaling domain (Eshhar et al. 1993). While this initial design had demonstrable effector function, proliferation and expansion were greatly enhanced by the incorporation of signal transmembrane co-stimulatory domains into later-generation constructs (Hombach et al. 2001). This translated into marked improvement of antitumor efficacy in early animal models (Brentjens et al. 2003). The clinical experience of 19-CAR-T for relapsed and/or refractory (rel/ref) B-NHL and Hodgkin lymphoma (HL) reviewed in this chapter will largely focus on "second-generation" 19-CAR-T constructs with TCR/CD3 signal 1 coupled to signal 2 co-stimulation with either CD28 or 4-1BB. Additionally, there will be brief mention of data with other tumor targets including kappa light chain and CD30 as well as later-generation constructs.

6.1.1 Clinical Studies: 19-CAR-T for Patients with Rel/Ref B-NHL

The initial clinical experience in 19-CAR-T for patients with rel/ref follicular lymphoma (FL) $n = 2$ and diffuse large B-cell lymphoma (DLBCL) $n = 2$ was with a first-generation construct from the City of Hope (Jensen et al. 2010). The two DLBCL patients received 19-CAR-T 1 month following high-dose therapy and autologous stem cell transplantation (HDT-ASCT), and one of the two patients had progressive disease following CAR-T infusion. The two patients with FL experienced disease progression following therapy. Interleukin-2 (IL-2) was infused adjunctively in the two patients with FL with the intent of providing proliferative stimulus to the CAR-T cell. Significant toxicity was not observed, and 19-CAR-T failed to persist with only one of four patients demonstrating persistence of 19-CAR-T in the peripheral blood at 1 week post-infusion.

The National Cancer Institute (NCI) was the first group to publish a case report of a second-generation 19-CAR-T incorporating a CD28 co-stimulatory domain (along with exogenous IL-2) in a patient with FL (Kochenderfer et al. 2010). The patient experienced a partial remission (PR) lasting approximately 10 months, and the 19-CAR-T product was noted to persist for >6 months. This group subsequently updated their prospective experience of 19-CAR-T incorporating CD28 co-stimulation for re/ref B-NHL preceded by lymphodepleting chemotherapy consisting of cyclophosphamide 60–120 mg/kg and fludarabine at a total dose of 125 mg/m^2 (Kochenderfer et al. 2015). All six patients with indolent B-NHL (including splenic marginal zone lymphoma $n = 1$ and CLL/SLL $n = 4$) responded with either a partial (PR, $n = 2$) or complete remission (CR, $n = 4$). Six of the seven evaluable patients with DLBCL, including three patients with primary mediastinal B NHL, responded with either a PR ($n = 2$) or CR ($n = 4$). Two of the patients were not evaluable for a response and one patient experienced stable disease. The longest durations of responses were 12 and 23 months from treatment for DLBCL and indolent B-NHL, respectively. Peripheral expansion of the 19-CAR-T product peaked at 7–17 days. Because of toxicity, predominately in the form of cytokine-release syndrome (CRS), the dose of 19-CAR-T was subsequently lowered from 5×10^6/kg to 1×10^6/kg. Greater than or equal to grade 3 toxicity, again predominately CRS, was observed in 13 of 15 patients. A subsequent study by the same group of lower-dose chemotherapy (cyclophosphamide 900 mg/m^2 and fludarabine 90 mg/m^2) presented at the American Society of Hematology (ASH) meeting in 2014, noted less toxicity related to severe CRS with six of nine patients responding to 19-CAR-T therapy (Kochenderfer et al. 2014). They have subsequently updated their experience reporting increased IL-15 post-infusion correlated to CAR-T expansion and clinical response (Kochenderfer et al. 2017a) with remissions lasting greater than 4 years (Kochenderfer et al. 2017b). Following these studies, this CAR-T construct was licensed to Kite Pharma as KTE-C19 and subsequently axicabtagene ciloleucel (axi-cel), a 19-CAR-T with CD28 co-stimulation following fludarabine and cyclophosphamide conditioning, for rel/ref B-NHL with initial presentation by Locke et al. at ASH 2015 wherein six patients had been treated and three patients experienced >grade 3 toxicity including a grade 4 encephalopathy and grade 4 CRS. Three patients were evaluable for response, in short follow-up at 1 month, with ORR of 100% (CR, $n = 2$; PR, $n = 1$) (Locke et al. 2015). This leads to the multicenter phase II, Zuma-1 trial that led to FDA approval of the first CAR-T-cell therapy for the treatment of adult patients with rel/ref large B-cell lymphoma after at least two lines of standard therapy. In this study, axi-cel was administered to 101 patients with DLBCL ($n = 77$), primary mediastinal B-cell lymphoma, or transformed FL ($n = 24$) following low-dose fludarabine and cyclophosphamide conditioning. At 6-month follow-up, ORR was 82% (CR, $n = 55$ [54%]; PR, $n = 28$ [28%]. At median follow-up period (15.4 months), 42% of patients maintained a response (CR, 40%). The overall rate of survival at 18 months was 52%. Ninety-three percent of all patients experienced CRS, while 64% experienced neurotoxicity (NT), which were all resolved. Forty-three percent of patients were treated with tocilizumab, and 27% received glucocorticoids for the management of CRS and/or NT with no apparent effect on response rates (Neelapu et al. 2017).

The group at the University of Pennsylvania recently published their phase IIa study treating chemorefractory FL and DLBCL patients with 19-CAR-T (Schuster et al. 2017a). In contrast to a CD28 second-signal co-stimulatory domain, their construct incorporates a 4-1BB co-stimulatory transmembrane molecule. Patients were treated with variable lymphodepleting chemotherapy per treating physician prior to administration of 19-CAR-T. This report included 14 evaluable patients with FL and 14 evaluable patients with DLBCL. Of the 28 patients treated with 19-CAR-T, 18 (64%) had a response. CR was achieved with 6 of the 14 patients (43%) with DLBCL and 10 of the 14 patients (71%) with FL. Continuous response was observed at the median follow-up of 28.6 months in 86% of patients with DLBCL and in 89% of patients with FL. Following infusion, median peak expansion of 19-CAR-T cells was 8 days in patients with a response and 10 days in patients without a response.

Fourteen of 16 patients who achieved CR had PCR-detectable levels of 19-CAR-T DNA between 6 and 24 months after infusion. Eight of 16 patients in CR proceeded to sustained B-cell recovery at median of 6.7 months. The investigators observed severe CRS in five patients (18%) and severe encephalopathy in three patients (11%) among which two cases were self-limiting and one case was fatal. This treatment was further explored in a multicenter, multinational phase II study (The JULIET Trial) presented at ASH 2017 (Schuster et al. 2017b). The investigators reported best ORR of 53% with 39.5% CR rate in 81 patients infused and evaluable. The CR rate at 6 months was 30% with CTL019 detectable in the peripheral blood up to 1 year post-infusion. CRS occurred in 58% of patient and 23% grade 3–4. They reported a 12% incidence of neurotoxicity. This study led to FDA approval of Novartis Pharmaceuticals licensed, tisagenlecleucel, on May 1, 2018 for rel/ref adult DLBCL following at least two lines of chemotherapy.

The group from the Fred Hutchinson Cancer Research Center (FHCRC) published their experience of treating rel/ref B-NHL with lentivirus transduced 19-CAR-T with a secondary 4-1BB co-stimulatory molecule in a fixed 1:1 ratio of CD4:CD8, based largely upon preclinical modeling of improved persistence and efficacy of the 19-CAR-T product (Riddell et al. 2014). These investigators tested the effects of adding fludarabine to conditioning regimen preceding variable doses of 19-CAR-T infusion. In the cyclophosphamide and fludarabine conditioning arm, 18 B-NHL patients achieved an ORR of 72% (CR, $n = 9$; PR, $n = 4$). In the cyclophosphamide-based conditioning without fludarabine arm, 12 B-NHL patients achieved an ORR of 50% (CR, $n = 1$; PR, $n = 5$) (Turtle et al. 2016). Of the total 32 evaluable patients, 20 developed any grade CRS, and 9 developed severe NT associated with treatment. Severe CRS was observed in four patients, all of whom had received cyclophosphamide and fludarabine conditioning. There was also a correlation between 19-CAR-T dose and severe CRS and NT. Thus, adding fludarabine to the conditioning regimen and treatment with higher doses of 19-CAR-T correlated with increasing toxicities. Three of six patients (50%) treated at the highest dose (2×10^7/kg) after cyclophosphamide and fludarabine conditioning developed severe CRS, and four of six patients (67%) developed severe NT. Of note, peak serum concentrations of IL-6, interferon gamma (IFN-γ), ferritin, and C-reactive protein correlated with development and severity of CRS. The highest IL-6 and IFN-γ levels were seen in patients who received cyclophosphamide and fludarabine conditioning followed by infusion of the highest 19-CAR-T dose. This technology was subsequently licensed to Juno Therapeutics, and a multi-institutional trial was initiated. In a preliminary update at the 2017 ASH meeting, investigators reported all grade CRS rate at 30% (12/69), severe CRS rate at 1% (1/69), and NT rate at 20% (14/69) (Abramson et al. 2017). At the time of the report, best ORR was 75% (51/68), with a CR at 56% (38/68).

A complete summary of the clinical studies for rel/ref B-NHL with second-generation 19-CAR-T is summarized in Table 6.1.

Table 6.1 Clinical studies of 19-CAR-T for relapsed or refractory B-NHL

Institution	Viral vector	Co-stimulatory molecule	Conditioning	Patients	Clinical responses	Notes
NCI (Kochenderfer et al. 2015)	Gamma retrovirus	CD28	Cyc 60–120 mg/kg Flu 125 mg/m^2	iB-NHL $n = 6$, aB-NHL $n = 9$	iB-NHL 6/6 (CR = 4, PR = 2) aB-NHL 6/7 (CR = 4, PR = 2) inevaluable $n = 3$	13/15 ≥grade 3 toxicity
NCI (Kochenderfer et al. 2014)	Gamma retrovirus	CD28	Cyc 90 mg/m^2 flu 90 mg/m^2	FL $n = 1$ DLBCL $n = 8$	FL PR DLBCL 6/8 (CR = 1, PR = 5)	No patients required vasopressor or MV
NCI (Kochenderfer et al. 2017a, b)	Gamma retrovirus	CD28	Cyc 900-1500 mg/m^2 flu 90 mg/m^2	DLBCL $n = 19$ FL $n = 2$ MCL $n = 1$	73% ORR (55% CR; 18% PR)	IL-15 levels correlated with response
UPenn (Schuster et al. 2017a)	Lentivirus	4-1BB	Variable	FL $n = 14$ DLBCL $n = 14$	FL and DLBCL 64% ORR (FL 71% CR DLBCL 43% CR)	8/28 ≥grade 3 toxicity
FHCRC (Turtle et al. 2016)	Gamma retrovirus	4-1BB	cyc 2–4 g/m^2 cyc 2–4 g/m^2 + VP-16 300–600 mg/m^2 cyc 60 mg/kg + flu 75 mg/m^2	B-NHL flu(+) $n = 18$ flu(−) $n = 12$	flu(+) 72% ORR flu(−) 50% ORR	Improved efficacy and increased toxicity with fludarabine
Moffitt (Locke et al. 2015)	Gamma retrovirus	CD28	cyc + flu	$n = 6$	All 3 evaluable at one month (CR = 2, PR = 1)	$n = 3$ ≥grade 3 toxicity attributable to CAR-T

(continued)

Table 6.1 (continued)

Institution	Viral vector	Co-stimulatory molecule	Conditioning	Patients	Clinical responses	Notes
Multicenter (Novartis) (Neelapu et al., 2017)	Gamma retrovirus	CD28	cyc + flu	*n* = 101	82% ORR (54% CR; 28% PR)	93% CRS; 64% neurotoxicity, all of which resolved
Multicenter (Kite) (Schuster et al. 2017b)	Lentivirus	4-1BB	Variable	*n* = 81	53.1 % ORR (39.5% CR, 13.6% PR)	58% CRS; 12% neurotoxicity
Multicenter (Juno) (Abramson et al. 2017)	Gamma retrovirus	4-1BB	cyc + flu	*n* = 68	75% ORR (56% CR)	30% CRS; 20% neurotoxicity

aB-NHL aggressive B-NHL, *CRS* cytokine-release syndrome, *cyc* cyclophosphamide, *flu* fludarabine, *MV* mechanical ventilation, *ORR* overall response rate, *VP-16* etoposide

6.1.2 Clinical Studies: 19-CAR-T Following Hematopoietic Cell Transplantation (HCT)

6.1.2.1 19-CAR-T in Consolidation Following High-Dose Therapy and Autologous HCT (HDT-AHCT)

Investigators at the NCI initially leveraged microenvironmental biologic optimization of adoptive cellular therapy demonstrating improved antitumor efficacy with increasing intensity of chemo-/radiotherapy conditioning for patients with metastatic melanoma (Dudley et al. 2008). Additionally, elegant animal experiments suggest reinfusion of hematopoietic progenitor cells potentiates proliferative expansion of adoptive cellular therapy by providing lymphoproliferative cytokines including IL-7 and IL-15 (Wrzesinski et al. 2007). DLIs as adoptive therapy have improved efficacy in a minimal residual state (Chang and Huang 2013). These aforementioned lines of evidence provide rationale for exploring 19-CAR-T in consolidation following standard-of-care HDT-AHCT wherein historically approximately 40–50% of patients experience progression of disease following transplantation for rel/ref DLBCL, the most common indication (Gisselbrecht et al. 2010; Vose et al. 2013). These studies are summarized in Table 6.2. The first large prospective published experience was recently reported in manuscript form by investigators at the City of Hope (Wang et al. 2016). The authors report on two sequential clinical trials of 19-CAR-T following HDT-AHCT for B-NHL. In the first study, NHL-1, eight patients were treated with a first-generation 19-CAR-T transduced into CD8+ enriched central memory cells, and in the second study, NHL-2, the 19-CAR-T product was a fixed 1:1 CD4:CD8 with a second-generation construct containing a CD28 co-stimulatory transmembrane domain. Most of the patients on study were in a functional imaging complete metabolic remission (Barrington et al. 2014) at the time of HDT-AHCT. In the NHL-1 study, with a median follow-up of approximately 2 years in the nonprogressors, a 2-year progression-free survival (PFS) was observed in 50% of the patients (95%CI: 16–84%). In the NHL-2 study, wherein all eight patients treated were in a chemosensitive remission (7/8 in complete metabolic remission) at the time of HDT-AHCT, at a median follow-up of 12 months, the 1-year PFS was 75% (95% CI, 35–97%). The authors noted improved persistence of the second-generation 19-CAR-T product in NHL-2. No CRS or other >grade 3 toxicity was attributable to the 19-CAR-T product on either study.

Two additional centers have presented their prospective experience, of 19-CAR-T following HDT-AHCT for B-NHL, MD Anderson Cancer Center (MDACC) and Memorial Sloan Kettering Cancer Center (MSKCC). The group from MDACC published their prospective experience with 19-CAR-T constructed by the *Sleeping Beauty* transposon with two phase 1 studies that enrolled 26 patients with advanced NHL or ALL (Kebriaei et al. 2016). Patients underwent HCT in autologous ($n = 7$) or allogenic ($n = 19$) settings followed by 19-CAR-T infusion as an adjuvant therapy. Patients who underwent auto-AHCT experienced progression-free and overall survival rates of 83% and 100% at 30 months, while the same end points for patients who received allo-HSCT were 53% and 63%, respectively, at 12 months. Three patients that received allo-HCT developed GvHD. One patient that developed

Table 6.2 Clinical studies of 19-CAR-T for relapsed or refractory B-NHL in consolidation following HDT-ASCT

Institution	Viral vector	Co-stimulatory molecule	Conditioning	Patients	PFS	Notes
City of Hope (Wang et al. 2016)	Lentivirus	"NHL1," none "NHL2," CD28	BEAM	"NHL1" DBLCL *n* = 7, MCL *n* = 1 "NHL2" DLBCL *n* = 4, MCL *n* = 4	"NHL1" 50% at 1-year "NHL2" 75% at 2 years	Improved expansion with second-generation "NHL2" 19-CAR-T
MDACC (Kebriaei et al. 2016)	Transposon system	CD28	Auto: BEAM Allo: variable	FL *n* = 3, DLBCL *n* = 4, HL *n* = 1, MCL *n* = 1, B-ALL *n* = 17 (auto, *n* = 7; allo, *n* = 19)	Auto-HSCT, 83% at 30 mos Allo-HSCT, 53% at 12 mos	19-CAR-T persisted in blood on average 201 d (auto), 51 d (allo)
MSKCC (Sauter et al. 2015)	Gamma retrovirus	CD28	BEAM	*n* = 11 rel/ref DLBCL/ transformed B-NHL in PR or marrow involvement	40% at 12 months	7/11 patients with ≥grade 3 neurotoxicity

BEAM carmustine, etoposide, cytarabine, melphalan

GvHD died of preexisting conditions, while GvHD of the other two patients was resolved. Genomic analysis of 19-CAR-T cells generated by transposition showed uniform and stable insertion events through the genome with low rates of aberrant recombination. Of note, investigators could detect 19-CAR-T cells in blood for an average of 201 days in auto-HCT and 51 days in allo-HCT recipients.

Lastly, investigators from MSKCC have tested CAR-T in consolidation for high-risk rel/ref DLBCL/aggressive histology B-NHL in partial chemosensitive remission following a HDT-AHCT (Sauter et al. 2015). All patients on this study had either functional imaging-positive disease and/or bone marrow involvement characterizing them as high-risk per phase I study eligibility criteria. The 19-CAR-T utilized by this group includes a CD28 co-stimulatory molecule. Interim data presented at the 2015 ASCO meeting revealed 4 of 10 evaluable patients in continuous complete remission at a median of 14 months post-HDT-ASCT and 19-CAR-T and up to nearly 2 years in two patients, following study treatment (Sauter et al. 2015). The most common grade >3 toxicity attributable to 19-CAR-T was NT in 7/11 patients that was fully reversible.

6.1.2.2 19-CAR-T Following Allogeneic (Allo-HCT)

To test safety of 19-CAR-T post-allo-HCT, the group at the NCI reported a phase I dose escalation trial in B-NHL patients that progressed following allo-HCT (Brudno et al. 2016). The protocol did not include a lymphodepleting conditioning regimen before infusion. Of 20 patients, none developed GvHD after 19-CAR-T infusion, and an ORR of 40% (CR, $n = 6$; PR, $n = 2$) was achieved. The response rate was highest for ALL, and the longest ongoing CR was greater than 30 months in a patient with CLL. Anti-malignancy response of 19-CAR-T infusion was rapid; blood B-lymphocytes decreased from 3372 to 0/μl over 11 days in a case of CLL, compared to several weeks observed in standard donor lymphocyte infusion (DLI) treatment. Of note, after infusion 19-CAR-T cells had a significant elevation in programmed cell death protein 1 (PD-1) expression before reaching peak blood levels.

6.1.2.3 Later-Generation CAR Products

Two abstracts were presented at ASH 2015 with third- and fourth-generation constructs, respectively. Investigators from Sweden reported short interim follow-up on a phase I/II study testing a third-generation 19-CAR-T construct incorporating CD28 and IL-2 for rel/ref B-cell malignancies (including CLL and ALL). They reported 6/14 initial complete responses in lymphoma ($n = 11$) and ALL ($n = 3$) with investigation ongoing (Enblad et al. 2015). Lastly, investigators from China reported on a phase I/II clinical trial of a fourth-generation 19-CAR-T construct consisting of CD28/CD137/CD27 and iCasp9 apoptosis-inducible safety switch (4SCAR19) (Chang et al. 2015). Thirteen patients with rel/ref B-NHL (including 12 with either DLBCL or Burkitt's lymphoma) were treated with 4SCAR19 preceded by fludarabine and cyclophosphamide conditioning, and eight experienced a CR at 3–10 months post-4SCAR19 treatment. Three patients died of non-disease-related causes with or without severe CRS, and two patients died of progressive lymphoma with a 120-day disease-free survival of 53% (95% CI: 36–69%) (Chang et al. 2015).

6.1.3 Clinical Studies: Alternate Tumor Antigen Targets for CAR Therapy (CD20, Kappa Light Chain, CD30, and CD22)

The earliest clinical experience with CAR-T therapy for B-NHL was with a scFv targeting CD20 in a first-generation construct (Till et al. 2008). In conjunction with adjunctive IL-2, the 20-CAR-T persisted in vivo up to 9 weeks post-infusion. Of the seven patients treated with MCL or FL, two patients achieved a CR, one patient a PR, and four had experienced stable disease. A second study utilized a first-generation neomycin-resistance selected 20-CAR-T following HDT-ASCT detected 20-CAR-T up to only 1 week post-infusion by quantitative polymerase chain reaction (qPCR), and no clinical responses were detected (Jensen et al. 2010). Given that B cell NHL is clonally restricted to either kappa (κ) or lambda (λ) immunoglobulin light chain, the group from Baylor College of Medicine investigated targeting κ-light chain with CAR-T and presented results on seven patients with rel/ref B-NHL at the 2013 ASH meeting (Ramos et al. 2013). Per PCR, the κ-CAR-T peaked in the periphery at 1–2 weeks post-infusion and persisted for up to 6 months. Three of the seven patients responded to κ-CAR-T (CR, $n = 2$, PR, $n = 1$).

With the success of the antibody-drug conjugate brentuximab vedotin (BV) targeting CD30 in patients with CD30+ hematologic malignancies including Hodgkin lymphoma (HL) and anaplastic large cell lymphoma (ALCL) (Younes et al. 2010), the group from Baylor has developed a CAR construct targeting CD30 (30-CAR-T) in conjunction with a functional CD3ζ and CD28 co-stimulatory domain transduced via a retrovirus. They reported interim results of a prospective phase I study of 30-CAR-T wherein 18 products were transduced and 9 patients were treated (HL, $n = 7$, ALCL, $n = 2$). Eight of the patients had previously failed BV. Importantly, no patients received lymphodepleting chemotherapy prior to infusion of 30-CAR-T on study. Following safe administration to dose level #3 on the phase I study, at 6-week evaluation post-infusion, $n = 1$ CR and $n = 1$ PR, four patients with stable disease and three patients with progression of disease (Ramos et al. 2015). Given the safe administration, the Baylor investigators plan to incorporate 30-CAR-T following HDT-ASCT in the subsequent study.

CD22 emerged as a target tumor antigen for CAR-T therapy in B-ALL, as its expression is largely restricted to B-cell lineage. Recently, the first clinical experience of 22-CAR-T therapy in 21 patients (age range 7–30 years) with B-ALL was reported by the investigators at the NIH (Fry et al. 2018). The 22-CAR-T construct included a 4-1BB co-stimulatory domain, and patients were administered doses $\geq 1 \times 10^6$ per kg. All patients had at least one bone marrow transplantation, and notably 17 patients had received CD19-targeted immunotherapy wherein 15 had received 19-CAR-T therapy prior to this trial. A dose-dependent anti-malignant response was observed. Of 21 patients, 12 (57%) achieved CR, 9 of whom had received prior CD19-directed immunotherapy and had CD19 diminished or CD19-negative B-cell populations. Eight patients in CR experienced relapse at a median of 6 months following 22-CAR-T infusion. Given their experience with CD22 as a valid CAR-T therapy antigen, the investigators plan to extend their studies to CD19-CD22 multispecific CAR therapy to decrease the possibility of relapses associated with antigen escape.

6.2 Expert Point of View

Despite the above encouraging data, 19-CAR-T therapy for B-NHL appears less active than in B-ALL wherein the vast majority of patients achieve CR (Davila et al. 2014; Maude et al. 2014). Whether this is due to differences in the microenvironment (marrow- versus nodal-based disease) or other biologic features between B-ALL and B-NHL histologies remains unknown. Most recently, to analyze the genomic, phenotypic, and functional mechanisms of success or failure of CAR-T-cell therapy, the group at the University of Pennsylvania presented a trial of 41 patients with advanced and high-risk CLL, who received at least one dose of 19-CAR-T cells (Fraietta et al. 2018). They reported that intrinsic properties of 19-CAR-T isolated from patients who responded to CAR-T-cell therapy were markedly different than 19-CAR-T cells isolated from patients who were unresponsive. 19-CAR-T cells of the responders had elevated expression profiles of early memory differentiation, as well as comparatively enriched IL-6 signatures, and these cells had superior expansion during clinical manufacturing, while the 19-CAR-T cells of the unresponsive patients had elevated expression of late memory, apoptosis, and aerobic glycosylation that are associated with T-cell exhaustion, as well as poor expansion profiles. Of note, $CD27^{+}PD1^{-}CD8^{+}$ 19-CAR-T-cell population expressing high levels of the IL-6 receptor correlated with a therapeutic response.

Currently, the two major toxicities of 19-CAR-T therapy include CRS and NT manifestations including, but not limited to, seizures, seizure-like activity, focal motor deficits, aphasia, and global encephalopathy (Lee et al. 2014). These toxicities temper the encouraging activity of this treatment modality, and strategies to abrogate the associated morbidity (and potential mortality) are mentioned in the section below. Lastly, it is important to note that many of the previously reviewed studies are in short follow-up. To this end, it is important to await longer follow-up from phase II studies. Given the time and resource necessary for autologous leukapheresis and CAR-T production, it will be imperative to analyze forthcoming efficacy data in later phase studies by intention to treat. This is particularly relevant in the rel/ref setting of aggressive histology disease, i.e., DLBCL, wherein patients' disease phenotype and natural history may preclude proceeding to CAR-T treatment.

6.3 Future Directions

Much of the clinical development around CAR-T therapy is strategies to prevent or treat toxicity related to treatment, most notably the use of anti-IL-6 receptor blockade to abrogate CRS (Davila et al. 2014). Additionally, engineering suicide genetic elements to "turn off" the activated cellular product when toxicity is observed are being developed (Di Stasi et al. 2011). Safety and management cohort of the ZUMA-1 trial reported results of an IL-6 receptor blocker, tocilizumab, used as CRS prophylaxis at day 2 of infusion. Rates of patients with grade ≥3 CRS were lower in the prophylaxis cohort, 1 of 34 (3%), compared to 13 of 101 (13%) in the main cohort (Locke et al. 2017). However, a concern of potentially greater severe NT in the experimental group may provide insight into the pathophysiology of NT in the setting of IL-6 receptor blockade. A recent report from MSKCC described factors associated with NT in ALL patients receiving 19-28z CAR-T including cytokines such as IL-6, as well as others that may be produced by other cellular lineages (Santomasso et al. 2018). Another complication of CAR-T therapy are infections that are potentially related to prior cytotoxic treatments and/or lymphodepleting conditioning regimens. A recent phase I/II study that enrolled 133 patients reported that incidence of infections after 19-CAR-T-cell therapy was comparable to other salvage chemo-immunotherapies. Prior cytotoxic treatments, 19-CAR-T dose, CRS severity, and ALL malignancy were associated with more frequent infections (Hill et al. 2018).

Future investigation toward improvement in 19-CAR-T efficacy for B-NHL may involve additional pharmacologic adjuncts to catalyze the therapeutic potential of this adoptive cellular therapy. The Bruton's tyrosine kinase inhibitor ibrutinib, which has demonstrated impressive single-agent activity in many histologies of B-NHL (Smith 2015), has been found to inhibit Th2 responses while enhancing Th1-based immunity via inhibition of the interleukin-2-inducible kinase (ITK) in preclinical models. Subsequent to this discovery, CLL patients previously exposed to ibrutinib demonstrated enhanced ex vivo and in vivo expansion of 19-CAR-T in addition to decreased expression of programmed cell death 1 (PD-1) on the product (Fraietta et al. 2016; Long et al. 2017). PD-1 is a T-cell exhaustion receptor serving as a downregulator of T cells upon engagement of PD-1 ligand-1 (PD-L1) or PD-L2 and is upregulated on adoptive transfer of CAR-T (Abate-Daga et al. 2013). This receptor is pharmacologically targetable by checkpoint inhibitors in active clinical investigation for various lymphoma histologies (Matsuki and Younes 2016). Clinical trials combining checkpoint inhibitors and 19-CAR-T are being designed. A clinical experience of 19-CAR-T in CLL patients that had received ibrutinib was reported by the FHCRC investigators wherein 24 patients achieved an ORR of 71% (Turtle et al. 2017). Furthermore, in a case report, ongoing treatment with a PD-1 inhibitor antibody after 19-CAR-T therapy resulted in a durable CR response in a DLBCL patient that was otherwise unresponsive to 19-CAR-T (Chong et al. 2017). Ibrutinib has also been shown to enhance 19-CAR-T cytotoxic killing of MCL in cell lines, in vivo, as well as in xenograft mouse models (Ruella et al. 2016). Additional potential combinatorial strategies could include immune modulatory agents, such as lenalidomide, which has previously been shown to enhance T-cell synapse formation and downregulation of tumor cell inhibitory molecules (Ramsay et al. 2012) and has demonstrated enhanced antitumor efficacy of 19-CAR-T and 20-CAR-T in animal models (Otahal et al. 2016).

Lastly, active development of third- and later-generation CAR-T is ongoing. Included in these investigations is development of constructs with co-stimulatory elements and/or lymphoproliferative cytokine genes engineered into the 19-CAR product (Pegram et al. 2012). Additionally, combinatorial antigen specificity is under active investigation (Kloss et al. 2013; Zah et al. 2016) toward the goal of circumnavigating antigen escape (Jackson and Brentjens 2015; Gardner et al. 2016).

References

Abate-Daga D, Hanada K, Davis JL et al (2013) Expression profiling of TCR-engineered T cells demonstrates overexpression of multiple inhibitory receptors in persisting lymphocytes. Blood 122:1399–1410

Abramson JSPM, Gordon LI, Lunning MA, Arnason JE, Wang M, Forero A, Maloney DG, Albertson T, Garcia J, Li D, Xie B, Siddiqi T (2017) High durable CR rates in relapsed/refractory (R/R) aggressive B-NHL treated with the CD19-directed CAR T cell product JCAR017 (TRANSCEND NHL 001): defined composition allows for dose-finding and definition of pivotal cohort. Blood 130(Suppl 1):581

Barrington SF, Mikhaeel NG, Kostakoglu L et al (2014) Role of imaging in the staging and response assessment of lymphoma: consensus of the international conference on malignant lymphomas imaging working group. J Clin Oncol 32:3048–3058

Brentjens RJ, Latouche JB, Santos E et al (2003) Eradication of systemic B-cell tumors by genetically targeted human T lymphocytes co-stimulated by CD80 and interleukin-15. Nat Med 9:279–286

Brudno JN, Somerville RP, Shi V et al (2016) Allogeneic T cells that express an anti-CD19 chimeric antigen receptor induce remissions of B-cell malignancies that progress after allogeneic hematopoietic stem-cell transplantation without causing graft-versus-host disease. J Clin Oncol 34:1112–1121

Chang YJ, Huang XJ (2013) Donor lymphocyte infusions for relapse after allogeneic transplantation: when, if and for whom? Blood Rev 27:55–62

Chang LJ, Dong L, Zhu J, Ying Z, Kuo HH, Liu Y, Song YQ, Wang XP, Jia YQ, Niu T, Liu T, Pan L, Liu ZG, Li T, Li YC, Yao K, Ke X, Jing H, Bao F (2015) 4SCAR19 chimeric antigen receptor-modified T cells as a breakthrough therapy for highly chemotherapy-resistant late-stage B cell lymphoma patients with bulky tumor mass. Blood 126:264

Chong EA, Melenhorst JJ, Svoboda J, Nasta SD, Landsburg DJ, Mato AR, Tian L, Parakandi H, Lacey SF, June CH, Schuster SJ (2017) Phase I/II study of pembrolizumab for progressive diffuse large B cell lymphoma after anti-CD19 directed chimeric antigen receptor modified T cell therapy. Blood 130(Suppl 1):4121

Davila ML, Riviere I, Wang X et al (2014) Efficacy and toxicity management of 19-28z CAR T cell therapy in B cell acute lymphoblastic leukemia. Sci Transl Med 6:224ra25

Di Stasi A, Tey SK, Dotti G et al (2011) Inducible apoptosis as a safety switch for adoptive cell therapy. N Engl J Med 365:1673–1683

Dudley ME, Yang JC, Sherry R et al (2008) Adoptive cell therapy for patients with metastatic melanoma: evaluation of intensive myeloablative chemoradiation preparative regimens. J Clin Oncol 26:5233–5239

Enblad GKH, Wikstrom K, Essand M, Savoldo B, Brenner MK, Dotti G, Hallbook H, Hoglund M, Hagberg H, Loskog A (2015) Third generation CD19-CAR T cells for relapsed and refractory lymphoma and leukemia report from the Swedish phase I/IIa trial. Blood 126:1534

Eshhar Z, Waks T, Gross G et al (1993) Specific activation and targeting of cytotoxic lymphocytes through chimeric single chains consisting of antibody-binding domains and the gamma or zeta subunits of the immunoglobulin and T-cell receptors. Proc Natl Acad Sci U S A 90:720–724

Fraietta JA, Beckwith KA, Patel PR et al (2016) Ibrutinib enhances chimeric antigen receptor T-cell engraftment and efficacy in leukemia. Blood 127:1117–1127

Fraietta JA, Lacey SF, Orlando EJ et al (2018) Determinants of response and resistance to CD19 chimeric antigen receptor (CAR) T cell therapy of chronic lymphocytic leukemia. Nat Med 24:563–571

Fry TJ, Shah NN, Orentas RJ et al (2018) CD22-targeted CAR T cells induce remission in B-ALL that is naive or resistant to CD19-targeted CAR immunotherapy. Nat Med 24:20–28

Gardner R, Wu D, Cherian S et al (2016) Acquisition of a CD19-negative myeloid phenotype allows immune escape of MLL-rearranged B-ALL from CD19 CAR-T-cell therapy. Blood 127:2406–2410

Gisselbrecht C, Glass B, Mounier N et al (2010) Salvage regimens with autologous transplantation for relapsed large B-cell lymphoma in the rituximab era. J Clin Oncol 28:4184–4190

Hill JA, Li D, Hay KA et al (2018) Infectious complications of CD19-targeted chimeric antigen receptor-modified T-cell immunotherapy. Blood 131:121–130

Hombach A, Wieczarkowiecz A, Marquardt T et al (2001) Tumor-specific T cell activation by recombinant immunoreceptors: CD3 zeta signaling and CD28 costimulation are simultaneously required for efficient IL-2 secretion and can be integrated into one combined CD28/CD3 zeta signaling receptor molecule. J Immunol 167:6123–6131

Jackson HJ, Brentjens RJ (2015) Overcoming antigen escape with CAR T-cell therapy. Cancer Discov 5:1238–1240

Jensen MC, Popplewell L, Cooper LJ et al (2010) Antitransgene rejection responses contribute to attenuated persistence of adoptively transferred CD20/CD19-specific chimeric antigen receptor redirected T cells in humans. Biol Blood Marrow Transplant 16:1245–1256

Kebriaei P, Singh H, Huls MH et al (2016) Phase I trials using sleeping beauty to generate CD19-specific CAR T cells. J Clin Investig 126:3363–3376

Kloss CC, Condomines M, Cartellieri M et al (2013) Combinatorial antigen recognition with balanced signaling promotes selective tumor eradication by engineered T cells. Nat Biotechnol 31:71–75

Kochenderfer JN, Wilson WH, Janik JE et al (2010) Eradication of B-lineage cells and regression of lymphoma in a patient treated with autologous T cells genetically engineered to recognize CD19. Blood 116:4099–4102

Kochenderfer JN, Somerville R, Lu L et al (2014) Anti-CD19 CAR T cells administered after low-dose chemotherapy can induce remissions of chemotherapy-refractory diffuse large B-cell lymphoma. Blood 124:550

Kochenderfer JN, Dudley ME, Kassim SH et al (2015) Chemotherapy-refractory diffuse large B-cell lymphoma and indolent B-cell malignancies can be effectively treated with autologous T cells expressing an anti-CD19 chimeric antigen receptor. J Clin Oncol 33:540–549

Kochenderfer JN, Somerville RPT, Lu T et al (2017a) Lymphoma remissions caused by anti-CD19 chimeric antigen receptor T cells are associated with high serum interleukin-15 levels. J Clin Oncol 35:1803–1813

Kochenderfer JN, Somerville RPT, Lu T et al (2017b) Long-duration complete remissions of diffuse large B cell lymphoma after anti-CD19 chimeric antigen receptor T cell therapy. Mol Ther 25:2245–2253

Lee DW, Gardner R, Porter DL et al (2014) Current concepts in the diagnosis and management of cytokine release syndrome. Blood 124:188–195

Locke FLNS, Bartlett NL, Siddiqi T, Chavez JC, Hosing CM, Ghobadi A, Budde LE, Navale L, Aycock JS, Wiezorek J, Go WY (2015) Phase 1 clinical results of the ZUMA-1 (KTE-C19-101) study: a phase 1-2 multi-center study evaluating the safety and efficacy of anti-CD19 CAR T cells (KTE-C19) in subjects with refractory aggressive non-Hodgkin lymphoma (NHL). Blood 126:3991

Locke FL, Neelapu S, Bartlett NL, Lekakis LJ, Jacobson CA, Braunschweig I, Oluwole OO, Siddiqi T, Lin Y, Timmerman JM, Reagan PM, Bot A, Rossi JM, Sherman M, Navale L, Jiang Y, Aycock JS, Elias M, Wiezorek JS, Go WY, Miklos DB (2017) Preliminary results of prophylactic Tocilizumab after Axicabtagene ciloleucel (axi-cel; KTE-C19) treatment for patients with refractory, aggressive non-Hodgkin lymphoma (NHL). Blood 130(Suppl 1):1547

Long M, Beckwith K, Do P et al (2017) Ibrutinib treatment improves T cell number and function in CLL patients. J Clin Investig 127:3052–3064

Matsuki E, Younes A (2016) Checkpoint inhibitors and other immune therapies for Hodgkin and non-Hodgkin lymphoma. Curr Treat Options Oncol 17:31

Maude SL, Frey N, Shaw PA et al (2014) Chimeric antigen receptor T cells for sustained remissions in leukemia. N Engl J Med 371:1507–1517

Neelapu SS, Locke FL, Bartlett NL et al (2017) Axicabtagene ciloleucel CAR T-cell therapy in refractory large B-cell lymphoma. N Engl J Med 377:2531–2544

Otahal P, Prukova D, Kral V et al (2016) Lenalidomide enhances antitumor functions of chimeric antigen receptor modified T cells. Oncoimmunology 5:e1115940

Pegram HJ, Lee JC, Hayman EG et al (2012) Tumor-targeted T cells modified to secrete IL-12 eradicate systemic tumors without need for prior conditioning. Blood 119:4133–4141

Ramos CASB, Liu E, Gee AP, Mei Z, Grilley BJ, Rooney CM, Heslop HE, Brenner MK, Dotti G (2013) Clinical responses in patients infused with T lymphocytes redirected to target κ-light immunoglobulin chain. Blood 122:506

Ramos CA, Ballarad B, Liu E, Dakhova O, Mei Z, Liu H, Grilley B, Rooney CM, Gee AP, Chang BH, Bollard CM, Brenner MK, Dotti G, Heslop HE, Savoldo B (2015) Chimeric T cells for therapy of CD30+ Hodgkin and non-Hodgkin lymphomas. Blood 126:185

Ramsay AG, Clear AJ, Fatah R et al (2012) Multiple inhibitory ligands induce impaired T-cell immunologic synapse function in chronic lymphocytic leukemia that can be blocked with lenalidomide: establishing a reversible immune evasion mechanism in human cancer. Blood 120:1412–1421

Riddell SR, Sommermeyer D, Berger C et al (2014) Adoptive therapy with chimeric antigen receptor-modified T cells of defined subset composition. Cancer J 20:141–144

Ruella M, Kenderian SS, Shestova O et al (2016) The addition of the BTK inhibitor Ibrutinib to anti-CD19 chimeric antigen receptor T cells (CART19) improves responses against mantle cell lymphoma. Clin Cancer Res 22(11):2684–2696

Santomasso BD, Park JH, Salloum D et al (2018) Clinical and biologic correlates of neurotoxicity associated with CAR T cell therapy in patients with B-cell acute lymphoblastic leukemia (B-ALL). Cancer Discov 8(8):958–971. https://doi.org/10.1158/2159-8290.CD-17-1319

Sauter CS, Riviere I, Bernal Y et al (2015) Phase I trial of 19-28z chimeric antigen modified T cells (19-28z CAR-T) post-high dose therapy and autologous stem cell transplant (HDT-ASCT) for relapsed and refractory (rel/ref) aggressive B-cell non-Hodgkin lymphoma (B-NHL). J Clin Oncol 33:8515

Schuster SJ, Svoboda J, Chong EA et al (2017a) Chimeric antigen receptor T cells in refractory B-cell lymphomas. N Engl J Med 377:2545–2554

Schuster SJ, Bishop MR, Tam CS, Waller EK, Borchmann P, McGuirk JP, Jaeger U, Jaglowski S, Andreadis C, Westin JR, Fleury I, Bachanova V, Ronan Foley S, Ho PJ, Mielke S, Magenau JM, Holte H, Van Besien K, Kersten MJ, Teshima T, Tobinai K, Corradini P, Anak O, Bubuteishvili Pacaud L, del Corral C, Awasthi R, Tai F, Salles G, Maziarz RT (2017b) Primary analysis of Juliet: a global, pivotal, phase 2 trial of CTL019 in adult patients with relapsed or refractory diffuse large B-cell lymphoma. Blood 130(Suppl 1):577

Smith MR (2015) Ibrutinib in B lymphoid malignancies. Expert Opin Pharmacother 16:1879–1887

Till BG, Jensen MC, Wang J et al (2008) Adoptive immunotherapy for indolent non-Hodgkin lymphoma and mantle cell lymphoma using genetically modified autologous CD20-specific T cells. Blood 112:2261–2271

Turtle CJ, Hanafi LA, Berger C et al (2016) Immunotherapy of non-Hodgkin's lymphoma with a defined ratio of CD8+ and CD4+ CD19-specific chimeric antigen receptor-modified T cells. Sci Transl Med 8:355ra116

Turtle CJ, Hay KA, Hanafi LA et al (2017) Durable molecular remissions in chronic lymphocytic leukemia treated with CD19-specific chimeric antigen receptor-modified T cells after failure of Ibrutinib. J Clin Oncol 35:3010–3020

Vose JM, Carter S, Burns LJ et al (2013) Phase III randomized study of rituximab/carmustine, etoposide, cytarabine, and melphalan (BEAM) compared with iodine-131 tositumomab/BEAM with autologous hematopoietic cell transplantation for relapsed diffuse large B-cell lymphoma: results from the BMT CTN 0401 trial. J Clin Oncol 31:1662–1668

Wang X, Popplewell LL, Wagner JR et al (2016) Phase I studies of central-memory-derived CD19 CAR T cell therapy following autologous HSCT in patients with B-cell NHL. Blood 127(24):2980–2990

Wrzesinski C, Paulos CM, Gattinoni L et al (2007) Hematopoietic stem cells promote the expansion and function of adoptively transferred antitumor CD8 T cells. J Clin Investig 117:492–501

Younes A, Bartlett NL, Leonard JP et al (2010) Brentuximab vedotin (SGN-35) for relapsed CD30-positive lymphomas. N Engl J Med 363:1812–1821

Zah E, Lin MY, Silva-Benedict A et al (2016) T cells expressing CD19/CD20 Bispecific chimeric antigen receptors prevent antigen escape by malignant B cells. Cancer Immunol Res 4(6):498–508

T Cell Receptors-Gene-Modified T Cells for Cancer: Methods, Data, and Challenges

7

Aaron P. Rapoport and Jean A. Yared

7.1 Introduction

The potential for cellular immunotherapy to offer significant therapeutic benefit to patients suffering from advanced forms of cancer was highlighted by the success of allogeneic blood and marrow hematopoietic cell transplants (HCTs) for hematologic malignancies and tumor-infiltrating lymphocytes (TIL) therapy for solid tumors, especially melanoma. These forms of therapy carry risks and technical challenges including potentially lethal graft-versus-host disease (GvHD) in the case of allogeneic HCTs and the inability to isolate and successfully prepare TIL for up to 50% of patients (Tran et al. 2008). Furthermore while the high frequency of clinical responses to TIL therapy amply demonstrated that autologous T cell therapy of cancer was possible, the cure rates from TIL were very low and likely limited by the prevalence of tumor-reactive T cells bearing low-affinity TCRs for tumor-associated antigens (TAA) as a result of thymic selection as well as the reestablishment of immunosuppressive mechanisms. For tumors characterized by genomic instability which display higher levels of patient tumor-specific neoantigens, the therapeutic potential for TIL may be greater (Maby et al. 2015). The identification of key immune checkpoints (e.g., CTLA-4/CD80 and PD-1/PDL-1) and the development of antibodies (e.g., ipilimumab, nivolumab, pembrolizumab) which block these inhibitory receptors and pathways have led to durable systemic responses in patients with a variety of advanced solid tumors including melanoma, lung cancer, and head and neck cancer—an unprecedented occurrence in the history of cancer therapy (Hodi et al. 2010; Brahmer et al. 2015; Seiwert et al. 2016). Nonetheless, the overall impact of such therapies may still be limited by the restricted repertoire and low

A. P. Rapoport (✉) J. A. Yared
University of Maryland School of Medicine, Greenebaum Comprehensive Cancer Center, Department of Medicine, Hematology/Oncology, Baltimore, MD, USA
e-mail: arapoport@umm.edu; jyared@umm.edu

M.-A. Perales et al. (eds.), *Cell and Gene Therapies*, Advances and Controversies in Hematopoietic Transplantation and Cell Therapy,
https://doi.org/10.1007/978-3-319-54368-0_7

affinity of the naturally occurring endogenous T cells present in the patient. Therefore, there remains a strong rationale for the engineering of tumor specificity into a patient's own T cells, in order to overcome these limitations.

Progress in the understanding of TCR structure and function and advancements in synthetic biology and cell transduction methodologies have converged to make it feasible to engineer patient-derived T cells to express novel receptors or receptor constructs which can redirect the T cells to known tumor targets. Eshhar and colleagues were among the first to demonstrate that T cells could be redirected to tumors by introducing tumor-specific "T-body" or "CAR (chimeric antigen receptor)" constructs by gene modification (Gross et al. 1989). Through a series of elegant experimental advancements, these and other investigators have generated second- and third-generation CARs against the B cell antigen CD19 which exert a high frequency of durable responses in patients with advanced and refractory chronic lymphocytic leukemia, B cell lymphoma, and perhaps most impressively relapsed and resistant pediatric and adult acute lymphoblastic leukemia (ALL) (Maus et al. 2014; Porter et al. 2011; Grupp et al. 2013; Kochenderfer et al. 2015). While the CAR approach offers a cellular immunotherapy strategy that is not HLA-restricted and thereby expands the scope of patients who can be treated with each construct while avoiding the problem of MHC downregulation in tumors (Gross and Eshhar 1992), several limitations and clinical challenges exist: The tumor antigens for CAR-engineered T cells must be expressed on the cell surface and absent from critical non-tumor target organs and tissues. Also, the "non-physiologic" signaling mechanisms for CARs which are composed of the CD3-zeta cytoplasmic domain and one or more costimulatory domains (e.g., CD28 or 41BB or both) may lead to rapid proliferation and cytokine release syndrome (CRS) which requires careful clinical management and sometimes can be fatal (Barrett et al. 2014). However other factors including the density and accessibility of target antigen and the distribution of tumor cells may also contribute to the magnitude of T cell proliferation and the occurrence of CRS following adoptive transfer of both CAR T cells and TCR-engineered T cells.

Immunotherapy using TCR-engineered T cells involves the transfer of gene constructs encoding TCR alpha and beta chains which recognize 8–10 amino acid peptides processed from TAA and expressed in the context of HLA molecules. To date, the most common HLA-restricted TCRs tested in humans have been specific for HLA-A*02:01 which is found in about 50% of Caucasians, about 40% of Hispanics, and about 20–24% of African-Americans (Ellis et al. 2000; Gonzalez-Galarza et al. 2015). The frequency of HLA-A*02:01 is about 22% among Japanese, about 18% among US Asians, and highly variable in Chinese (0–24%). Because these peptides can be drawn from both the intracellular and extracellular proteins, the range of TAA which can be recognized by TCR-engineered T cells is estimated to be five- to tenfold higher than that for CARs based in part on the fact that only about 28% of all cellular proteins are expressed on the cell membrane in whole or in part (Uhlen et al. 2015). Furthermore, these TCR-engineered T cells typically employ physiological signaling pathways which may offer a safety advantage with respect to CRS. In this chapter, we will discuss the development of tumor-specific TCRs, their clinical applications and safety considerations, and future directions.

7.2 TCR Structure and Function

Physiologic T cell responses are primarily dependent upon the intermolecular interaction between the clonotypic alpha-beta TCR and the cognate peptide-MHC (major histocompatibility complex). This interaction is stabilized by CD4 and CD8 which bind to specific constant regions of the MHC class II and class I molecules, respectively, as well as by interactions between CD2 and CTLA-4 and CD28 on the T cells and CD58 (for CD2) and CD80 (for CTLA-4 and CD28) on the antigen-presenting or tumor target cells (Bridgeman et al. 2012). The interface between the TCR and the peptide-MHC complex (pMHC) involves the pMHC surface and the three hypervariable complementarity determining regions (CDRs) of the alpha and beta chains (Rudolph et al. 2006). The CDR1α and CDR2α regions are encoded by one of 47 TCR-α germline variable genes, while the CDR1β and CDR2β regions are encoded by one of 57 TCR-β germline variable genes. The CDR2 loops mainly contact the MHC molecule, while the CDR1 loops can contact both the MHC and the peptide. On the other hand, the CDR3α and CDR3β loops of the alpha and beta chains are encoded by variable (V), diversity (D, β chains only), and joining (J) segments and further diversified enzymatically by random nucleotide insertions at the junctional regions of the V-D-J gene segments. As predicted, the hypervariable CDR3α and CDR3β loops mainly contact the antigen peptide. Altogether the TCR generation mechanism can produce ~10^{15} to 10^{20} unique alpha and beta pairs able to recognize an enormous range of antigenic structures (Miles et al. 2011). TCRs on the surface of T cells bind to the pMHC with a certain affinity which is determined during T cell ontogeny. During T cell development and maturation in the thymus, T cells bearing TCRs that bind to cognate antigens too strongly are eliminated by negative selection, while T cells that bind too weakly are eliminated by apoptosis (Jameson et al. 1995). More specifically, early-stage double-positive ($CD4^+/CD8^+$) T cells are first positively selected through interaction with peptide-MHC molecules expressed by thymic cortical epithelial cells, while in the medulla of the thymus, single-positive ($CD4^+/CD8^-$ or $CD4^-/CD8^+$) T cells encounter medullary epithelial cells which express an abundance of peptides derived from genes expressed in all somatic tissues (Nitta et al. 2010; Groettrup et al. 2010). As a result of this interaction, T cells which bear TCRs which exhibit high-affinity interactions with self-peptides are negatively selected. This affinity maturation process results in a vast repertoire of TCRs that bind to their cognate antigens in the context of the MHC, strongly if derived from nonself (e.g., microbial) antigens but weakly if derived from self-antigens (dissociation constant or K_D ~ 0.1 to 500 μM or greater). Of note, antibodies typically bind their cognate antigens with K_D values in the nM or pM range (van der Merwe and Davis 2003).

This editing mechanism significantly reduces the risk of autoimmune disease but conversely also limits the ability of the native immune system to recognize TAA since in most cases these are peptides that are derived from self-proteins that have been re-expressed or overexpressed in the tumor. This model of T cell ontogeny helps to explain the lack of success of cancer vaccination strategies which have thus far yielded limited clinical benefits with an objective response rate of 3.3% among more than 1300 patients who received a variety of cancer vaccines both at the NIH Surgery Branch and in the published literature (Rosenberg et al. 1994, 2004). It also explains the differential affinity ranges that have been observed for virus and cancer-specific TCRs with markedly higher affinities for TCRs that bind viral antigens than cancer-related antigens (Aleksic et al. 2012). In general the binding affinity of TCRs for cancer-related antigens that are "self"-antigens is about tenfold lower than the binding affinity of TCRs for nonself and microbial antigens.

Another important principle is that the avidity of a TCR for its cognate pMHC and the kinetics of the interaction are major determinants of T cell activation (Zoete et al. 2013; Davis et al. 1998; Irving et al. 2012; Stone et al. 2009). Using techniques such as surface plasmon resonance (SPR) and isothermal titration calorimetry, the biophysical characteristics have been calculated for dozens of TCR-pMHC interactions (Bridgeman et al. 2012). On the basis of this work, two major models of T cell activation have been developed: the "affinity model" which proposes that the level of T cell activation depends on the total number of TCRs bound to peptide-MHC complexes and the "half-life model" whereby optimal T cell activation requires that the TCR engage the peptide-MHC complex with sufficient binding strength and time to induce signaling (Zoete et al. 2013). It follows that strategies which generate TCRs with higher affinity for cognate tumor antigens could lead to superior therapeutic effect especially when combined with forced expression of those affinity-enhanced TCRs on cytotoxic T cells. Indeed multiple investigators have shown that affinity enhancement of TCRs for cognate peptide-MHC complex within the physiologic TCR affinity range (K_D ~ 200 μM to 1 μM) and in the presence of low levels of peptide-MHC complexes which is typical for most tumors results in improved T cell function (Robbins et al. 2008; Zhao et al. 2007). On the other hand, affinity enhancement into the supraphysiologic range ($K_D < 1$ μM) often led to functional impairment due in part to diminished expression of costimulatory molecules accompanied by increased PD-1 expression and upregulation of SHP-1 and SHP-2 phosphatases which serve to downregulate T cell function (Irving et al. 2012; Hebeisen et al. 2013, 2015). Further enhancement of affinity to K_D levels of <1 nM may lead to cross-reactivity with other peptide-MHC complexes. Thus an overarching principle has emerged that optimal function (including T cell activation and target specificity) of a given TCR occurs within a certain window of binding affinities. Within the physiologic range of TCR affinity mentioned above, the specific affinity for optimal T cell function is not possible to predict for each TCR-p-MHC complex and must be empirically determined in each case.

7.3 Isolation of Therapeutic TCRs and Strategies for Functional Enhancement

Candidate TCRs for therapeutic applications have generally been identified initially by isolating TIL from patient tumors. To illustrate the process of generating a TCR for therapeutic application, the steps taken to generate an affinity-enhanced TCR for a naturally processed peptide that is derived from the cancer-testis antigens (CTAgs) NY-ESO-1 and LAGE-1 is described in some detail. This process involved both experimental iteration and serendipity. Among the various classes of TAA which could be targeted by T cells, the CTAgs or cancer-germline antigens (CGs) are attractive because of their relatively clean expression profiles, being mainly restricted to germ cells and cancers (Ilyas and Yang 2015; Kvistborg et al. 2013). In addition, these antigens are shared by a variable but significant proportion of patients who develop specific cancers, and some may promote cancer cell survival and confer chemotherapy resistance (Monte et al. 2006), thus increasing the potential clinical benefit from targeting these antigens with TCR-modified T cells. Other classes of TAA including tissue differentiation or lineage-specific antigens and neoantigens derived from patient-specific mutations may be less desirable targets for TCR-engineered T cells due to "off-tumor" expression leading to damage of normal tissues and application to very small numbers of patients, respectively.

NY-ESO-1 was originally identified as a putative human tumor antigen by a method called serological expression cloning of recombinant cDNA libraries from human tumors (SEREX) using tissue obtained from a patient with squamous cell carcinoma of the esophagus (Chen et al. 1997). The function of NY-ESO-1 is unknown. NY-ESO-1 expression is detected in testis, ovary, and weakly in uterus specimens, but no mRNA can be detected by reverse transcription-polymerase chain reaction (RT-PCR) in any other normal tissue. NY-ESO-1 (CTAG-1B) is an immunogenic cancer-testis antigen (CTA) associated with spontaneous and vaccine-induced immunity that can lead to clinical cancer responses (Hunder et al. 2008; Yuan et al. 2008). Up to 60% of advanced myelomas have been reported to express NY-ESO-1, a feature correlated to tumor proliferation and high-risk features (van Baren et al. 1999; Jungbluth et al. 2005; Condomines et al. 2007; Atanackovic et al. 2007; van Rhee et al. 2005).

In addition to myeloma, multiple solid tumors express NY-ESO-1 at rates of up to 50% including melanoma and cancers of the bladder, lung, ovary, uterus, and esophagus (Chen et al. 1997). Reported expression rates vary between different studies; RT-PCR is more sensitive than immunohistochemistry (IHC) and tends to give higher figures for NY-ESO-1 expression. Figures derived from IHC are more reliable, since this technique detects protein rather than RNA. A feature of CTAgs like NY-ESO-1 is that they can have heterogenous expression in the tumor and so it is informative to measure both aspects in tissue sections by RNA- or protein-based approaches. CTLs recognizing the HLA-A*0201-restricted epitope NY-ESO$_{157–165}$ (SLLMWITQC) have been grown from the blood and lymph nodes of myeloma patients by several different groups (Atanackovic et al. 2007; van Rhee et al. 2005).

LAGE-1, a highly homologous TAA with a very similar expression pattern as NY-ESO-1, also shares the same epitope, and T cell clones specific for this epitope also kill antigen-positive tumor cells (van Rhee et al. 2005).

TCR gene cDNA sequences were isolated from the NY-ESO-1 *HLA-A*0201-SLLMWITQC*-restricted T cell clone 1G4 (Jager et al. 1998). This CTL clone was cultured from a metastatic lymph node derived from an 81-year-old woman with melanoma who exhibited both strong serologic and cytolytic reactivities against autologous tumor cells. The CTL clone (1G4) was found to recognize the SLLMWITQC peptide corresponding to amino acids 157–165 of NY-ESO-1 in an HLA-A*02:01-restricted manner. Note that the SLLMWITQC peptide sequence is the identical sequence derived and expressed from the LAGE-1 antigen, and therefore LAGE-1 antigen-positive tumors are also targeted by the 1G4 T cell clone.

The cDNA coding sequences for the mature extracellular regions of the α and β chain TCR proteins were cloned into separate *E. coli* plasmid vectors and expressed as protein inclusion bodies. These inclusion bodies were purified, solubilized, and then refolded as soluble α/β heterodimeric TCR proteins (sTCR). Both TCR chains were genetically truncated at the C terminus immediately before the native intra-chain cysteine residues and joined together by means of an artificial disulfide bond engineered between the α and β chain TCR constant regions. The 1G4 sTCR protein was purified, and its HLA-peptide antigen-binding kinetics were analyzed by surface plasmon resonance (SPR) using a BIAcore 3000. The 1G4 gene sequences also served as a platform to generate variants with enhanced antigen-binding affinity using bacteriophage display of large numbers of mutated 1G4 TCR proteins.

The HLA-A*0201-SLLMWITQC-peptide antigen complex was required for validation of antigen binding of the 1G4 T cell clone and the soluble version, as well as for testing and selection of affinity-enhanced variants generated by phage display. This complex was made by cloning the HLA-A*0201 protein and β2 microglobulin into *E. coli* expression vectors. These proteins were then expressed separately as protein inclusion bodies prior to solubilization, mixing with the SLLMWITQC peptide and refolding. The refolded pMHC antigen complex was then purified by ion exchange and size exclusion chromatography.

A 1G4 sTCR phage-display library was constructed with mutations covering the hypervariable complementarity determining region (CDR3 region) of the β chain. Three rounds of selection/enrichment for high-affinity TCR clones were performed. Competition ELISA assays for high-affinity mutant TCR phage identified several candidate TCR β-chain CDR3 mutations. These high-affinity β chain mutants then formed the basis of a library where the CDR3 α chain was also mutated in a similar manner (Li et al. 2005). This complex library was then used to isolate still higher affinities. Later, mutations were introduced into the CDR2 regions of both chains, and these libraries were then reselected (Dunn et al. 2006).

7.4 Biochemical Validation and Efficacy Testing of the Affinity-Enhanced NY-ESO-1 sTCR Clones

High-affinity mutant TCR alpha and beta chain genes were cloned separately into *E. coli* expression vectors. These mutant TCR chains were expressed and refolded in various paired combinations including with wild-type chains. They were then purified and analyzed for binding to HLA-A*0201-SLLMWITQC antigen by SPR. As mentioned, earlier studies using T cells transfected with high-affinity TCRs indicated that TCRs with very high affinities could exhibit diminished function and altered target specificity suggesting that TCRs with moderately increased affinity should be preferentially evaluated (Zhao et al. 2007). Thus, the high-affinity mutant CDR3α chain TCR sequences (Li et al. 2005) and mutant CDR2β chain TCR sequences (Dunn et al. 2006) were partially back-mutated to the wild-type 1G4 TCR sequence. A panel of these phage-derived 1G4 TCR mutants was then assessed in TCR-transfected T cells (Robbins et al. 2008). From these data TCRs with single or dual amino acid substitutions in the antigen-binding region and which were anticipated to have optimal cellular properties were selected for comparison in lentiviral T cell transduction and functional studies. These studies consisted of cytokine release assays and cytotoxicity assays against a panel of NY-ESO-1 positive and negative tumor cell lines. From these studies, an affinity-enhanced NY-ESO-1-TCR construct emerged as the "winner" based on enhanced binding properties, enhanced cytokine release, and target cell killing as well as retention of antigen specificity. This construct consisted of an alpha-chain variant (c259) carrying amino acid substitutions at positions 95 (threonine → leucine) and 96 (serine → tyrosine) of the CDR3 region of the 1G4 NY-ESO-1 TCR clone combined with the wild-type beta chain of the 1G4 NY-ESO-1 TCR clone. This affinity-enhanced TCR had a $T_{1/2}$ of 19 s and K_D of 730 nM vs 2.2 seconds and 9.3 μM for the wild-type 1G4 TCR, indicating about tenfold higher "dwell" time and binding strength for the 1G4 NY-ESO-1 TCR variant known as c259 (Robbins et al. 2008).

It should be noted that other investigators have taken a structural approach starting with crystallographic structures of TCR-peptide-MHC complexes in order to elucidate points of contact. Amino acid substitutions can then be made logically rather than randomly based on structure compatibilities in order to achieve affinity enhancements (Zoete et al. 2013; Haidar et al. 2009; Malecek et al. 2014). This approach has also led to development of affinity-enhanced variants of the HLA-A*02:01-restricted TCR for NY-ESO-$1_{157–165}$ (Schmid et al. 2010). Furthermore, a high-throughput TCR gene-capture methodology has also been developed to more rapidly isolate and identify tumor antigen-specific TCR sequences from human tumor tissue both with and without prior knowledge of antigen specificities. This methodology was used to develop a library of CTAg-specific TCRs and may also facilitate TCR-engineered T cell immunotherapy against private neoantigens which are expressed by individual patient tumors (Linnemann et al. 2013).

The cytotoxic effects of T cells transduced with the affinity-enhanced variant of the HLA-A*02:01-restricted TCR for NY-ESO-1$_{157–165}$ were then evaluated in the immunodeficient NSG (NOD/*scid*/γ_c^{null}) mouse model using the human B cell precursor acute lymphoblastic leukemia cell line (NALM-6) as the tumor target. The immunodeficient NOD/*scid*/γ_c^{null} (NOG) mouse is an excellent xenotransplantation model to measure the in vivo repopulation of human CD4 T cells (Ito et al. 2009). Following engraftment, the human hematopoietic cells can be maintained in NSG mice for at least 2 months or until fatal xenogeneic GvHD. Intravenous injection of NALM-6 into NSG mice provides a systemic tumor model with rapid evolution toward animal death within 20–23 days. Parental NALM-6 cells express both HLA-A1 and HLA-A2 molecules and also low levels of certain cancer-testis antigens including MAGE A3, but no NY-ESO-1 antigen. To achieve higher expression of this antigen, NALM-6 cells were transduced with lentiviruses expressing NY-ESO-1 proteins in conjunction with the green fluorescent (GFP) protein (NALM6-GFP-NY-ESO1). As a control cell line, NALM-6 cells were transduced with GFP only (NALM6-GFP). In previous experiments, the NALM6-GFP-NY-ESO1 cells induced mouse death within 23 days, similar to the parental NALM-6 cells.

The efficacy study used parental and transduced NALM-6 cell lines and evaluated the impact of CD4 and CD8 T cells which were genetically modified by lentiviral transfection to express NY-ESO-1 TCR on animal survival. The infused study cell number was 5×10^6 CD4 and CD8 T cells. This dose was chosen based on pilot data in the NALM-6 model which indicated that this is the effective dose required to observe an antitumor effect. Since a human is on average 3000-fold larger than an average mouse, a cell dose of 5×10^6 cells in a mouse roughly corresponds to a human dose of ~10 billion cells. The starting dose in human trials was expected to be about 1×10^9, and so the dose evaluated in the preclinical murine experiments represented about ten times greater than the human dose that would be administered in phase I trials.

As expected, all the control mice (injected with saline and mock/untransduced T cells) died between day 19 and 23. Also, the high-affinity NY-ESO1 TCR (c259)-transduced T cells did not give the mice any survival advantage when mice were inoculated with the NY-ESO-1-*negative* NALM6 tumor cells. However when mice carrying the NALM6-NY-ESO-1 *positive* tumor cells were treated with the NY-ESO-1-TCR-transduced T cells, a significant survival advantage was seen regardless of the TCR affinity (wt or the affinity-enhanced c259 TCR variant). These data suggested that both NY-ESO-1 TCRs were effective against tumor cells expressing the cognate antigen.

7.5 Clinical Translation of the Affinity-Enhanced NY-ESO-1 (c259) TCR

In the course of translating the affinity-enhanced NY-ESO-1 (c259) TCR to the bedside, several additional considerations merited attention including optimization of function by the transduced T cells and preclinical testing to minimize the risk of off-tumor effects. Two potential impediments to tumor targeting and killing by TCR-modified T cells include the potential problem of "mispairing" of transduced alpha and beta chains with the native T cell alpha and beta chains as well as the limited availability of components of the CD3 signaling complex. Second, both mispairing and the physiological redundancy of any TCR to potentially recognize a large number different peptides in the context of HLA molecules can lead to "off-target" recognition and off-tumor toxicities. The formation and surface expression of a functional TCR requires pairing of the new alpha and beta chains followed by association with the four invariant chains of the CD3 complex, namely, CD3γ, CD3δ, CD3ε (two subunits), and CD3ζ (two subunits). Furthermore, the availability of the CD3 subunits particularly CD3ζ is limited and partially formed TCR-CD3 complexes that undergo degradation in the endoplasmic reticulum (Minami et al. 1987, Mallabiabarrena et al. 1992). Ex vivo studies have shown that introduction of a novel TCR into a lymphocyte which expresses its native TCR results in mispairing between exogenous alpha and beta chains and endogenous beta and alpha chains sufficient to generate neoreactivities which are either HLA class I or class II restricted and directed against both allogeneic and autologous targets (van Loenen et al. 2010). Furthermore, such mispairing with generation of autoreactive T cells was thought to contribute to lethal GvHD in a mouse model which utilized an unusually intensive conditioning regimen (Bendle et al. 2010). It should be noted that to date, no known immunotoxicity has been demonstrated to occur in humans on the basis of mispairing between native and exogenous TCR chains. Potential strategies for reducing mispairing and enhancing the surface expression and function of transduced therapeutic TCRs include the optimization of equimolar translation of the introduced alpha and beta chains using the internal ribosome entry site (IRES) sequence of the encephalomyocarditis virus or more recently the "self-cleaving" 2A sequences from picornaviruses or porcine teschovirus which allows the ribosome to skip from one chain sequence to an adjacent one in order to achieve nearly equivalent translation and production of each peptide chain (Furler et al. 2001; Szymczak et al. 2004). Two other strategies to augment preferential pairing of the exogenous TCR chains include introduction of a second cysteine residue to generate an extra disulfide bond between the introduced alpha and beta chains and use of murine TCR sequences to facilitate species-specific pairing (van Loenen et al. 2010; Cohen et al. 2006, 2007). The molecular techniques which promote equimolar synthesis of the exogenous TCR alpha and beta chains have already been employed in the development of therapeutic TCRs for human studies.

The issues of "on-target, off-tumor" and "off-target, off-tumor" toxicities whereby adoptively transferred TCR gene-modified T cells recognize cognate peptide antigen on non-tumor cells and elicit damage to normal tissues or recognize unintended, "cross-reactive" peptides or HLA molecules on non-tumor cells and elicit normal tissue injury are likely more common causes of TCR-engineered T cell toxicities. These toxicities will also be discussed further in the context of the clinical studies. Steps taken during preclinical development to mitigate against these toxicities include the following: (i) alanine substitution scanning to identify which amino acid residues in the antigen peptide are critical for TCR binding and thereby identify structurally similar peptide sequences in other genes which the TCR could potentially recognize, followed by binding assays to test for potential cross-reactivity; (ii) testing of the TCR against an "alloreactivity panel" to search for cross-reactivity with other HLA molecules in addition to the one that the TCR is known to bind; (iii) testing of the TCR against a large panel of primary cells and tissues; and (iv) careful assessment of the true distribution of the target antigen to minimize the risk of "on-target/off- tumor" effects. As mentioned, on-target/off-tumor toxicity and off-target/off-tumor toxicity will also be discussed further in the context of the clinical studies.

7.6 Early Clinical Studies of TCR-Engineered Lymphocytes

The first clinical trial of TCR-engineered T cells for cancer immunotherapy focused on the melanocyte differentiation antigen MART-1 which is expressed in 80–90% melanoma cases and frequently recognized by melanoma TIL. Using a TCR isolated from a melanoma TIL which was HLA-A*02:01 restricted and recognized the MART-1:27-35 epitope AAGIGILTV, investigators cloned a cDNA for this TCR into a retrovirus and then transduced autologous peripheral blood lymphocytes from 15 HLA-A*02:01+ patients with advanced melanoma (Morgan et al. 2006). After myeloablative therapy to enhance the impact of the T cell immunotherapy through various mechanisms, these patients received the transduced T cells followed by maintenance therapy using IL-2. Of the 15 patients who were treated, 1 had a complete regression that lasted for 23 months, while a second patient exhibited a complete regression of an axillary mass and a 90% reduction in the size of a liver lesion which was resected 10 months later, and the patient remained disease-free 9 years after treatment.

To augment response rates, a higher-affinity TCR for the MART was identified and tested. TCRs for the MART-1:27-35 AAGIGILTV were isolated from TIL derived from 24 melanoma patients and tested for avidity for the HLA-peptide complex and IFN-γ production by transduced lymphocytes. A specific TCR termed DMF5 exhibited the strongest response and was selected for further clinical development (Johnson et al. 2006). Similar preclinical studies for another melanocyte differentiation antigen gp100 led to development and selection of a relatively high-affinity TCR directed against the gp100:154-162 epitope KTWGQYWQV which was isolated from a T cell clone generated from an HLA-A*02:01+-transgenic mouse that had been immunized with the gp100:154-162 epitope. Treatment of patients with autologous T cells engineered to express the high-affinity MART-1 TCR (DMF5) led to objective responses in 6 of 20 patients (30%) with advanced melanoma and in 3 of 16 patients (17%) who received autologous lymphocytes transduced with the high-affinity gp100 TCR (Johnson et al. 2009). Of the 36 total patients treated in these two studies, 34 eventually relapsed, while 1 patient was an ongoing partial responder nearly 8 years after receiving treatment with the MART-1:27-35 TCR, and a second patient had an ongoing complete response nearly 8 years after receiving treatment with the gp100:154-162 TCR.

Importantly, severe "on-target, off-tumor" toxicities were observed in most of the patients who were treated with cells engineered to express both the MART-1 and the gp100 TCRs including skin rash in 29 of 36 patients which culminated in loss of the majority of epidermal melanocytes (Robbins 2015). In addition, uveitis developed in 11/20 patients who received the MART-1 TCR-modified T cells and 4/16 patients who received the gp100 TCR gene-modified T cells; 13 of the 15 affected patients were successfully treated with steroid eye drops. Acute hearing loss developed in 10/20 patients who received MART-1 TCR-expressing T cells and 5/16 patients treated with gp100 TCR-expressing T cells, while 9 of the 36 total patients developed vertigo presumably due to engineered T cell attack on inner ear melanocytes; all patients responded to intratympanic steroid injections (Robbins 2015). The higher objective response rates and also the on-target/off-tumor toxicity rates in these latter studies suggest that affinity enhancement may increase the potency of TCR-modified T cells.

Another clinical trial was conducted involving the adoptive transfer of T cells engineered to express an affinity-enhanced TCR for an HLA-A*02:01 restricted immunogenic peptide composed of amino acids 691–699 from the carcinoembryonic antigen (CEA) found on most colon cancers but also normal colonic epithelial cells found in the crypts. This TCR also contained a serine → threonine substitution at codon 112 in the CDR3 region of the TCR-α which seemed to augment recognition of the CEA peptide on colon cancer cell lines (Parkhurst et al. 2009). Treatment of HLA-A*02:01+ patients with metastatic colon cancer who had high levels of circulating CEA using $CEA_{691-699}$-directed TCR-expressing T cells elicited a 6-month partial response in one of three patients but predictably led to severe inflammatory colitis and grade 1 diarrhea in one patient but grade 3 diarrhea in two patients requiring administration of oral corticosteroids in two of the three patients (Robbins 2015; Parkhurst et al. 2009). While these autoimmune toxicities resolved in 4–6 weeks, the trial was terminated early. The clinical experience with autologous T cells engineered to express TCRs directed against lineage-specific or "differentiation" antigens which are expressed on tumors but also normal tissue counterparts suggests that occasional clinical responses can be obtained which are sometimes durable, but the benefits seem more than offset by "on-target, off-tumor" immunotoxicities. The lack of selectivity against tumor tissue may be explained in part by the presence of immuno-inhibitory factors which are operative in the tumor bed but not in the normal tissue. This has led to studies using T cells engineered to carry TCRs which are directed against antigens that are mainly or exclusively expressed by tumors including the cancer-testis antigens (CTAs) or cancer-germ line antigens (CGs), most notably NY-ESO-1.

7.7 Clinical Studies of NY-ESO-1 TCR-Expressing T Cells in Solid Tumors

The NY-ESO-1 cancer-testis or cancer-germline antigen is widely expressed in solid tumors including melanoma, lung, breast, ovarian, prostate, and bladder tumors where the expression frequency ranges between 10 and 50% (Chen et al. 1997). NY-ESO-1 is abundantly and even more frequently expressed in synovial cell sarcomas where it is found in approximately 60–70% of tumors (Jungbluth et al. 2001). Based on the higher frequency and selectivity of expression in synovial cell sarcoma and melanoma, a clinical trial was conducted using autologous T cells engineered to express the affinity-enhanced HLA-A*02:01-restricted (c259) variant of the 1G4 NY-ESO-1 TCR carrying amino acid substitutions at positions 95 (threonine → leucine) and 96 (serine → tyrosine) of the alpha-chain CDR3 region combined with the wild-type beta chain of the 1G4 NY-ESO-1 TCR clone. After lymphodepleting chemotherapy consisting of fludarabine and cyclophosphamide, patients received retrovirally transduced autologous T cells carrying the affinity-enhanced NY-ESO-1 TCR followed by IL-2 maintenance therapy (Robbins et al. 2011). Four of six HLA-A*02:01+ patients with synovial cell sarcoma and five of eleven advanced melanoma patients exhibited clinical responses by RECIST criteria; 2/11 melanoma patients had complete responses that persisted for more than 1 year, while a partial response in one patient with synovial sarcoma lasted for 18 months. A recent report using a similar experimental design with expanded cohorts of patients and longer follow-up included 18 patients with progressive synovial cell sarcoma, 11 of whom had objective responses, and 20 patients with advanced melanoma, 11 of whom had objective responses (Robbins et al. 2015). The projected 3- and 5-year overall survival rates for the synovial cell sarcoma patients were 38% and 14%, respectively, while the projected survivals for the melanoma patients were 33% at both timepoints. Using this larger study, the investigators sought to identify predictors of response. Although some patients in this study were also immunized with a peptide vaccine derived from the NY-ESO-$1_{157–165}$ epitope, receipt of this vaccine did not correlate with response, while higher T cell numbers and one measure of enhanced functionality (IFNγ production in response to peptide-pulsed EBV-transformed lymphocyte targets) did seem to correlate to better clinical response. Importantly, no toxicities attributable to the transduced T cells were observed in accordance with the restricted expression of NY-ESO-1 to tumors and germ cells.

7.8 Clinical Studies of NY-ESO-1 TCR-Expressing T Cells in Myeloma

Up to 60% of advanced myelomas have also been reported to express NY-ESO-1, a feature which is correlated to enhanced tumor proliferation and other high-risk features including relapsed and extramedullary disease (van Baren et al. 1999; Jungbluth et al. 2005; Condomines et al. 2007; Atanackovic et al. 2007; van Rhee et al. 2005). High-dose chemotherapy followed by autologous stem cell transplantation (AHCT) has been a mainstay of therapy for myeloma and better clinical outcomes following AHCT for myeloma and other hematologic neoplasms that may be associated with rapid post-transplant lymphocyte recovery (Porrata et al. 2001; Porrata and Markovic 2004). In addition, tumor-reactive T cells are present at low frequencies in the marrow and blood of myeloma patients which may target myeloma cells upon activation (Dhodapkar et al. 2002; Noonan et al. 2005). Thus autologous immune-mediated control of myeloma may be possible.

We and other investigators have studied whether cancer vaccines administered post-AHCT could be immunogenic and improve outcomes. Our studies involved combined cellular and vaccine strategies under the hypothesis that transfers of ex vivo costimulated autologous T cells will improve functional T cell recovery, thereby providing a platform for enhanced vaccine-directed immune responses. For these studies autologous T cells were stimulated by coculture with immunomagnetic beads conjugated with anti-CD3 and anti-CD28 monoclonal antibodies to prevent T cell anergy through combined CD3 and CD28 signaling (Li et al. 1999; Boussiotis et al. 2000). Using microbial vaccines including a pneumococcal conjugate vaccine (Prevnar®) and an influenza vaccine as well as a cancer antigen vaccine based on peptides derived from hTERT and survivin, these studies showed that an early post-transplant infusion of 1–5 × 10^{10} in vivo vaccine-primed and ex vivo costimulated T cells followed by booster immunizations led to protective antimicrobial antibody responses in a majority of patients and cancer vaccine-directed T cell responses in about 1/3 of patients (Rapoport et al. 2005, 2011; Stadtmauer et al. 2011). The addition of novel adjuvants such as the toll-like receptor-3 (TLR3) agonist Poly-ICLC (Hiltonol®) to a MAGE-A3 tumor antigen vaccine led to functional T cell responses in more than 2/3 of patients and a marginally significant better EFS for patients who developed IFN-γ responses on both $CD4^+$ and $CD8^+$ T cells (Rapoport et al. 2014). Furthermore, a pattern of schedule-dependent T cell expansion was observed, whereby the most robust $CD4^+$ and $CD8^+$ T cell recoveries post-AHCT occurred when the ex vivo costimulated T cells were infused very early after high-dose chemotherapy (on day +2 after autologous stem cell transplantation rather than day +14 or day +100) presumably as a result of the homeostatic expansion mechanisms (e.g., unbound IL-15) that prevail after lymphodepleting chemotherapy (Rapoport et al. 2009). Using this platform of high-dose, lymphodepleting chemotherapy followed by AHCT and then adoptive transfer of ex vivo costimulated autologous T cells, we conducted and reported a phase I/II clinical trial (NCT01352286) designed to evaluate the safety and activity of autologous T cells genetically engineered to express the affinity-enhanced TCR (NY-ESO^{c259}) that recognizes the NY-ESO-1/LAGE-1 peptide complex HLA-A*0201-SLLMWITQC (NY-ESO-$1_{157-165}$) and infused post-AHCT (Rapoport et al. 2015). Patients with high-risk or relapsed multiple myeloma (MM), who were HLA-A*0201 positive and whose myeloma was positive for NY-ESO-1 and/or LAGE-1 by quantitative qRT-PCR, were eligible. Figure 7.1 shows a flow diagram for this clinical trial. Briefly, autologous CD25-depleted CD4 and CD8 T cells were activated and expanded using anti-CD3/anti-CD28 antibody-conjugated microbeads, and genetically modified with a self-inactivating (SIN) lentiviral vector encoding the affinity-enhanced NY-ESO/LAGE-1 TCR. Engineered T cells were administered 4 days after high-dose melphalan and 2 days following auto-HCT (day +2 of AHCT), at a dose range of 1–10 billion total cells. We hypothesized that adoptive transfer of NY-ESO^{c259} TCR-engineered T cells would improve the duration and depth of post-AHCT clinical responses in HLA-A201-positive patients with advanced NY-ESO-1/LAGE-1-expressing MM.

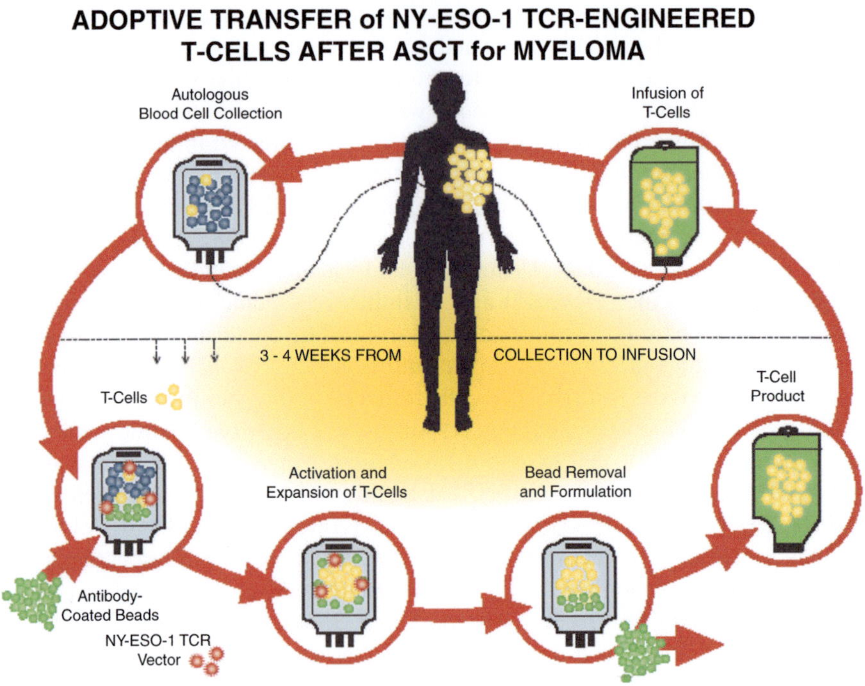

Fig. 7.1 Autologous leukapheresis is performed. CD25-depleted CD4 and CD8 T cells are activated and expanded using anti-CD3/anti-CD28 antibody-conjugated microbeads, and genetically modified with a self-inactivating (SIN) lentiviral vector encoding the affinity-enhanced NY-ESO/LAGE-1 TCR. Engineered T cells are administered 4 days after high-dose melphalan or 2 days following auto-HCT (day +2 of AHCT), at a dose range of 1–10 billion total cells

Prior to enrollment on study, patients had received a median of three prior therapies (range 1–4) including five with prior AHCT. Sixty percent (12/20) of tumors contained cytogenetic abnormalities most of which were considered high risk. Twenty patients (median age of 58, range 44–72 years) received a mean of 8 billion total CD3 T cells (range 1–10 billion) which were genetically modified at an average of 33% (range 18–49%, study minimum was 10%). Thus a mean of 2.4 billion transduced CD3 T cells (range 0.45–3.9 billion) were infused. Infusions were well-tolerated, and no clinically apparent CRS was detected although significant elevations of serum IL-6 were detected in all patients (median 22-fold increase; range 8- to 2272-fold) within 7–28 days post infusion which overlapped with the period of maximum T cell expansion. A subset of responding patients with high levels of engineered T cells were evaluated by flow cytometry for cytokine production (IFN-γ) and cytotoxic potential (granzyme B production and CD107α surface expression) in response to peptide-loaded targets. The data showed that polyfunctional T cells which were generated during manufacturing engrafted in the patients where they remained functional in the peripheral blood for up to a year after infusion.

The majority of adverse events were related to the high-dose melphalan. Importantly, there were no treatment-related fatalities. All serious adverse events (SAEs) (5) were resolved, and the 17 adverse events which were at least probably related to the treatment were grade 3 or lower. Notably a skin rash with lymphocytosis occurred in 3/20 patients, and some patients had a diarrheal syndrome that occurred later than expected for melphalan-induced mucositis, and three cases were confirmed by biopsy to be autologous graft-versus-host disease (autoGvHD). However, analysis of engineered T cells in inflamed and normal colonic tissue and peripheral blood was performed in patients who developed autoGvHD, and while engineered T cells were present in inflamed tissue, they were diluted at sites of inflammation compared to adjacent non-inflamed tissues, suggesting that they were not driving the event. Also we previously observed acute GvHD (aGvHD) involving the GI tract after adoptive transfer of activated but non-gene-modified T cells (Rapoport et al. 2009).

The median progression-free survival (PFS) of this high-risk cohort was 19.1 months (the lower bound of the 95% CI was 8.5 months, upper bound has not been reached yet), while 15/20 (75%) patients remained alive at the time of the initial report. Engineered T cells were found to expand, traffick to marrow, and persist for at least 6 months in all but one patient as determined by Q-PCR and/or flow cytometry. Engineered cells were detected in the blood or marrow by flow cytometry for as long as 2 years after infusion in two patients. This length of persistence is unusual for TCR gene-modified T cells and for gene-modified T cells in general and may reflect adoptive transfer in the setting of AHCT (after intensive lymphodepleting chemotherapy), the use of ex vivo costimulation of the transduced T cells and/or properties of the NY-ESO-1-TCR, and expression vector. Evidence for specific targeting of antigen-positive myeloma cells came from several directions: Compared to enrollment levels, loss of NY-ESO-1 and LAGE-1 transcripts by qRT-PCR analysis on marrow specimens was observed in 12/15 evaluable patients at day 100 and in 11/13 evaluable patients at day 180. Conversely, the 3/15 patients who had detectable levels of NY-ESO-1 and LAGE-1 transcripts in the marrow at day 100 also had very low or undetectable levels of engineered T cells in the peripheral blood which was followed by a relapse in two patients. Four patients had an increase in CD138 transcripts (as a measure of plasma cells in general) in the absence of NY-ESO-1/LAGE-1 transcripts, suggesting that pressure from the immune response was potentially selecting for tumor escape subclones that lacked target tumor antigen. Two patients with prolonged persistence of gene-modified T cells developed durable partial responses associated with residual NY-ESO-1/LAGE-1-*negative* myeloma cells also consistent with the phenomenon of antigen-negative tumor escape. Furthermore, on a statistical basis, between days 0 through 180 post-transplant, the persistence of gene-modified T cells in peripheral blood was inversely correlated with the level of NY-ESO-1 expression in the marrow ($p = 0.022$) and possibly with LAGE-1 ($p = 0.098$). In contrast, there was no relationship over time between T cell persistence in blood and CD138 expression (reflecting total plasma cells) in the marrow. Altogether, these data suggest induction of a robust and tumor antigen-specific memory immune response.

7.9 Risks of TCR-Engineered T Cell Therapy: The MAGE-A3 and MART-1 Experiences

The three major categories of toxicity resulting from TCR-modified T cell therapy include (1) on-target/off-tumor toxicity, (2) off-target/off-tumor toxicity, (3) and CRS presumably resulting from excessive T cell activation. The clinical studies using affinity-enhanced MART-1 (DMF5) and gp100 TCR-engineered T cells that were described earlier amply illustrated examples of "on-target/off-tumor toxicity" resulting from T cell attack on normal melanocytes in the skin and inner ear. These studies suggest that further development of TCR immunotherapy against lineage-specific or tissue differentiation antigens may be difficult. The following studies provide examples of "off-target/off-tumor toxicity."

A companion myeloma trial involving post-AHCT adoptive transfers of autologous T cells engineered to express an affinity-enhanced TCR for the HLA-A*01-restricted MAGE-A3 peptide (EVDPIGHLY) complex was also developed and implemented. This high-affinity MAGE-A3 TCR (MAGE-A3^{a3a} TCR) carried four substitutions in the alpha chain of the CDR2 region, while the beta chain remained wild type. As with the NY-ESO-1 affinity-enhanced TCR, this MAGE-A3 TCR underwent extensive preclinical development involving synthetic biology, biophysical and immunological testing, and extensive screening of normal tissues and cells. After high-dose melphalan (day 2), AHCT (day 0), and T cell infusion (day +2), the first patient treated on this study developed cardiogenic shock accompanied by fever, hypoxia, and hypotension on days +3 to +5 and died 5 days after T cell transfer (day +7) (Linette et al. 2013). PCR analysis of the peripheral blood for the MAGE-A3^{a3a} TCR sequences revealed robust in vivo gene-modified T cell expansion which was >400 cells/μl just 3 days after T cell transfer. By the time of the patient's death, the transduced T cells were estimated to have expanded ~200-fold in vivo. The transduced T cells localized to the bone marrow, lung, heart, and liver, but the highest concentrations were in the blood and pericardial fluid. At autopsy, there was extensive myocardial necrosis with a striking CD3$^+$ lymphoid cellular infiltration in the myocardium; similar infiltration was not observed in the skeletal muscle or other examined organs. Cytokine analysis of the blood and pericardial fluid was consistent with immune cell activation (including ~100-fold increases in IFN-γ and ~1000-fold increases in IL-6). A similar clinical course and cardiac histopathology were observed in a second patient who had melanoma and received MAGE-A3^{a3a} TCR-transduced T cells after conditioning with high-dose cyclophosphamide (Linette et al. 2013). Elegant post-SAEs in vitro studies using an alanine-scanning methodology to delineate critical TCR-binding residues in the MAGE-A3 peptide EVDPIGHLY ultimately identified a peptide (ESDPIVAQY) derived from the very large (3-megadalton) cardiac muscle protein titin as the likely target of off-tumor, off-target TCR cross-reactivity (Cameron et al. 2013). Interestingly extensive preclinical testing revealed no concerns for off-target activity, and post-SAEs testing of 38 cardiac-derived primary cells (including 10 which were HLA-A*01+) showed no evidence for activation of MAGE-A3^{a3a} TCR-transduced T cells by IFN-γ ELISpot analysis. The only model which demonstrated robust reactivity with the affinity-enhanced TCR was an iCell cardiomyocyte culture system which was derived from induced pluripotent stem cells and included a mixture of spontaneously electrically active atrial, nodal, and ventricular-like myocytes which may be more representative of normal heart tissue.

In another clinical trial using an affinity-enhanced HLA-A*2:01 TCR against the MAGEA3: 112-120 peptide (KVAELVHFL), two of seven melanoma patients who received chemotherapy conditioning followed by adoptive transfer of transduced autologous T cells along with IL-2 had complete responses, one lasting more than 4 years, and two additional patients had objective partial responses (Morgan et al. 2013). A single patient with synovial cell sarcoma also had a partial response which lasted for 5 months. However severe neurological toxicity occurred in three patients characterized by mental status changes in all, seizures in two, and white matter vacuolation in one. A possible explanation was cross-reactivity of the affinity-enhanced TCR against a peptide derived from MAGE-A12 which is expressed at low levels in brain tissue. Nonetheless it is unclear why this neurological toxicity was observed in only a subset of treated patients. These studies highlight both the clinical potency of affinity-enhanced TCR-engineered T cells as well as the potential danger of serious and even fatal off-tumor and off-target toxicities. Improvements in the margin of safety for these reagents may require more complex preclinical testing using (i) amino acid (alanine) scanning methodologies to identify critical binding residues and thereby expand the search for potentially cross-reactive peptides in the human genome as well as (ii) more relevant human tissue models such as organ-like structures derived from induced pluripotent stem cells.

Although not thought to be as common as in CAR T cell trials, a fatality apparently due to CRS from excessive T cell activation was recently reported in a study of autologous T cells engineered to express a TCR for the HLA-A*0201-restricted 26-35 epitope of MART-1, which was not affinity enhanced (van den Berg et al. 2015). A patient with very bulky and widely metastatic melanoma (including an 18 cm retroperitoneal mass, a 16 cm pelvic mass, malignant abdominal ascites, and brain and pulmonary metastases) was treated with MART-1 TCR-modified T cells after conditioning with cyclophosphamide and fludarabine. Six days after T cell infusion, the patient had seizures, cerebral hemorrhage, and cardiac arrest and died several days later with multi-organ failure and irreversible brain injury. Following T cell infusion, levels of IL-6, IFN-γ, C-reactive protein (CRP), and procalcitonin were extremely elevated suggestive of CRS or excessive T cell activation. Although the gene-modified T cells were widely distributed in known tumor sites as well as in multiple vital organs including the heart, there was no evidence for any cross-reactivity with any experimental models of cardiac tissue including beating heart cardiomyocyte cultures.

7.10 Current Clinical Trials Using TCR Gene-Modified T Cells

A number of clinical trials have demonstrated the feasibility and efficacy of genetically modified TCR therapies for different types of cancer as reported above, with clinical activity including tumor regression being reported in a significant subset of patients. These early studies have spawned an outgrowth of promising TCR trials directed against an increasing array of tumor-associated targets. Table 7.1 below

Table 7.1 Active clinical trials using TCR-engineered T cells

Target antigen	Target malignancy	Clinical phase	Sponsor/collaborators	NCT trial ID#
NY-ESO-1	Melanoma	Phase ½	Adaptimmune	NCT01350401
NY-ESO-1	Multiple solid cancers	Phase 2	NCI	NCT00670748
MART-1	Melanoma	Phase 2	NCI	NCT00910650
Gp100	Melanoma	Phase 1	Immunocore	NCT01211262
NY-ESO-1	Multiple myeloma	Phase ½	Adaptimmune	NCT01352286
NY-ESO-1	Ovarian cancer	Phase ½	Adaptimmune	NCT01567891
Tyrosinase	Melanoma	Phase 1	Loyola University/NCI	NCT01586403
WT1	AML/CML	Phase ½	Cell Therapy Catapult|Leukemia-lymphoma research|Department of Health, United Kingdom|University College, London	NCT01621724
WT1	Hematological malignancies	Phase ½	Fred Hutchinson Cancer Research Center|NCI	NCT01640301
MAGE-A4	Solid tumors	Phase 1	Tianjin Medical University Cancer Institute and Hospital	NCT01694472
NY-ESO-1	Solid tumors	Phase 2	Jonsson Comprehensive Cancer Center	NCT01697527
CEA	Adenocarcinoma	Phase 2	Roger Williams Medical Center	NCT01723306
NY-ESO-1	Multiple myeloma	Phase ½	Adaptimmune	NCT01892293
NY-ESO-1	Solid tumors	Phase 1	Jonsson Comprehensive Cancer Center|NCI	NCT02070406
MAGE-A4	Solid tumors	Phase 1	Mie University|Takara Bio Inc.|Shionogi|Fiverings Co., Ltd.|Statcom Co. Ltd.	NCT02096614
NY-ESO-1	Solid tumors	Phase 1	Mie University|Takara Bio Inc.|Shionogi|Fiverings Co., Ltd.|Statcom Co. Ltd.	NCT02366546
WT1	NSCLC/ mesothelioma	Phase 1/2	Fred Hutchinson Cancer Research Center|NCI	NCT02408016
NY-ESO-1	Multiple solid tumors	Phase 1	Shenzhen Second People's Hospital|Shenzhen Institute for Innovation and Translational Medicine	NCT02457650
Gp100	Melanoma	Phase 1/2	Immunocore Ltd.|MedImmune LLC	NCT02535078
WT1	AML/MDS	Phase ½	Cell Therapy Catapult|Leukemia-lymphoma research|Department of Health, United Kingdom|University College, London	NCT02550535
Gp100	Uveal melanoma	Phase 1	Immunocore Ltd	NCT02570308

Table 7.1 (continued)

Target antigen	Target malignancy	Clinical phase	Sponsor/collaborators	NCT trial ID#
NY-ESO-1	NSCLC	Phase 1/2	Adaptimmune	NCT02588612
MART-1	Melanoma	Phase 1/2	The Netherlands Cancer Institute	NCT02654821
HBV	HCC	Phase 1	Lion TCR Pte. Ltd.|First Affiliated Hospital, Sun Yat-sen University|Agency for Science, Technology and Research|Sun Yat-sen Memorial Hospital of Sun Yat-sen University	NCT02686372
HBV	HCC	Phase 1/2	Lion TCR Pte. Ltd.|First Affiliated Hospital, Sun Yat-sen University|Agency for Science, Technology and Research|Sun Yat-sen Memorial Hospital of Sun Yat-sen University	NCT02719782

AML acute myeloid leukemia, *CEA* carcinoembryonic antigen, *CML* chronic myeloid leukemia, *Gp100* glycoprotein 100, *HBV* hepatitis B virus, *HCC* hepatocellular carcinoma, *MART-1* melanoma antigen recognized by T cells 1, *NCI* National Cancer Institute, *TCR* T cell receptor, *WT1* Wilms tumor 1

lists current clinical trials that are registered with the National Cancer Institute. Notably, some of these new trials also target epitopes of TAA such as WT1 that are expressed at low levels in normal hematopoietic stem cells but at much higher levels in leukemia.

7.11 Expert Point of View and Future Directions

A therapeutic "proof of principle" for affinity-enhanced TCR-engineered autologous T cells has been amply demonstrated for both certain hematological malignancies (e.g., myeloma) and solid tumors (e.g., melanoma, synovial sarcoma). Several challenges remain before this form of therapy can be more widely applicable. High-affinity TCRs will need to be developed against a greater variety of new targets including peptides derived from established tumor-specific genes such as the widely expressed cancer-testis or cancer-germline antigens. Other candidates could be peptides derived from recurring cancer-specific mutations (e.g., IDH-1/IDH-2 in acute leukemia or KRAS in solid tumors) or the common breakpoint regions of cancer-specific fusion genes (e.g., BCR-ABL in CML) since these mutations may also generate "shared" tumor-associated antigenic peptides. Investigators will need to address the inherent problem of HLA-restriction by offering TCRs that reach a wider range of HLA molecules beyond the traditional and common targets of HLA-A*2:01 and HLA-A*01. As noted above preclinical testing will need to expand significantly beyond studying cell lines and normal tissue arrays to ensure a greater margin of safety for these powerful cell-based therapies. Additional barriers to successful cellular immunotherapy using TCR-modified T cells and CAR T cells include the myriad of mechanisms that cancers (particularly solid tumors) and the tumor microenvironment deploy to suppress effector immune responses including surface expression of PDL-1, PDL-2, and CTLA-4 and elaboration of indoleamine-2,3-dioxygenase (IDO) which depletes tryptophan, increases kynurenine, and thereby promotes formation of T_{regs} and myeloid-derived suppressor cells (MDSCs). In this regard, the advent of the checkpoint inhibitors including PD-1, PDL-1, and CTLA-4 antibodies and the small molecule inhibitors of the IDO enzyme may provide a logical pathway for developing novel combination approaches.

Acknowledgments The authors warmly thank Gwendolyn Binder-Scholl for critical review of the manuscript and Kris Rifkin for assistance with Fig. 7.1.

References

Aleksic M, Liddy N, Molloy PE, Pumphrey N, Vuidepot A, Chang KM, Jakobsen BK (2012) Different affinity windows for virus and cancer-specific T-cell receptors: implications for therapeutic strategies. Eur J Immunol 42(12):3174–3179

Atanackovic D, Arfsten J, Cao Y, Gnjatic S, Schnieders F, Bartels K, Schilling G, Faltz C, Wolschke C, Dierlamm J, Ritter G, Eiermann T, Hossfeld DK, Zander AR, Jungbluth AA, Old LJ, Bokemeyer C, Kroger N (2007) Cancer-testis antigens are commonly expressed in multiple myeloma and induce systemic immunity following allogeneic stem cell transplantation. Blood 109(3):1103–1112

Barrett DM, Teachey DT, Grupp SA (2014) Toxicity management for patients receiving novel T-cell engaging therapies. Curr Opin Pediatr 26(1):43–49

Bendle GM, Linnemann C, Hooijkaas AI, Bies L, de Witte MA, Jorritsma A, Kaiser AD, Pouw N, Debets R, Kieback E, Uckert W, Song JY, Haanen JB, Schumacher TN (2010) Lethal graft-versus-host disease in mouse models of T cell receptor gene therapy. Nat Med 16(5):565–570

Boussiotis VA, Freeman GJ, Taylor PA, Berezovskaya A, Grass I, Blazar BR, Nadler LM (2000) p27kip1 functions as an anergy factor inhibiting interleukin 2 transcription and clonal expansion of alloreactive human and mouse helper T lymphocytes. Nat Med 6(3):290–297

Brahmer J, Reckamp KL, Baas P, Crino L, Eberhardt WE, Poddubskaya E, Antonia S, Pluzanski A, Vokes EE, Holgado E, Waterhouse D, Ready N, Gainor J, Aren Frontera O, Havel L, Steins M, Garassino MC, Aerts JG, Domine M, Paz-Ares L, Reck M, Baudelet C, Harbison CT, Lestini B, Spigel DR (2015) Nivolumab versus docetaxel in advanced squamous-cell non-small-cell lung cancer. N Engl J Med 373(2):123–135

Bridgeman JS, Sewell AK, Miles JJ, Price DA, Cole DK (2012) Structural and biophysical determinants of alphabeta T-cell antigen recognition. Immunology 135(1):9–18

Cameron BJ, Gerry AB, Dukes J, Harper JV, Kannan V, Bianchi FC, Grand F, Brewer JE, Gupta M, Plesa G, Bossi G, Vuidepot A, Powlesland AS, Legg A, Adams KJ, Bennett AD, Pumphrey NJ, Williams DD, Binder-Scholl G, Kulikovskaya I, Levine BL, Riley JL, Varela-Rohena A, Stadtmauer EA, Rapoport AP, Linette GP, June CH, Hassan NJ, Kalos M, Jakobsen BK (2013) Identification of a Titin-derived HLA-A1-presented peptide as a cross-reactive target for engineered MAGE A3-directed T cells. Sci Transl Med 5(197):197ra103

Chen YT, Scanlan MJ, Sahin U, Tureci O, Gure AO, Tsang S, Williamson B, Stockert E, Pfreundschuh M, Old LJ (1997) A testicular antigen aberrantly expressed in human cancers detected by autologous antibody screening. Proc Natl Acad Sci U S A 94(5):1914–1918

Cohen CJ, Zhao Y, Zheng Z, Rosenberg SA, Morgan RA (2006) Enhanced antitumor activity of murine-human hybrid T-cell receptor (TCR) in human lymphocytes is associated with improved pairing and TCR/CD3 stability. Cancer Res 66(17):8878–8886

Cohen CJ, Li YF, El-Gamil M, Robbins PF, Rosenberg SA, Morgan RA (2007) Enhanced antitumor activity of T cells engineered to express T-cell receptors with a second disulfide bond. Cancer Res 67(8):3898–3903

Condomines M, Hose D, Raynaud P, Hundemer M, De Vos J, Baudard M, Moehler T, Pantesco V, Moos M, Schved JF, Rossi JF, Reme T, Goldschmidt H, Klein B (2007) Cancer/testis genes in multiple myeloma: expression patterns and prognosis value determined by microarray analysis. J Immunol 178(5):3307–3315

Davis MM, Boniface JJ, Reich Z, Lyons D, Hampl J, Arden B, Chien Y (1998) Ligand recognition by alpha beta T cell receptors. Annu Rev Immunol 16:523–544

Dhodapkar MV, Krasovsky J, Olson K (2002) T cells from the tumor microenvironment of patients with progressive myeloma can generate strong, tumor-specific cytolytic responses to autologous, tumor-loaded dendritic cells. Proc Natl Acad Sci U S A 99(20):13009–13013

Dunn SM, Rizkallah PJ, Baston E, Mahon T, Cameron B, Moysey R, Gao F, Sami M, Boulter J, Li Y, Jakobsen BK (2006) Directed evolution of human T cell receptor CDR2 residues by phage display dramatically enhances affinity for cognate peptide-MHC without increasing apparent cross-reactivity. Protein Sci 15(4):710–721

Ellis JM, Henson V, Slack R, Ng J, Hartzman RJ, Katovich Hurley C (2000) Frequencies of HLA-A2 alleles in five U.S. population groups. Predominance of A*02011 and identification of HLA-A*0231. Hum Immunol 61(3):334–340

Furler S, Paterna JC, Weibel M, Bueler H (2001) Recombinant AAV vectors containing the foot and mouth disease virus 2A sequence confer efficient bicistronic gene expression in cultured cells and rat substantia nigra neurons. Gene Ther 8(11):864–873

Gonzalez-Galarza FF, Takeshita LY, Santos EJ, Kempson F, Maia MH, da Silva AL, Teles e Silva AL, Ghattaoraya GS, Alfirevic A, Jones AR, Middleton D (2015) Allele frequency net 2015 update: new features for HLA epitopes, KIR and disease and HLA adverse drug reaction associations. Nucleic Acids Res 43:D784–D788

Groettrup M, Kirk CJ, Basler M (2010) Proteasomes in immune cells: more than peptide producers? Nat Rev Immunol 10(1):73–78

Gross G, Eshhar Z (1992) Endowing T cells with antibody specificity using chimeric T cell receptors. FASEB J 6(15):3370–3378

Gross G, Waks T, Eshhar Z (1989) Expression of immunoglobulin-T-cell receptor chimeric molecules as functional receptors with antibody-type specificity. Proc Natl Acad Sci U S A 86(24):10024–10028

Grupp SA, Kalos M, Barrett D, Aplenc R, Porter DL, Rheingold SR, Teachey DT, Chew A, Hauck B, Wright JF, Milone MC, Levine BL, June CH (2013) Chimeric antigen receptor-modified T cells for acute lymphoid leukemia. N Engl J Med 368(16):1509–1518

Haidar JN, Pierce B, Yu Y, Tong W, Li M, Weng Z (2009) Structure-based design of a T-cell receptor leads to nearly 100-fold improvement in binding affinity for pepMHC. Proteins 74(4):948–960

Hebeisen M, Baitsch L, Presotto D, Baumgaertner P, Romero P, Michielin O, Speiser DE, Rufer N (2013) SHP-1 phosphatase activity counteracts increased T cell receptor affinity. J Clin Invest 123(3):1044–1056

Hebeisen M, Allard M, Gannon PO, Schmidt J, Speiser DE, Rufer N (2015) Identifying individual T cell receptors of optimal avidity for tumor antigens. Front Immunol 6:582

Hodi FS, O'Day SJ, McDermott DF, Weber RW, Sosman JA, Haanen JB, Gonzalez R, Robert C, Schadendorf D, Hassel JC, Akerley W, van den Eertwegh AJ, Lutzky J, Lorigan P, Vaubel JM, Linette GP, Hogg D, Ottensmeier CH, Lebbe C, Peschel C, Quirt I, Clark JI, Wolchok JD, Weber JS, Tian J, Yellin MJ, Nichol GM, Hoos A, Urba WJ (2010) Improved survival with ipilimumab in patients with metastatic melanoma. N Engl J Med 363(8):711–723

Hunder NN, Wallen H, Cao J, Hendricks DW, Reilly JZ, Rodmyre R, Jungbluth A, Gnjatic S, Thompson JA, Yee C (2008) Treatment of metastatic melanoma with autologous $CD4^+$ T cells against NY-ESO-1. N Engl J Med 358(25):2698–2703

Ilyas S, Yang JC (2015) Landscape of tumor antigens in T cell immunotherapy. J Immunol 195(11):5117–5122

Irving M, Zoete V, Hebeisen M, Schmid D, Baumgartner P, Guillaume P, Romero P, Speiser D, Luescher I, Rufer N, Michielin O (2012) Interplay between T cell receptor binding kinetics and the level of cognate peptide presented by major histocompatibility complexes governs CD8+ T cell responsiveness. J Biol Chem 287(27):23068–23078

Ito R, Katano I, Kawai K, Hirata H, Ogura T, Kamisako T, Eto T, Ito M (2009) Highly sensitive model for xenogenic GvHD using severe immunodeficient NOG mice. Transplantation 87(11):1654–1658

Jager E, Chen YT, Drijfhout JW, Karbach J, Ringhoffer M, Jager D, Arand M, Wada H, Noguchi Y, Stockert E, Old LJ, Knuth A (1998) Simultaneous humoral and cellular immune response against cancer-testis antigen NY-ESO-1: definition of human histocompatibility leukocyte antigen (HLA)-A2-binding peptide epitopes. J Exp Med 187(2):265–270

Jameson SC, Hogquist KA, Bevan MJ (1995) Positive selection of thymocytes. Annu Rev Immunol 13:93–126

Johnson LA, Heemskerk B, Powell DJ Jr, Cohen CJ, Morgan RA, Dudley ME, Robbins PF, Rosenberg SA (2006) Gene transfer of tumor-reactive TCR confers both high avidity and tumor reactivity to nonreactive peripheral blood mononuclear cells and tumor-infiltrating lymphocytes. J Immunol 177(9):6548–6559

Johnson LA, Morgan RA, Dudley ME, Cassard L, Yang JC, Hughes MS, Kammula US, Royal RE, Sherry RM, Wunderlich JR, Lee CC, Restifo NP, Schwarz SL, Cogdill AP, Bishop RJ, Kim H, Brewer CC, Rudy SF, Van Waes C, Davis JL, Mathur A, Ripley RT, Nathan DA, Laurencot CM, Rosenberg SA (2009) Gene therapy with human and mouse T-cell receptors mediates cancer regression and targets normal tissues expressing cognate antigen. Blood 114(3):535–546

Jungbluth AA, Antonescu CR, Busam KJ, Iversen K, Kolb D, Coplan K, Chen YT, Stockert E, Ladanyi M, Old LJ (2001) Monophasic and biphasic synovial sarcomas abundantly express cancer/testis antigen NY-ESO-1 but not MAGE-A1 or CT7. Int J Cancer 94(2):252–256

Jungbluth AA, Ely S, DiLiberto M, Niesvizky R, Williamson B, Frosina D, Chen YT, Bhardwaj N, Chen-Kiang S, Old LJ, Cho HJ (2005) The cancer-testis antigens CT7 (MAGE-C1) and MAGE-A3/6 are commonly expressed in multiple myeloma and correlate with plasma-cell proliferation. Blood 106(1):167–174

Kochenderfer JN, Dudley ME, Kassim SH, Somerville RP, Carpenter RO, Stetler-Stevenson M, Yang JC, Phan GQ, Hughes MS, Sherry RM, Raffeld M, Feldman S, Lu L, Li YF, Ngo LT, Goy A, Feldman T, Spaner DE, Wang ML, Chen CC, Kranick SM, Nath A, Nathan DA, Morton KE, Toomey MA, Rosenberg SA (2015) Chemotherapy-refractory diffuse large B-cell lymphoma and indolent B-cell malignancies can be effectively treated with autologous T cells expressing an anti-CD19 chimeric antigen receptor. J Clin Oncol Off J Am Soc Clin Oncol 33(6):540–549

Kvistborg P, van Buuren MM, Schumacher TN (2013) Human cancer regression antigens. Curr Opin Immunol 25(2):284–290

Li L, Yee C, Beavo JA (1999) CD3- and CD28-dependent induction of PDE7 required for T cell activation. Science 283(5403):848–851

Li Y, Moysey R, Molloy PE, Vuidepot AL, Mahon T, Baston E, Dunn S, Liddy N, Jacob J, Jakobsen BK, Boulter JM (2005) Directed evolution of human T-cell receptors with picomolar affinities by phage display. Nat Biotechnol 23(3):349–354

Linette GP, Stadtmauer EA, Maus MV, Rapoport AP, Levine BL, Emery L, Litzky L, Bagg A, Carreno BM, Cimino PJ, Binder-Scholl GK, Smethurst DP, Gerry AB, Pumphrey NJ, Bennett AD, Brewer JE, Dukes J, Harper J, Tayton-Martin HK, Jakobsen BK, Hassan NJ, Kalos M, June CH (2013) Cardiovascular toxicity and titin cross-reactivity of affinity-enhanced T cells in myeloma and melanoma. Blood 122(6):863–871

Linnemann C, Heemskerk B, Kvistborg P, Kluin RJ, Bolotin DA, Chen X, Bresser K, Nieuwland M, Schotte R, Michels S, Gomez-Eerland R, Jahn L, Hombrink P, Legrand N, Shu CJ, Mamedov IZ, Velds A, Blank CU, Haanen JB, Turchaninova MA, Kerkhoven RM, Spits H, Hadrup SR, Heemskerk MH, Blankenstein T, Chudakov DM, Bendle GM, Schumacher TN

(2013) High-throughput identification of antigen-specific TCRs by TCR gene capture. Nat Med 19(11):1534–1541

Maby P, Tougeron D, Hamieh M, Mlecnik B, Kora H, Bindea G, Angell HK, Fredriksen T, Elie N, Fauquembergue E, Drouet A, Leprince J, Benichou J, Mauillon J, Le Pessot F, Sesboue R, Tuech JJ, Sabourin JC, Michel P, Frebourg T, Galon J, Latouche JB (2015) Correlation between density of $CD8^+$ T-cell infiltrate in microsatellite unstable colorectal cancers and Frameshift mutations: a rationale for personalized immunotherapy. Cancer Res 75(17):3446–3455

Malecek K, Grigoryan A, Zhong S, Gu WJ, Johnson LA, Rosenberg SA, Cardozo T, Krogsgaard M (2014) Specific increase in potency via structure-based design of a TCR. J Immunol 193(5):2587–2599

Mallabiabarrena A, Fresno M, Alarcon B (1992) An endoplasmic reticulum retention signal in the CD3 epsilon chain of the T-cell receptor. Nature 357(6379):593–596

Maus MV, Grupp SA, Porter DL, June CH (2014) Antibody-modified T cells: CARs take the front seat for hematologic malignancies. Blood 123(17):2625–2635

Miles JJ, Douek DC, Price DA (2011) Bias in the alphabeta T-cell repertoire: implications for disease pathogenesis and vaccination. Immunol Cell Biol 89(3):375–387

Minami Y, Weissman AM, Samelson LE, Klausner RD (1987) Building a multichain receptor: synthesis, degradation, and assembly of the T-cell antigen receptor. Proc Natl Acad Sci U S A 84(9):2688–2692

Monte M, Simonatto M, Peche LY, Bublik DR, Gobessi S, Pierotti MA, Rodolfo M, Schneider C (2006) MAGE-A tumor antigens target p53 transactivation function through histone deacetylase recruitment and confer resistance to chemotherapeutic agents. Proc Natl Acad Sci U S A 103(30):11160–11165

Morgan RA, Dudley ME, Wunderlich JR, Hughes MS, Yang JC, Sherry RM, Royal RE, Topalian SL, Kammula US, Restifo NP, Zheng Z, Nahvi A, de Vries CR, Rogers-Freezer LJ, Mavroukakis SA, Rosenberg SA (2006) Cancer regression in patients after transfer of genetically engineered lymphocytes. Science 314(5796):126–129

Morgan RA, Chinnasamy N, Abate-Daga D, Gros A, Robbins PF, Zheng Z, Dudley ME, Feldman SA, Yang JC, Sherry RM, Phan GQ, Hughes MS, Kammula US, Miller AD, Hessman CJ, Stewart AA, Restifo NP, Quezado MM, Alimchandani M, Rosenberg AZ, Nath A, Wang T, Bielekova B, Wuest SC, Akula N, McMahon FJ, Wilde S, Mosetter B, Schendel DJ, Laurencot CM, Rosenberg SA (2013) Cancer regression and neurological toxicity following anti-MAGE-A3 TCR gene therapy. J Immunother 36(2):133–151

Nitta T, Murata S, Sasaki K, Fujii H, Ripen AM, Ishimaru N, Koyasu S, Tanaka K, Takahama Y (2010) Thymoproteasome shapes immunocompetent repertoire of $CD8^+$ T cells. Immunity 32(1):29–40

Noonan K, Matsui W, Serafini P, Carbley R, Tan G, Khalili J, Bonyhadi M, Levitsky H, Whartenby K, Borrello I (2005) Activated marrow-infiltrating lymphocytes effectively target plasma cells and their clonogenic precursors. Cancer Res 65(5):2026–2034

Parkhurst MR, Joo J, Riley JP, Yu Z, Li Y, Robbins PF, Rosenberg SA (2009) Characterization of genetically modified T-cell receptors that recognize the CEA:691-699 peptide in the context of HLA-A2.1 on human colorectal cancer cells. Clin Cancer Res 15(1):169–180

Porrata LF, Markovic SN (2004) Timely reconstitution of immune competence affects clinical outcome following autologous stem cell transplantation. Clin Exp Med 4(2):78–85

Porrata LF, Gertz MA, Inwards DJ, Litzow MR, Lacy MQ, Tefferi A, Gastineau DA, Dispenzieri A, Ansell SM, Micallef IN, Geyer SM, Markovic SN (2001) Early lymphocyte recovery predicts superior survival after autologous hematopoietic stem cell transplantation in multiple myeloma or non-Hodgkin lymphoma. Blood 98(3):579–585

Porter DL, Levine BL, Kalos M, Bagg A, June CH (2011) Chimeric antigen receptor-modified T cells in chronic lymphoid leukemia. N Engl J Med 365(8):725–733

Rapoport AP, Stadtmauer EA, Aqui N, Badros A, Cotte J, Chrisley L, Veloso E, Zheng Z, Westphal S, Mair R, Chi N, Ratterree B, Pochran MF, Natt S, Hinkle J, Sickles C, Sohal A, Ruehle K, Lynch C, Zhang L, Porter DL, Luger S, Guo C, Fang HB, Blackwelder W, Hankey K, Mann D, Edelman R, Frasch C, Levine BL, Cross A, June CH (2005) Restoration of immunity in

lymphopenic individuals with cancer by vaccination and adoptive T-cell transfer. Nat Med 11(11):1230–1237
Rapoport AP, Stadtmauer EA, Aqui N, Vogl D, Chew A, Fang HB, Janofsky S, Yager K, Veloso E, Zheng Z, Milliron T, Westphal S, Cotte J, Huynh H, Cannon A, Yanovich S, Akpek G, Tan M, Virts K, Ruehle K, Harris C, Philip S, Vonderheide RH, Levine BL, June CH (2009) Rapid immune recovery and graft-versus-host disease-like engraftment syndrome following adoptive transfer of costimulated autologous T cells. Clin Cancer Res 15(13):4499–4507
Rapoport AP, Aqui NA, Stadtmauer EA, Vogl DT, Fang HB, Cai L, Janofsky S, Chew A, Storek J, Akpek G, Badros A, Yanovich S, Tan MT, Veloso E, Pasetti MF, Cross A, Philip S, Murphy H, Bhagat R, Zheng Z, Milliron T, Cotte J, Cannon A, Levine BL, Vonderheide RH, June CH (2011) Combination immunotherapy using adoptive T-cell transfer and tumor antigen vaccination on the basis of hTERT and survivin after AHCT for myeloma. Blood 117(3):788–797
Rapoport AP, Aqui NA, Stadtmauer EA, Vogl DT, Xu YY, Kalos M, Cai L, Fang HB, Weiss BM, Badros A, Yanovich S, Akpek G, Tsao P, Cross A, Mann D, Philip S, Kerr N, Brennan A, Zheng Z, Ruehle K, Milliron T, Strome SE, Salazar AM, Levine BL, June CH (2014) Combination immunotherapy after AHCT for multiple myeloma using MAGE-A3/poly-ICLC immunizations followed by adoptive transfer of vaccine-primed and costimulated autologous T cells. Clin Cancer Res 20(5):1355–1365
Rapoport AP, Stadtmauer EA, Binder-Scholl GK, Goloubeva O, Vogl DT, Lacey SF, Badros AZ, Garfall A, Weiss B, Finklestein J, Kulikovskaya I, Sinha SK, Kronsberg S, Gupta M, Bond S, Melchiori L, Brewer JE, Bennett AD, Gerry AB, Pumphrey NJ, Williams D, Tayton-Martin HK, Ribeiro L, Holdich T, Yanovich S, Hardy N, Yared J, Kerr N, Philip S, Westphal S, Siegel DL, Levine BL, Jakobsen BK, Kalos M, June CH (2015) NY-ESO-1-specific TCR-engineered T cells mediate sustained antigen-specific antitumor effects in myeloma. Nat Med 21(8):914–921
Robbins PF (2015) T-cell receptor-transduced T cells: clinical experience. Cancer J 21(6):480–485
Robbins PF, Li YF, El-Gamil M, Zhao Y, Wargo JA, Zheng Z, Xu H, Morgan RA, Feldman SA, Johnson LA, Bennett AD, Dunn SM, Mahon TM, Jakobsen BK, Rosenberg SA (2008) Single and dual amino acid substitutions in TCR CDRs can enhance antigen-specific T cell functions. J Immunol 180(9):6116–6131
Robbins PF, Morgan RA, Feldman SA, Yang JC, Sherry RM, Dudley ME, Wunderlich JR, Nahvi AV, Helman LJ, Mackall CL, Kammula US, Hughes MS, Restifo NP, Raffeld M, Lee CC, Levy CL, Li YF, El-Gamil M, Schwarz SL, Laurencot C, Rosenberg SA (2011) Tumor regression in patients with metastatic synovial cell sarcoma and melanoma using genetically engineered lymphocytes reactive with NY-ESO-1. J Clin Oncol Off J Am Soc Clin Oncol 29(7):917–924
Robbins PF, Kassim SH, Tran TL, Crystal JS, Morgan RA, Feldman SA, Yang JC, Dudley ME, Wunderlich JR, Sherry RM, Kammula US, Hughes MS, Restifo NP, Raffeld M, Lee CC, Li YF, El-Gamil M, Rosenberg SA (2015) A pilot trial using lymphocytes genetically engineered with an NY-ESO-1-reactive T-cell receptor: long-term follow-up and correlates with response. Clin Cancer Res 21(5):1019–1027
Rosenberg SA, Yang JC, Topalian SL, Schwartzentruber DJ, Weber JS, Parkinson DR, Seipp CA, Einhorn JH, White DE (1994) Treatment of 283 consecutive patients with metastatic melanoma or renal cell cancer using high-dose bolus interleukin 2. JAMA 271(12):907–913
Rosenberg SA, Yang JC, Restifo NP (2004) Cancer immunotherapy: moving beyond current vaccines. Nat Med 10(9):909–915
Rudolph MG, Stanfield RL, Wilson IA (2006) How TCRs bind MHCs, peptides, and coreceptors. Annu Rev Immunol 24:419–466
Schmid DA, Irving MB, Posevitz V, Hebeisen M, Posevitz-Fejfar A, Sarria JC, Gomez-Eerland R, Thome M, Schumacher TN, Romero P, Speiser DE, Zoete V, Michielin O, Rufer N (2010) Evidence for a TCR affinity threshold delimiting maximal CD8 T cell function. J Immunol 184(9):4936–4946
Seiwert TY, Burtness B, Mehra R, Weiss J, Berger R, Eder JP, Heath K, McClanahan T, Lunceford J, Gause C, Cheng JD, Chow LQ (2016) Safety and clinical activity of pembrolizumab for treatment of recurrent or metastatic squamous cell carcinoma of the head and neck (KEYNOTE-012): an open-label, multicentre, phase 1b trial. Lancet Oncol 17(7):956–965

Stadtmauer EA, Vogl DT, Luning Prak E, Boyer J, Aqui NA, Rapoport AP, McDonald KR, Hou X, Murphy H, Bhagat R, Mangan PA, Chew A, Veloso EA, Levine BL, Vonderheide RH, Jawad AF, June CH, Sullivan KE (2011) Transfer of influenza vaccine-primed costimulated autologous T cells after stem cell transplantation for multiple myeloma leads to reconstitution of influenza immunity: results of a randomized clinical trial. Blood 117(1):63–71

Stone JD, Chervin AS, Kranz DM (2009) T-cell receptor binding affinities and kinetics: impact on T-cell activity and specificity. Immunology 126(2):165–176

Szymczak AL, Workman CJ, Wang Y, Vignali KM, Dilioglou S, Vanin EF, Vignali DA (2004) Correction of multi-gene deficiency in vivo using a single 'self-cleaving' 2A peptide-based retroviral vector. Nat Biotechnol 22(5):589–594

Tran KQ, Zhou J, Durflinger KH, Langhan MM, Shelton TE, Wunderlich JR, Robbins PF, Rosenberg SA, Dudley ME (2008) Minimally cultured tumor-infiltrating lymphocytes display optimal characteristics for adoptive cell therapy. J Immunother 31(8):742–751

Uhlen M, Fagerberg L, Hallstrom BM, Lindskog C, Oksvold P, Mardinoglu A, Sivertsson A, Kampf C, Sjostedt E, Asplund A, Olsson I, Edlund K, Lundberg E, Navani S, Szigyarto CA, Odeberg J, Djureinovic D, Takanen JO, Hober S, Alm T, Edqvist PH, Berling H, Tegel H, Mulder J, Rockberg J, Nilsson P, Schwenk JM, Hamsten M, von Feilitzen K, Forsberg M, Persson L, Johansson F, Zwahlen M, von Heijne G, Nielsen J, Ponten F (2015) Proteomics. Tissue-based map of the human proteome. Science 347(6220):1260419

van Baren N, Brasseur F, Godelaine D, Hames G, Ferrant A, Lehmann F, Andre M, Ravoet C, Doyen C, Spagnoli GC, Bakkus M, Thielemans K, Boon T (1999) Genes encoding tumor-specific antigens are expressed in human myeloma cells. Blood 94(4):1156–1164

van den Berg JH, Gomez-Eerland R, van de Wiel B, Hulshoff L, van den Broek D, Bins A, Tan HL, Harper JV, Hassan NJ, Jakobsen BK, Jorritsma A, Blank CU, Schumacher TN, Haanen JB (2015) Case report of a fatal serious adverse event upon administration of T cells transduced with a MART-1-specific T-cell receptor. Mol Ther 23(9):1541–1550

van der Merwe PA, Davis SJ (2003) Molecular interactions mediating T cell antigen recognition. Annu Rev Immunol 21:659–684

van Loenen MM, de Boer R, Amir AL, Hagedoorn RS, Volbeda GL, Willemze R, van Rood JJ, Falkenburg JH, Heemskerk MH (2010) Mixed T cell receptor dimers harbor potentially harmful neoreactivity. Proc Natl Acad Sci U S A 107(24):10972–10977

van Rhee F, Szmania SM, Zhan F, Gupta SK, Pomtree M, Lin P, Batchu RB, Moreno A, Spagnoli G, Shaughnessy J, Tricot G (2005) NY-ESO-1 is highly expressed in poor-prognosis multiple myeloma and induces spontaneous humoral and cellular immune responses. Blood 105(10):3939–3944

Yuan J, Gnjatic S, Li H, Powel S, Gallardo HF, Ritter E, Ku GY, Jungbluth AA, Segal NH, Rasalan TS, Manukian G, Xu Y, Roman RA, Terzulli SL, Heywood M, Pogoriler E, Ritter G, Old LJ, Allison JP, Wolchok JD (2008) CTLA-4 blockade enhances polyfunctional NY-ESO-1 specific T cell responses in metastatic melanoma patients with clinical benefit. Proc Natl Acad Sci U S A 105(51):20410–20415

Zhao Y, Bennett AD, Zheng Z, Wang QJ, Robbins PF, Yu LY, Li Y, Molloy PE, Dunn SM, Jakobsen BK, Rosenberg SA, Morgan RA (2007) High-affinity TCRs generated by phage display provide $CD4^+$ T cells with the ability to recognize and kill tumor cell lines. J Immunol 179(9):5845–5854

Zoete V, Irving M, Ferber M, Cuendet MA, Michielin O (2013) Structure-based, rational design of T cell receptors. Front Immunol 4:268

Part II

Beyond Chimeric Antigen Receptor and T-Cell Receptors: Data, Consensus and Challenges

Cytotoxic T Cells for Infections: From Donor Specific to "Off the Shelf"

8

Maria A. V. Marzolini and Karl S. Peggs

8.1 Introduction

Allogeneic haematopoietic cell transplantation (HCT) results in a period of profound immunosuppression, with both quantitative and functional deficiencies in virus-specific T cells, rendering recipients susceptible to opportunistic and latent viruses. These infections can cause significant morbidity and contribute to mortality post-transplant. The main viral pathogens causing life-threatening disease in the post-transplant period include *Cytomegalovirus* (CMV) and Epstein-Barr viruses (EBV), both of which are often asymptomatic in immunocompetent hosts. Although there are pharmacological antiviral therapies available, these have significant side-effects, may not be effective for each virus, do not reconstitute viral immunity and may provoke drug resistance. Therefore, research has focused on developing adoptive cellular therapies, consisting of virus-specific cytotoxic T lymphocytes (CTLs), to correct the deficiencies in viral immunity post-transplant. In this review, we begin by detailing the advances made in producing single-virus-specific T cells, in particular for CMV and EBV, and then proceed to describe the progress in developing multi-virus-specific T cells and in broadening the repertoire of available donor sources with the generation of virus-specific T cells from virus-naïve individuals and the use of third-party donors.

M. A. V. Marzolini · K. S. Peggs (✉)
UCL Cancer Institute, University College London, London, UK
e-mail: m.marzolini@ucl.ac.uk; karl.peggs@ucl.ac.uk

M.-A. Perales et al. (eds.), *Cell and Gene Therapies*, Advances and Controversies in Hematopoietic Transplantation and Cell Therapy,
https://doi.org/10.1007/978-3-319-54368-0_8

8.2 *Cytomegalovirus*-Specific T Cells

Cytomegalovirus (CMV), also known as human herpesvirus 5 (HHV-5), is a member of the *Betaherpesvirinae* family. It is an opportunistic, ubiquitous virus. The seroprevalence rate in the general population is between 50 and 80%, although in some high-risk subgroups it can be as high as 90% and is influenced by birthplace and age, being positively associated with lower household income and increasing age (Zhang et al. 1995; Bate et al. 2010; Staras et al. 2006). In the majority of immunocompetent individuals, primary CMV infection is asymptomatic although in a small minority of people a syndrome similar to infectious mononucleosis may occur (Peggs 2009). Following primary infection, the virus has a period of clinical latency whereby it resides in mononuclear leucocytes, evading immune surveillance and being controlled by the composite immune cells of the innate and adaptive systems (Hanley and Bollard 2014). The complications of CMV infection are seen acutely in patients who are severely immunocompromised when an absolute and functional deficiency in CMV-reactive T lymphocytes can lead to viral dissemination and the development of CMV disease, including pneumonitis, retinitis, colitis, encephalitis and hepatitis.

The importance of the recovery of protective CMV-specific immune responses post-allogeneic HCT was initially identified by Reusser et al. (1991) who observed that none of the patients with a detectable CMV-specific CTL response post-transplant developed CMV pneumonitis compared with a 60% mortality rate from CMV pneumonitis in those without a detectable response. Despite advances in antiviral therapies, which are associated with an improved outcome when instigated early in the reactivation process, CMV pneumonia post-HCT still has a reported overall survival of 30% at 6 months after diagnosis (Erard et al. 2015). CMV serostatus is an independent risk factor for outcome following unrelated donor transplant (Boeckh and Ljungman 2009), and having a CMV-seropositive donor has also been identified as a risk factor for bacterial and fungal infection (Nichols et al. 2002).

Although there are a number of active pharmacological antiviral therapies, treatment is often accompanied by undesirable side-effects such as nephrotoxicity and myelosuppression, the drugs do not offer a long-term solution to the deficiency in CMV-reactive T cells and they may provoke drug resistance in some cases.

The foundation for CMV-specific adoptive cellular therapy was established in proof-of-concept research performed by Riddell et al. (1992) with the demonstration that adoptive cellular therapy (ACT) using donor-derived CMV-specific $CD8^+$ T-cell clones could effectively restore immunity to CMV. Three patients were given ACT weekly for 4 weeks in escalating doses, following which CTL responses were detected and none of the patients subsequently developed CMV disease. An expanded Phase I clinical study was reported in 14 recipients of matched related CMV-seropositive donor allogeneic HCT (Walter et al. 1995). The cells were infused as a prophylactic therapy with no major side-effects and all of the patients reconstituted CMV-specific CTLs.

Following this initial research, a number of Phase I–II studies were performed to assess the safety and efficacy of CMV-specific T cells as adoptive cellular therapy (Table 8.1). These studies were heterogeneous in design, hindering direct comparison between studies, particularly with respect to the indication for therapy, cellular selection techniques, cell doses and transplant conditioning regimens. Early studies examined the use of CMV-specific T cells as a prophylactic therapy (Walter et al. 1995; Blyth et al. 2013; Micklethwaite et al. 2007), whilst, with the advent of polymerase chain reaction (PCR)-guided CMV surveillance, other studies examined their usage as a pre-emptive therapy to prevent the development of CMV disease once CMV reactivation had been detected (Cobbold et al. 2005; Peggs et al. 2009, 2011). A minority of studies focused on those with refractory CMV viraemia or disease (Feuchtinger et al. 2010; Einsele et al. 2002). One Phase II study (Peggs et al. 2009) which investigated the use of CMV-specific T cells in both the prophylactic and pre-emptive setting included 30 patients, 10 of whom received the cells as prophylaxis. Only three patients, in the prophylactic group, developed a primary infective episode that required additional antiviral therapy, whereas the remaining patients in the study experienced no secondary episodes of viral reactivation following the initial clearance, suggesting the effectiveness of the therapy in different indicative settings.

Graft-versus-host disease (GvHD) is a potentially serious complication following allogeneic HCT and is a known side effect following therapy with donor lymphocyte infusions (DLIs) (Nikiforow and Alyea 2014; Tomblyn and Lazarus 2008). Therefore, there was concern that the adoptive transfer of virus-specific cytotoxic T lymphocytes could cause or worsen GvHD in transplant recipients. The studies performed so far have reported only low rates of the induction of GvHD (Table 8.1) which are predominantly grades 1–2, including in those studies comprising of patients who would normally be at high risk for the development of GvHD (Perruccio et al. 2005). Notably, however, most studies have excluded patients with active GvHD, both because of the risk of exacerbation and because the enhanced immunosuppression would likely render the cells ineffective, and hence the patients at greatest risk for CMV complications are perhaps least well served by such approaches.

The largest published Phase II study to date was performed by Blyth et al. (2013). Fifty patients with CMV-seropositive donors received 2×10^7 cells/m^2 on or after day 28 post-transplant as prophylaxis and were compared with a contemporary control cohort who received pharmacotherapy. The median follow-up of 26 months was longer than most studies previously reported. There was no statistically significant difference in the development of acute GvHD between the 2 groups, despite the CMV T-cell group including more mismatched donors—12 out of 50 (24%) patients who received CMV T cells developed GvHD grades 2–4 (although 5 of these patients had developed acute GvHD prior to the CTL infusion) compared with 18% of the control group. Although there was no statistically significant difference in the cumulative incidence of CMV reactivation between the CMV T-cell group and cohort control group, there was a statistically significant difference in the peak CMV titre which was lower in the T-cell group (median peak CMV titre 0 vs 600

Table 8.1 Phase I/II studies of CMV-specific CTLs post-allogeneic HCT

Study name	No. of patients	Indication	Rate of aGvHD	CMV outcome	Donor type	Donor/recipient CMV status	Technique for production of CMV-specific CTLs	T-cell dose
Blyth et al. (2013)	50	Prophylaxis	7/50	26/50 CMV reactivation (14/26 developed CMV reactivation prior to ACT)	Sib = 36 MUD = 14	+/+ = 36 +/− = 14	Donor PBMCs—DCs pulsed with CMV pp65 peptide	2×10^7 cells/m^2
Walter et al. (1995)	14	Prophylaxis	3/14	0/14 had CMV viraemia or disease	Matched related donor	+/+ = 5 +/− = 9	Donor PBMCs cocultured with CMV fibroblasts. CD8+ CTL clones generated	4 escalating doses: 33 million to 1 billion cells /m^2
Peggs et al. (2003)	16	Previous episode of CMV viraemia	3/16 (grade 1 only)	8/16 cleared CMV without antivirals 2/14 evaluable pts had a second episode of CMV	Syn = 1 MUD = 4 MRD = 11	+/+ = 16	Donor PBMCs cocultures with DCs pulsed with CMV antigen	1×10^5 cells/kg
Perruccio et al. (2005)	25	Prophylaxis	1/25 (grade 2)	7/25 reactivated CMV	Haplos	+/+ = 23 +/− = 2	Donor PBMCs incubated with CMV peptide to produce T-cell clones specific for CMV	1×10^5 cells / kg to 3×10^6 cells/kg
Cobbold et al. (2005)	9	7 = after first episode 2 = persistent viraemia	2/9 grades 1–2 (both present before ACT)	8/9—CMV reactivation resolved 1 = marked reduction in viral load	Sib = 6 MUD = 3	Seropositive donors	Staining PBMCs with HLA-peptide tetramers containing peptides from CMV pp65 or I-1 followed by magnetic bead selection	1.2×10^3/kg to 3.3×10^4/kg

Peggs et al. (2011)	18	11 pre-emptive 7 prophylactic	8/18 (7/18 grades 1–2)	Prophylactic: none needed antiviral therapy within 6 months Pre-emptive: 9/11 needed antiviral therapy	Related donors	+/+ = 13 +/− = 5	Donor PBMCs incubated with recombinant pp65 or pool of overlapping peptides for CMVpp65. Cells labelled with IFN-γ capture reagent and warmed to reinitiate IFN secretion—magnetic beads	1 × 10^4 CD3+ cells/kg
Peggs et al. (2009)	30	10 pre-emptively 10 concurrent with antivirals 10 prophylactic	7/30 grade 1 4/30 grades 2–3	Prophylactic: 3/10 had a primary episode Pre-emptive: all needed antiviral drugs due to increasing viral titres	Sib = 17 MUD = 8 MMUD = 5	+/+ = 24 +/− = 6	T-cell lines generated from PBMCs with DCs pulsed with CMV cell lysate	1 × 10^5 cells/kg
Micklethwaite et al. (2007)	9	Prophylactic	3/9 (all had GvHD prior to ACT)	2 had CMV reactivation	MSD = 6 MUD = 1 MMRD = 2	+/+ = 6 +/− = 3	Donor PBMCs cocultured with DCs pulsed with HLA-A2 restricted nonapeptide NLV (derived from CMV-pp65 protein)	
Einsele et al. (2002)	8	Refractory to antiviral therapy	None	5/7 evaluable patients: viral DNA no longer detected	Sib = 2 MUD = 3 MMUD = 3	Seropositive donors	Donor PBMCs incubated for 10 days with CMV lysate	1 × 10^7 cells/m^2

(continued)

Table 8.1 (continued)

Study name	No. of patients	Indication	Rate of aGvHD	CMV outcome	Donor type	Donor/ recipient CMV status	Technique for production of CMV-specific CTLs	T-cell dose
Feuchtinger et al. (2010)	18	CMV disease or viraemia refractory to antiviral therapy	1/18	15/18 cases had clearance of CMV or a significant reduction of viral load	MUD = 3 Haplos =11 Cord = 2 MRD = 1 MMUD = 1	+/+ = 15 +/− = 1 −/+ = 2[a]	IFN-γ secretion—transfused on day of isolation	Mean dose: 21.3×10^3 CD3+/kg

PBMCs peripheral blood mononuclear cells, *Syn* syngeneic, *Haplos* haploidentical, *MUD* matched unrelated donor, *MRD* matched related donor, *MMRD* partially matched related donor, *Sib* sibling, + = CMV seropositive, − = CMV seronegative, *ACT* adoptive cellular therapy

[a]Third-party MMUD after cord-blood SCT

copies/ml, $P = 0.04$). Furthermore, in the CMV T-cell group, there was a decrease in the number of patients needing pharmacotherapy for CMV and also a decrease in the number of total treatment doses per patient. Although the study was non-randomised, it did demonstrate an acceptable safety profile of the therapy in comparison with those patients who received pharmacotherapy only.

8.3 Manufacturing Techniques to Directly Select CMV-Specific T Cells from Seropositive Donors

The practical clinical application of adoptive transfer of T-cell clones was hampered by the need for a prolonged in vitro expansion step, often requiring culture for up to 12 weeks, coupled with the associated financial expense. Advances in laboratory techniques to directly isolate antigen-specific T cells from the blood of seropositive donors have made a significant contribution to progress in the field of virus-specific adoptive cellular therapy. The two main techniques available are those based upon either HLA-multimer selection or the secretion of interferon gamma following peptide stimulation (Fig. 8.1).

An HLA multimer is composed of a number of HLA molecules which have been loaded with the antigenic peptide of interest, in this case a CMV peptide, and joined to a fluorophore or metal bead that can be detected by flow cytometry or selected magnetically (Ramirez and Olavarria 2013). The multimer binds to the T-cell

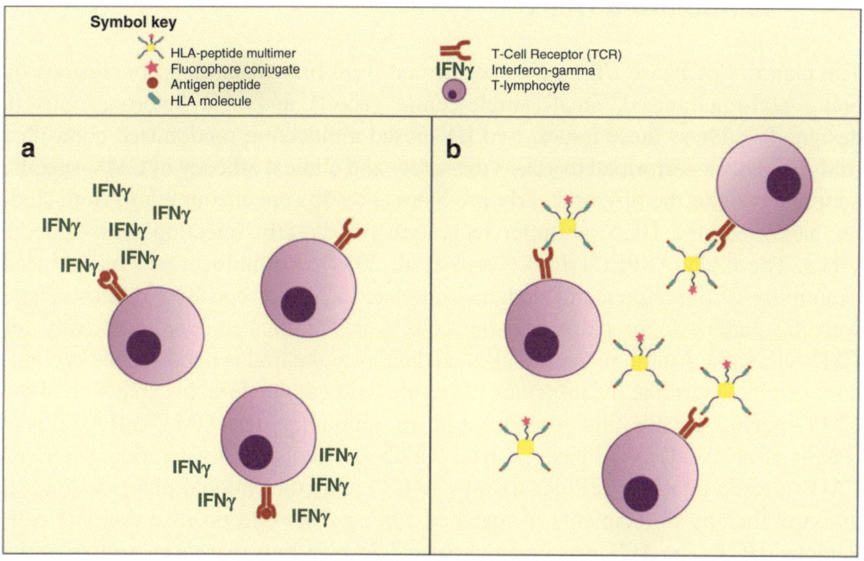

Fig. 8.1 Direct selection techniques for generating virus-specific T cells. (**a**) Gamma-capture technique based upon the secretion of interferon gamma following antigen stimulation. (**b**) The fluorophore-conjugated HLA-peptide multimer binds to T lymphocytes that are specific for the presenting viral peptide

receptor (TCR) of T cells that share a specificity for the antigenic peptide being presented. This allows for the detection and isolation of T cells which are specific for the relevant CMV peptide. The major limitation with this technique is that their use is restricted to those patients for whom there are viral peptides available for their HLA alleles and also that the product generated is limited to the class of HLA presentation, i.e. generally $CD8^+$ cells as generation of class II multimers is technically more challenging (Schmitt et al. 2011). Cobbold et al. (2005) used this technique to isolate CMV-specific $CD8^+$ T cells from seropositive donors. The cellular product was infused within 4 h to nine patients who had either had one episode of CMV reactivation or who had a persistent viraemia, and no prolonged ex vivo culture was required to obtain adequate numbers of cells. CMV viraemia levels reduced in all patients suggesting functionality of the CMV-specific CTLs.

The "gamma capture" technique involves the selection of T cells which release interferon gamma (IFN-γ) as a result of stimulation with a CMV peptide. The advantage of this technique is that it is applicable to all seropositive donors, irrespective of HLA type, thereby significantly widening applicability. The resultant product contains both $CD4^+$ and $CD8^+$ T cells. Zandvliet et al. (2010) reported the stimulation of donor PBMCs with a CMV-pp65 peptide pool, and the maximal IFN-γ production was seen at 4 h after stimulation. The technique has now been used successfully by a number of investigators (Peggs et al. 2011; Feuchtinger et al. 2010; Mackinnon et al. 2008).

8.4 Randomised Trials

The majority of Phase I/II studies performed were limited in their conclusions by being non-randomised, small single-centre reports and also heterogeneous in design. To address these issues, two UK-based multicentre randomised controlled trials have been performed to assess the safety and clinical efficacy of CMV-specific adoptive cellular therapy, and early provisional results are encouraging. Both studies have used the HLA-multimer technique for directly selecting virus-specific CTLs. The CMV-ASPECT trial (Chen et al. 2014) is a multicentre Phase II trial examining HCT recipients of matched unrelated CMV-seropositive donors. There were 52 patient-donor pairs, and the cells were administered pre-emptively for CMV viraemia. Although the full clinical data from the trial is pending, the preliminary results report that the infusions were safe with greater durable expansion of the CMV-specific T cells and reconstitution of immunity. The CMV-IMPACT trial (Peggs et al. 2014) is a Phase III trial which randomised between donor-derived CMV-specific adoptive cellular therapy (ACT) and conventional pharmacological antiviral therapy in recipients of matched sibling CMV-seropositive donor T cell-depleted HCT. The ACT was given at day 27/28 post-transplant irrespective of the CMV surveillance PCR results. There was no significant difference in the occurrence of GvHD or severe adverse events between the two groups. The preliminary analysis found that there were, however, fewer CMV reactivations in the ACT arm and a trend towards a decrease in the overall treatment duration.

8.5 Epstein-Barr Virus (EBV): Specific T Cells

Epstein-Barr virus (EBV), also known as human herpesvirus 4 (HHV-4), is a member of the human gamma-herpesvirus family and is highly prevalent in the community, with up to 90% of the adult population demonstrating evidence of previous infection. The primary infection may manifest clinically as infectious mononucleosis but may also be asymptomatic in immunocompetent individuals. Following the primary infection, the virus enters a phase of latency whereby it resides in B lymphocytes and the oropharyngeal lymphoid tissues and is kept quiescent by the host's EBV-specific cytotoxic T lymphocytes (Rickinson et al. 2014). In the post-transplant period, however, during which patients receive significant immunosuppressive therapy to minimise GvHD and prevent graft rejection or where immune reconstitution is delayed, EBV may reactivate from its latent phase and cause a rapid B-cell proliferation, resulting in post-transplant lymphoproliferative disease (PTLD). PTLD can manifest as fevers, lymphadenopathy, pharyngitis or extranodal involvement, including pulmonary complications, and symptoms which may mimic severe sepsis. Prompt diagnosis is required for rapid treatment as the doubling time of EBV has been estimated at 2–4 days (Styczynski et al. 2009; Carpenter et al. 2010) and the introduction of PCR surveillance has allowed for the early recognition of EBV reactivation. PTLD has been postulated to originate from donor-derived EBV-infected B lymphocytes in the majority of cases, usually occurring in the first 6–12 months post-transplant, and has an incidence of 0.5–17% in HCT recipients (Rasche et al. 2014; Rouce et al. 2014; Landgren et al. 2009; Gottschalk et al. 2005).

Current treatment strategies for PTLD are aimed at B-cell depletion and restoring the EBV-specific T-cell response. A reduction in immunosuppressants and the use of the monoclonal anti-CD20 antibody rituximab have improved the mortality post-PTLD, but, in those patients who fail to respond to this therapy, outcomes are poor (Styczynski et al. 2009). Papadopoulos et al. (1994) reported the use of unmanipulated donor lymphocyte infusions (DLIs) in five patients who developed PTLD post-T cell-depleted allogeneic HCT, and all patients achieved a complete pathological or clinical response within 30 days of receiving the infusion. There were, however, significant complications experienced including GvHD and also two deaths from pulmonary complications. This highlighted that unmanipulated DLIs contain alloreactive T cells as well as those that are EBV-specific, thereby increasing the risk of GvHD after infusion, and was followed by other reports of unmanipulated DLI causing severe GvHD when given as EBV-PTLD therapy (Heslop et al. 1994).

In view of the disadvantages associated with DLI therapy and the low levels of EBV-specific T cells contained in the product, research into T-cell therapy for EBV reactivation became focused on infusions of EBV-specific T cells. One of the largest studies for the use of EBV-specific T cells to prevent or treat EBV-PTLD was reported by Heslop et al. (2010) and examined 114 patients post-allogeneic HCT who had received the adoptive cellular therapy. The study was performed at three centres and had a median follow-up time of 10.5 years. The majority of the patients (101) received the cells as prophylaxis after being identified as high risk for

EBV-PTLD including 90 patients who received T cell-depleted transplants, and of these patients, none developed EBV-PTLD. Thirteen patients were treated for EBV-PTLD (either probable or biopsy proven), and 11/13 achieved a durable remission. Fifty-one patients had GvHD prior to the infusion, with 8/51 developing a recurrence of their GvHD post-infusion; however, no patient developed de novo GvHD. The estimated overall survival for all patients receiving EBV-specific T cells was 69% at 5 years and 67% at 10 years. Importantly, this study included 26 patients who had received infusions of donor-derived EBV-specific T cells which had been genetically marked to express the neo^R gene, allowing them to be tracked. Earlier studies of these genetically modified T cells had reported their persistence, their detection in the peripheral blood of patients which corresponds with a rise in the virus-specific activity and also their ability to elicit responses in patients with established EBV-PTLD (Rooney et al. 1995; Heslop et al. 1996; Rooney et al. 1998). In the study by Heslop et al. (2010), the genetically modified EBV-specific T cells showed persistence for up to 105 months post-infusion. This study confirmed the safety, durability and effectiveness of EBV-T cells.

Whereas the majority of published studies on EBV-T cells post-HCT focused mainly on patients receiving the therapy as prophylaxis, Doubrovina et al. (2012) reported a single-centre experience examining the fate of 49 patients who had biopsy-proven PTLD post-allogeneic HCT. The patients were treated primarily with either HLA-compatible DLI (30 patients) or EBV-specific T cells (19 patients). Durable remissions were reported in 73% of patients receiving DLI and 68% of those receiving EBV-CTLs. Whilst 17% of patients in the DLI group developed acute GvHD, which was reversible with therapy, none of the patients in the EBV-T-cell group developed GvHD. The investigators explored the reason for non-response in patients and identified that there was a lack of proliferation of the cells in vivo, and when examined in vitro, the cells were unable to lyse the donor-derived EBV-LCLs, suggesting that they failed to recognise the tumour antigens and thereby mount an effective immune response.

As these studies have shown, EBV-specific T-cell therapy is effective at restoring EBV-specific immunity post-transplant with an acceptable safety profile, which appears superior to the use of unmanipulated DLI therapy. Currently, however, this therapy is only available in the context of clinical trials due to the cost of manufacture with the associated need for specialist manufacturing techniques.

8.6 Multi-Virus-Specific T Cells

The success in generating efficacious virus-specific T-cell therapy for individual viruses is encouraging, but, on a practical level, the production of different single-virus-specific T cells for the infusion into the same patient would be costly and time-consuming and expose the patient to a variety of cellular products. In the period post-allogeneic HCT, recipients are susceptive to a multitude of viruses as a result of delayed immune reconstitution. Therefore, many research groups are now focusing their attentions on generating multi-virus-specific T cells from a single culture to allow for the infusion of a single product (Table 8.2). This was first shown to good effect by Leen et al. (2006) who succeeded in producing trivirus-specific T cells to the common viral pathogens, CMV, EBV and adenovirus. They generated EBV-LCLs from the donors and then genetically modified the EBV-transformed B-cell lines with a chimeric adenovirus vector integrating the CMV pp65 sequence (Ad5f35pp65). CTLs were generated in a two-step stimulation protocol, first with PBMCs transduced with the Ad5f35pp65 vector and then with EBV-LCL transduced with the same vector. This resulted in the generation of T cells specific for EBV, CMV and adenovirus antigens from a single culture. Of the 15 donor-derived $CD4^+$ and $CD8^+$ T-cell lines generated, 14 produced IFN-γ following stimulation with viral peptides from all three viruses, with the remaining cell line being bispecific for CMV and EBV but not responsive to adenovirus. They proceeded to test the T cells in 11 patients who had undergone a HCT. The T cells expanded post-infusion, with an associated reduction in viral levels and with no resultant GvHD at 3 months post-infusion. They demonstrated that the CMV-specific and EBV-specific T cells expanded within 4 weeks of infusion but that the adenovirus-specific cells only expanded in those patients who had a recent or active adenovirus infection. One of the main initial concerns with respect to generating multi-virus-specific T cells was that one of the immunodominant viral antigens may compete for presentation by antigen-presenting cells (APCs), thereby dominating the T-cell product. The trivirus T-cell product generated initially (Leen et al. 2006) was predominantly composed of CMV-specific T cells with a much smaller proportion of EBV- and adenovirus-specific T cells. Leen et al. attempted to address this question by removing the CMV component of the T cells, thereby eradicating the potential of competition from this antigen and generating a bispecific T-cell product for EBV and adenovirus (Leen et al. 2009). They studied the effect of these cells in 13 paediatric recipients of haploidentical and matched unrelated donor transplants. None of the patients developed de novo GvHD, and, when examining the patients' response, they identified that ten patients had a rise in EBV-specific T cells within 2 weeks of the infusion. In contrast, the only significant increase in the frequency of AdV-specific cells was seen in two patients who had an active AdV infection. Further analysis of the data identified that recipients of the T-cell product, who would usually be considered high risk for developing AdV infection, did not develop adenovirus infection, implying that the T-cell product may be providing a protective effect. Therefore, the peripheral blood from the recipients was examined both before and after the T-cell infusion, and the cells were expanded ex vivo. Adenovirus-specific T cells were detected but only from the post-infusion samples, suggesting that the cells were present but not being detected by conventional methods.

Following the generation of trivirus-specific T cells, the technique was further expanded to include more viruses. Papadopoulou et al. (2014) made a preparation of multi-virus T cells by stimulating PBMCs with overlapping libraries incorporating EBV, CMV, AdV, BK virus (BKV) and human herpesvirus 6 (HHV-6). They infused the product into 11 HCT recipients, 8 of whom already had established infection and 3 who received the cells as prophylaxis. Only one patient developed GvHD (stage II skin). The three patients receiving the product as prophylaxis all

Table 8.2 Reported studies of multi-virus-specific T cells

Study name	Number of patients	CTL-virus specificity	Rate of aGvHD	Outcome	Donor type	T-cell depletion	T-cell dose
Leen et al. (2009)	13	Adenovirus and EBV	No de novo GvHD post-CTL	*EBV*: 3 reactivations which resolved *AdV*: 11/13 had no AdV infection. 2/13 had active AdV at the time of infusion—both cleared the infection after CTL therapy	Haplo = 6 MUD = 7	13	$5 \times 10^6/m^2$ to $1.35 \times 10^8/m^2$
Leen et al. (2006)	11	CMV, EBV, AdV	None had GvHD at 3 months post-CTL	*CMV*: 3 reactivations which resolved *EBV*: 3 reactivation—2 cleared the infection. 1 developed PTLD but achieved remission without additional therapy *AdV*: 5 AdV positive before infusion—3/5 had reduction in AdV load post-CTLs	MRD = 4 MUD = 6 MMRD = 1	9/11	5×10^6 to 1×10^8 cells/m^2
Ma et al. (2015)	10	CMV, EBV, AdV, VZV	2 developed de novo GvHD (grades 2–3)	*VZV*: no reactivation *CMV*: 6 reactivated which resolved—no CMV disease *EBV*: no reactivation *AdV*: no infection	MSD	3/10	2×10^7 cells/m^2

Papadopoulou et al. (2014)	11	EBV, CMV, AdV, BKV, HHV-6 8 = already established viral infections 3 = prophylaxis	1 developed de novo GvHD post-CTL	Prophylaxis: all virus-free for >3 months *CMV*: 2 CR, 1 PR *EBV*: 5 CR *BKV*: 5 CR, 1 PR, 1 NR *AdV*: 1 CR *HHV-6*: 2 CR	MRD = 5 MUD = 3 MMUD = 2 Haplo = 1	Not specified	$5 \times 10^6/m^2$ to $2 \times 10^7/m^2$
Hanley et al. (2016, 2013)	34 PB-derived CTL 8 CB-derived CTL	CMV, EBV, AdV	None developed >grade 2 GvHD	*CMV*: 8/11 with viraemia cleared the infection *EBV*: 10/10 cleared viraemia *AdV*: 11/12 cleared viraemia	Not specified	Not specified	Median 5×10^7 cells/m^2

AdV adenovirus, *EBV* Epstein-Barr virus, *CMV* cytomegalovirus, *Haplo* haploidentical, *MUD* matched unrelated donor, *MRD* matched related donor, *MMRD* partially matched related donor, *MSD* matched sibling donor, *MMUD* partially matched unrelated donor, *PB* peripheral blood, *CB* cord blood, *aGvHD* acute graft-versus-host disease, *CR* complete response, *PR* partial response, *NR* no response, *PTLD* post-transplant lymphoproliferative disease

remained virus-free for more than 3 months, and, in the 8 patients who received the T cells as treatment (for 18 viral episodes), there was a response rate of 94% (15 complete response, 2 partial response). The spectrum of viruses included in the multi-virus-specific T cells (mVSTs) product has continued to be expanded, with reports of seven-virus-specific CTLs being generated, including against RSV and influenza (Gerdemann et al. 2012) and against VZV infection (Ma et al. 2015). The initial results, although encouraging, need to now be tested in larger, randomised studies.

8.7 Generation of Virus-Specific T Cells from Virus-Naïve Donors

Initially, the generation of donor-derived virus-specific T cells had a prerequisite that the donor should be seropositive for the relevant virus in order to successfully isolate virus-specific memory T cells. Inevitably, this restricted the widespread application of the product to a subgroup of transplant recipients and was not a viable treatment option for those patients with seronegative donors. Cord-blood transplants are often considered to be virus-naïve grafts, and the number of cord-blood transplants being performed has been increasing (Passweg et al. 2012). Therefore, the potential of producing virus-specific T cells from naïve donors was explored (Savoldo et al. 2002; Park et al. 2006; Jedema et al. 2011).

The process of generating virus-specific T cells from naïve donors was previously reported for EBV-specific CTLs. A comparison was made between generating EBV-T cells from EBV-seronegative adults and children (Savoldo et al. 2002). Two methods of generation of EBV-CTLs were adopted depending on the type of cell used as an APC. One method used EBV-LCLs as APCs, whereas the other method used dendritic cells (DCs) loaded with EBV antigen. They found that using EBV-LCLs as APCS effectively generated EBV-T cells from all seronegative adult donors but not from any of the seronegative children. The EBV antigen-loaded DCs expanded EBV-T cells in only a minority of the children indicating that different approaches may be needed depending on whether the donor is child or adult.

With the advent of multi-virus-specific T cells, Hanley et al. (2009) have explored the possibility of generating mVSTs from virus-naïve donors. Using cord blood, they developed a protocol to generate single cultures of T cells from cord blood by transducing EBV-LCLs with an Ad5f35CMVpp65 adenoviral vector, which recognised viral epitopes only after 2 weeks of expansion. They discovered that the recognition of adenovirus epitopes was the same for adult donor-derived T cells but that the pattern of CMV epitopes recognised appeared different to those recognised by adult donor-derived VSTs. Furthermore, they reported that the generation of CMV-specific T cells from cord blood did not depend upon the CMV serostatus of the mother.

The safety of multi-virus-specific T cells generated from naïve donors and used prophylactically has been reported in three consecutive cord-blood transplant patients (Hanley et al. 2015). The cells were generated from 20% of cord blood units where the remaining 80% were used as the transplanted graft. They reported no infusion-related toxicity or GvHD development post-infusion but confirmed the previous reports that the CMV-specific T cells generated from virus-naïve donors were specific for atypical epitopes for the CMV pp65 peptide (Hanley et al. 2009). The development of strategies to produce multi-virus-specific T cells from peripheral blood has also been explored. In a study where 34 patients were given peripheral blood-derived trivirus-specific T cells and 8 patients were given cord blood-derived CTLs, none of the patients developed GvHD greater than grade 2 (Hanley et al. 2013). Eleven patients had CMV reactivation detected prior to the infusion, and 8 of 11 became negative for the infection within 7 days of the infusion. All 10 of the patients with prior EBV reactivation and 11 of 12 patients with prior adenovirus infection cleared the virus infection after the cellular therapy.

The ability to generate virus-specific T-cell products also has an interesting application in those viruses where the donor will always be seronegative but for which the recipient may be seropositive, e.g. HIV, and there has been a recent report of HIV-specific T cells being generated from a HIV-naïve donor (Patel et al. 2016).

8.8 Virus-Specific T Cells from Third-Party Donors ("Off the Shelf")

The majority of virus-specific T-cell therapy research has been performed using the recipient's HCT donor as the source of the T cells. This is a logical approach as the donor has already been identified as the best available HLA-matched source, and it also serves to minimise the exposure of the recipient to allogeneic products. Returning to the original donor for additional cells is not an option that is available for all allogeneic HCT recipients and therefore limits the applicability of virus-specific T-cell therapy, particularly for those patients who have received a cord-blood transplant and for those patients whose donors are seronegative for specific viruses. Furthermore, the development of virus reactivation post-transplant frequently requires prompt therapy to prevent the development of virus-associated disease, and the time delay involved with contacting a donor and acquiring a cellular product can render the therapy impracticable for usage in routine clinical practice. Therefore, a number of research groups have developed banks of third-party donations of cellular products to enable the therapy to be picked "off the shelf" when it is required, thereby expediting the delivery of the product and also enabling those recipients without an available donor to receive therapy. Predictably, concerns have been raised regarding the potential degree of HLA mismatch which is acceptable for the donation, the prospect of a lack of persistence of the product due to allorejection by the host and the possibility for a subsequent induction or exacerbation of GvHD.

The majority of research has focused on EBV-specific T cells and the development of third-party banks of cells. Research initially focused on solid organ transplant recipients, whose donors may be deceased and in whom the stem cell compartment has not been rendered donor in origin, although the early studies did include small numbers of HCT recipients. Haque et al. (2002) developed a bank of cryopreserved EBV-specific T cells from the peripheral blood of healthy donors. They initially performed a Phase I/II trial in eight patients with refractory PTLD (seven patients were solid organ recipients and one received a HCT). They used the best available HLA-matched products in the bank, and the patients were given between one and six infusions. Of the five patients who completed the full therapy, three had a complete response, and two had no response. There were no reports of GvHD and no infusion-related adverse events. Following on from this, they performed a multicentre Phase II clinical trial (Haque et al. 2007) with 33 patients who had a diagnosis of biopsy-proven PTLD and had failed conventional therapy including 2 HCT recipients. The response rate of the whole cohort was 64% at 5 weeks and 52% at 6 months, and both of the HCT recipients achieved a complete response. This was similar to Barker et al. (2010) who reported two cases of patients diagnosed with EBV-PTLD post-allogeneic cord-blood transplantation being given partially HLA-matched EBV-T cells from third-party donors. Both of the patients achieved a CR which was maintained for at least 156 months.

The largest reported study so far using third-party virus-specific T cells for HCT recipients administered 18 virus-specific cell lines to 50 patients with refractory disease due to viral infections (Leen et al. 2013). The majority of patients (Schmitt et al. 2011) received them for CMV infection with 18 patients receiving adenovirus-specific T cells and 9 receiving EBV-specific T cells for refractory EBV-PTLD. At 6 weeks post-infusion, there was a 74% response rate (CR/PR) across all patients. With respect to the concerns regarding GvHD, only two patients developed de novo GvHD post-infusion, and this was grade 1 in both cases. The results above suggest that using virus-specific T cells from best available HLA-matched third-party donors may be safe and can induce durable remissions.

8.9 Expert Opinion

Significant research progress has been made in the field of virus-specific adoptive cellular therapy over the past two decades, resulting in safe and clinically effective products for a range of viruses (Table 8.3). New technological advances have allowed for the direct selection of virus-specific cells from seropositive donors, and this has eradicated the need for prolonged ex vivo expansion steps in the generation of single-virus-specific T cells, thereby accelerating the manufacturing process. The costs of generating virus-specific T cells, coupled with the regulations governing production of cellular products, have limited the widespread application of these products, and current availability is predominantly restricted to large specialist centres in the context of clinical trials. The advances in generating multi-virus-specific T-cell products, and the expansion of potential donor sources, have succeeded in broadening the clinical application to a wider range of recipients. Despite the progress made, further multicentre, randomised controlled trials are needed to compare these products with the available pharmacological therapies.

Table 8.3 Summary of key points

Key points
• Quantitative and qualitative deficiency in virus-reactive T cells post-allogeneic HCT renders the recipient susceptible to severe viral infections
• Virus-specific T cells have lower rates of inducible GvHD than unmanipulated CD3+ donor lymphocyte infusions (DLIs)
• Single-virus specific T-cell infusions for CMV and EBV are safe and efficient at restoring viral immunity in the post-transplant period
• Direct selection techniques, for example, gamma capture and the use of HLA-peptide multimers, have eradicated the need for prolonged ex vivo culture and accelerated the production process
• The generation of multi-virus-specific T cells from a single culture is possible and shows clinical efficacy in small studies
• The ability to generate cellular products from virus-naïve donors and third-party donors has resulted in an expansion of the availability of the product
• Phase III randomised controlled trials against current pharmacological therapies need to be performed
• Future directions of research include the genetic modification of virus-specific T cells to render them resistant to immunosuppressive therapies

8.10 Future Directions

Many of the clinical studies investigating virus-specific T cells have excluded patients who have concurrent GvHD requiring steroid therapy due to concerns regarding the survival of the cellular product in the presence of glucocorticoids. This subgroup of patients, however, are often at a higher risk of virus reactivation, and, thus far, they have been unable to benefit from the advances in virus-specific cellular therapy. Attempts have been made to address this issue using gene-editing strategies. Genetic engineering of CMV-specific T lymphocytes by inactivating the glucocorticoid receptor gene using TALEN (transcription activator-like effector nuclease) technology resulted in the production of steroid-resistant cells in preclinical models paving the way for clinical application (Menger et al. 2015). With respect to EBV-specific T cells, there have also been previous reports of the generation of EBV-specific CTLs resistant to the calcineurin inhibitor tacrolimus by transduction with a calcineurin mutant retroviral vector (Ricciardelli et al. 2013) and also EBV-specific T cells resistant to both tacrolimus and ciclosporin A (Brewin et al. 2009). The progress in gene therapy has also enabled Phase I clinical studies which are currently in progress to investigate the safety and toxicity of CMV TCR-transduced donor-derived T cells post-HCT (UK CRN 12518). Future directions in research into T cells for infections should be focused on optimising manufacturing techniques and examining the efficacy of multi-virus-specific T cells in larger, randomised cohorts of patients.

References

Barker JN, Doubrovina E, Sauter C, Jaroscak JJ, Perales MA, Doubrovin M et al (2010) Successful treatment of EBV-associated posttransplantation lymphoma after cord blood transplantation using third-party EBV-specific cytotoxic T lymphocytes. Blood 116(23):5045–5049

Bate SL, Dollard SC, Cannon MJ (2010) Cytomegalovirus seroprevalence in the United States: the national health and nutrition examination surveys, 1988–2004. Clin Infect Dis 50(11):1439–1447

Blyth E, Clancy L, Simms R, Ma CK, Burgess J, Deo S et al (2013) Donor-derived CMV-specific T cells reduce the requirement for CMV-directed pharmacotherapy after allogeneic stem cell transplantation. Blood 121(18):3745–3758

Boeckh M, Ljungman P (2009) How we treat cytomegalovirus in hematopoietic cell transplant recipients. Blood 113(23):5711–5719

Brewin J, Mancao C, Straathof K, Karlsson H, Samarasinghe S, Amrolia PJ et al (2009) Generation of EBV-specific cytotoxic T cells that are resistant to calcineurin inhibitors for the treatment of posttransplantation lymphoproliferative disease. Blood 114(23):4792–4803

Carpenter B, Haque T, Dimopoulou M, Atkinson C, Roughton M, Grace S et al (2010) Incidence and dynamics of Epstein-Barr virus reactivation after alemtuzumab-based conditioning for allogeneic hematopoietic stem-cell transplantation. Transplantation 90(5):564–570

Chen F, Peniket A, Tholouli E, Bloor A, Chakraverty R, Marks D et al (2014) CMV-specific T-cell therapy improves immune reconstitution following unrelated donor HCT: results of a randomized controlled trial. Biol Blood Marrow Transplant 20(2):S49

Cobbold M, Khan N, Pourgheysari B, Tauro S, McDonald D, Osman H et al (2005) Adoptive transfer of cytomegalovirus-specific CTL to stem cell transplant patients after selection by HLA-peptide tetramers. J Exp Med 202(3):379–386

Doubrovina E, Oflaz-Sozmen B, Prockop SE, Kernan NA, Abramson S, Teruya-Feldstein J et al (2012) Adoptive immunotherapy with unselected or EBV-specific T cells for biopsy-proven EBV+ lymphomas after allogeneic hematopoietic cell transplantation. Blood 119(11):2644–2656

Einsele H, Roosnek E, Rufer N, Sinzger C, Riegler S, Loffler J et al (2002) Infusion of cytomegalovirus (CMV)-specific T cells for the treatment of CMV infection not responding to antiviral chemotherapy. Blood 99(11):3916–3922

Erard V, Guthrie KA, Seo S, Smith J, Huang M, Chien J et al (2015) Reduced mortality of cytomegalovirus pneumonia after hematopoietic cell transplantation due to antiviral therapy and changes in transplantation practices. Clin Infect Dis 61(1):31–39

Feuchtinger T, Opherk K, Bethge WA, Topp MS, Schuster FR, Weissinger EM et al (2010) Adoptive transfer of pp65-specific T cells for the treatment of chemorefractory cytomegalovirus disease or reactivation after haploidentical and matched unrelated stem cell transplantation. Blood 116(20):4360–4367

Gerdemann U, Keirnan JM, Katari UL, Yanagisawa R, Christin AS, Huye LE et al (2012) Rapidly generated multivirus-specific cytotoxic T lymphocytes for the prophylaxis and treatment of viral infections. Mol Ther 20(8):1622–1632

Gottschalk S, Rooney CM, Heslop HE (2005) Post-transplant lymphoproliferative disorders. Annu Rev Med 56:29–44

Hanley PJ, Bollard CM (2014) Controlling cytomegalovirus: helping the immune system take the lead. Viruses 6(6):2242–2258

Hanley PJ, Cruz CR, Savoldo B, Leen AM, Stanojevic M, Khalil M et al (2009) Functionally active virus-specific T cells that target CMV, adenovirus, and EBV can be expanded from naive T-cell populations in cord blood and will target a range of viral epitopes. Blood 114(9):1958–1967

Hanley PJ, Leen A, Gee AP, Leung K, Martinez C, Krance RA et al (2013) Multi-virus-specific T-cell therapy for patients after hematopoietic stem cell and cord blood transplantation. Blood 122(21):140

Hanley PJ, Melenhorst JJ, Nikiforow S, Scheinberg P, Blaney JW, Demmler-Harrison G et al (2015) CMV-specific T cells generated from naive T cells recognize atypical epitopes and may be protective in vivo. Sci Transl Med 7(285):285ra63

Haque T, Wilkie GM, Taylor C, Amlot PL, Murad P, Iley A et al (2002) Treatment of Epstein-Barr-virus-positive post-transplantation lymphoproliferative disease with partly HLA-matched allogeneic cytotoxic T cells. Lancet 360(9331):436–442

Haque T, Wilkie GM, Jones MM, Higgins CD, Urquhart G, Wingate P et al (2007) Allogeneic cytotoxic T-cell therapy for EBV-positive posttransplantation lymphoproliferative disease: results of a phase 2 multicenter clinical trial. Blood 110(4):1123–1131

Heslop HE, Brenner MK, Rooney CM (1994) Donor T cells to treat EBV-associated lymphoma. N Engl J Med 331(10):679–680

Heslop HE, Ng CY, Li C, Smith CA, Loftin SK, Krance RA et al (1996) Long-term restoration of immunity against Epstein-Barr virus infection by adoptive transfer of gene-modified virus-specific T lymphocytes. Nat Med 2(5):551–555

Heslop HE, Slobod KS, Pule MA, Hale GA, Rousseau A, Smith CA et al (2010) Long-term outcome of EBV-specific T-cell infusions to prevent or treat EBV-related lymphoproliferative disease in transplant recipients. Blood 115(5):925–935

Jedema I, van de Meent M, Pots J, Kester MG, van der Beek MT, Falkenburg JH (2011) Successful generation of primary virus-specific and anti-tumor T-cell responses from the naive donor T-cell repertoire is determined by the balance between antigen-specific precursor T cells and regulatory T cells. Haematologica 96(8):1204–1212

Landgren O, Gilbert ES, Rizzo JD, Socie G, Banks PM, Sobocinski KA et al (2009) Risk factors for lymphoproliferative disorders after allogeneic hematopoietic cell transplantation. Blood 113(20):4992–5001

Leen AM, Myers GD, Sili U, Huls MH, Weiss H, Leung KS et al (2006) Monoculture-derived T lymphocytes specific for multiple viruses expand and produce clinically relevant effects in immunocompromised individuals. Nat Med 12(10):1160–1166

Leen AM, Christin A, Myers GD, Liu H, Cruz CR, Hanley PJ et al (2009) Cytotoxic T lymphocyte therapy with donor T cells prevents and treats adenovirus and Epstein-Barr virus infections after haploidentical and matched unrelated stem cell transplantation. Blood 114(19):4283–4292

Leen AM, Bollard CM, Mendizabal AM, Shpall EJ, Szabolcs P, Antin JH et al (2013) Multicenter study of banked third-party virus-specific T cells to treat severe viral infections after hematopoietic stem cell transplantation. Blood 121(26):5113–5123

Ma CK, Blyth E, Clancy L, Simms R, Burgess J, Brown R et al (2015) Addition of varicella zoster virus-specific T cells to cytomegalovirus, Epstein-Barr virus and adenovirus tri-specific T cells as adoptive immunotherapy in patients undergoing allogeneic hematopoietic stem cell transplantation. Cytotherapy 17(10):1406–1420

Mackinnon S, Thomson K, Verfuerth S, Peggs K, Lowdell M (2008) Adoptive cellular therapy for cytomegalovirus infection following allogeneic stem cell transplantation using virus-specific T cells. Blood Cells Mol Dis 40(1):63–67

Menger L, Gouble A, Marzolini MA, Pachnio A, Bergerhoff K, Henry JY et al (2015) TALEN-mediated genetic inactivation of the glucocorticoid receptor in cytomegalovirus-specific T cells. Blood 126(26):2781–2789

Micklethwaite K, Hansen A, Foster A, Snape E, Antonenas V, Sartor M et al (2007) Ex vivo expansion and prophylactic infusion of CMV-pp65 peptide-specific cytotoxic T-lymphocytes following allogeneic hematopoietic stem cell transplantation. Biol Blood Marrow Transplant 13(6):707–714

Nichols WG, Corey L, Gooley T, Davis C, Boeckh M (2002) High risk of death due to bacterial and fungal infection among cytomegalovirus (CMV)-seronegative recipients of stem cell transplants from seropositive donors: evidence for indirect effects of primary CMV infection. J Infect Dis 185(3):273–282

Nikiforow S, Alyea EP (2014) Maximizing GVL in allogeneic transplantation: role of donor lymphocyte infusions. Hematology 2014(1):570–575

Papadopoulos EB, Ladanyi M, Emanuel D, Mackinnon S, Boulad F, Carabasi MH et al (1994) Infusions of donor leukocytes to treat Epstein-Barr virus-associated lymphoproliferative disorders after allogeneic bone marrow transplantation. N Engl J Med 330(17):1185–1191

Papadopoulou A, Gerdemann U, Katari UL, Tzannou I, Liu H, Martinez C et al (2014) Activity of broad-spectrum T cells as treatment for AdV, EBV, CMV, BKV, and HHV6 infections after HCT. Sci Transl Med 6(242):242ra83

Park KD, Marti L, Kurtzberg J, Szabolcs P (2006) In vitro priming and expansion of cytomegalovirus-specific Th1 and Tc1 T cells from naive cord blood lymphocytes. Blood 108(5):1770–1773

Passweg JR, Baldomero H, Gratwohl A, Bregni M, Cesaro S, Dreger P et al (2012) The EBMT activity survey: 1990–2010. Bone Marrow Transplant 47(7):906–923

Patel S, Lam S, Cruz CR, Wright K, Cochran C, Ambinder RF et al (2016) Functionally active HIV-specific T cells that target gag and Nef can be expanded from virus-naive donors and target a range of viral epitopes: implications for a cure strategy after allogeneic hematopoietic stem cell transplantation. Biol Blood Marrow Transplant 22(3):536–541

Peggs KS (2009) Adoptive T cell immunotherapy for cytomegalovirus. Expert Opin Biol Ther 9(6):725–736

Peggs KS, Verfuerth S, Pizzey A, Khan N, Guiver M, Moss PA et al (2003) Adoptive cellular therapy for early cytomegalovirus infection after allogeneic stem-cell transplantation with virus-specific T-cell lines. Lancet 362(9393):1375–1377

Peggs KS, Verfuerth S, Pizzey A, Chow SL, Thomson K, Mackinnon S (2009) Cytomegalovirus-specific T cell immunotherapy promotes restoration of durable functional antiviral immunity following allogeneic stem cell transplantation. Clin Infect Dis 49(12):1851–1860

Peggs KS, Thomson K, Samuel E, Dyer G, Armoogum J, Chakraverty R et al (2011) Directly selected cytomegalovirus-reactive donor T cells confer rapid and safe systemic reconstitution of virus-specific immunity following stem cell transplantation. Clin Infect Dis 52(1):49–57

Peggs KS, Tholouli E, Chakraverty R, Nikolousis E, Bloor A, Devereux S et al (2014) CMV~IMPACT: results of a randomized controlled trial of Immuno-prophylactic adoptive cellular therapy following sibling donor allogeneic HCT. Blood 124(21):1109

Perruccio K, Tosti A, Burchielli E, Topini F, Ruggeri L, Carotti A et al (2005) Transferring functional immune responses to pathogens after haploidentical hematopoietic transplantation. Blood 106(13):4397–4406

Ramirez N, Olavarria E (2013) Viral-specific adoptive immunotherapy after allo-SCT: the role of multimer-based selection strategies. Bone Marrow Transplant 48(10):1265–1270

Rasche L, Kapp M, Einsele H, Mielke S (2014) EBV-induced post transplant lymphoproliferative disorders: a persisting challenge in allogeneic hematopoetic SCT. Bone Marrow Transplant 49(2):163–167

Reusser P, Riddell SR, Meyers JD, Greenberg PD (1991) Cytotoxic T-lymphocyte response to cytomegalovirus after human allogeneic bone marrow transplantation: pattern of recovery and correlation with cytomegalovirus infection and disease. Blood 78(5):1373–1380

Ricciardelli I, Brewin J, Lugthart G, Albon SJ, Pule M, Amrolia PJ (2013) Rapid generation of EBV-specific cytotoxic T lymphocytes resistant to calcineurin inhibitors for adoptive immunotherapy. Am J Transplant 13(12):3244–3252

Rickinson AB, Long HM, Palendira U, Munz C, Hislop AD (2014) Cellular immune controls over Epstein-Barr virus infection: new lessons from the clinic and the laboratory. Trends Immunol 35(4):159–169

Riddell SR, Watanabe KS, Goodrich JM, Li CR, Agha ME, Greenberg PD (1992) Restoration of viral immunity in immunodeficient humans by the adoptive transfer of T cell clones. Science 257(5067):238–241

Rooney CM, Smith CA, Ng CY, Loftin S, Li C, Krance RA et al (1995) Use of gene-modified virus-specific T lymphocytes to control Epstein-Barr-virus-related lymphoproliferation. Lancet 345(8941):9–13

Rooney CM, Smith CA, Ng CY, Loftin SK, Sixbey JW, Gan Y et al (1998) Infusion of cytotoxic T cells for the prevention and treatment of Epstein-Barr virus-induced lymphoma in allogeneic transplant recipients. Blood 92(5):1549–1555

Rouce RH, Louis CU, Heslop HE (2014) Epstein-Barr virus lymphoproliferative disease after hematopoietic stem cell transplant. Curr Opin Hematol 21(6):476–481
Savoldo B, Cubbage ML, Durett AG, Goss J, Huls MH, Liu Z et al (2002) Generation of EBV-specific CD4^{+} cytotoxic T cells from virus naive individuals. J Immunol 168(2):909–918
Schmitt A, Tonn T, Busch DH, Grigoleit GU, Einsele H, Odendahl M et al (2011) Adoptive transfer and selective reconstitution of streptamer-selected cytomegalovirus-specific CD8^{+} T cells leads to virus clearance in patients after allogeneic peripheral blood stem cell transplantation. Transfusion 51(3):591–599
Staras SA, Dollard SC, Radford KW, Flanders WD, Pass RF, Cannon MJ (2006) Seroprevalence of cytomegalovirus infection in the United States, 1988–1994. Clin Infect Dis 43(9):1143–1151
Styczynski J, Einsele H, Gil L, Ljungman P (2009) Outcome of treatment of Epstein-Barr virus-related post-transplant lymphoproliferative disorder in hematopoietic stem cell recipients: a comprehensive review of reported cases. Transpl Infect Dis 11(5):383–392
Tomblyn M, Lazarus HM (2008) Donor lymphocyte infusions: the long and winding road: how should it be traveled? Bone Marrow Transplant 42(9):569–579
Walter EA, Greenberg PD, Gilbert MJ, Finch RJ, Watanabe KS, Thomas ED et al (1995) Reconstitution of cellular immunity against cytomegalovirus in recipients of allogeneic bone marrow by transfer of T-cell clones from the donor. N Engl J Med 333(16):1038–1044
Zandvliet ML, van Liempt E, Jedema I, Veltrop-Duits LA, Willemze R, Guchelaar HJ et al (2010) Co-ordinated isolation of CD8(+) and CD4(+) T cells recognizing a broad repertoire of cytomegalovirus pp65 and IE1 epitopes for highly specific adoptive immunotherapy. Cytotherapy 12(7):933–944
Zhang LJ, Hanff P, Rutherford C, Churchill WH, Crumpacker CS (1995) Detection of human cytomegalovirus DNA, RNA, and antibody in normal donor blood. J Infect Dis 171(4):1002–1006

Regulatory T Cells: Broadening Applicability

9

Franziska Maria Uhl and Robert Zeiser

9.1 Introduction

Since their discovery in 1995 (Sakaguchi et al. 1995), regulatory T cells (T_{reg}) have been established as an anti-inflammatory T cell population which attenuates and modulates immune responses on multiple levels including initiation, progression, and termination (Campbell and Koch 2011). Over the past decades intensive research on this new T cell subtype led to deeper understanding of the intrinsic mechanisms of the immune system to contain and control inflammatory reactions. Graft-versus-host disease (GvHD) developing after allogeneic hematopoietic cell transplantation (allo-HCT) belongs to a variety of diseases, in which the immune system runs amok and attacks the own body in an autoreactive manner (Ferrara et al. 2009). As soon as the immense potential of T_{reg} to downregulate excessive autoimmune responses became evident, multiple translational approaches have been pursued in order to unravel the suppressive capability of T_{reg} in GvHD and be able to control or even prevent this fatal complication in the clinical setting. Ultimately, researchers and clinicians want to find a way to establish long-lasting tolerance within the graft without diminishing the beneficial graft-versus-tumor/graft-versus-leukemia (GvT/GvL) effect (Schneidawind et al. 2013).

The following chapter will give an overview of T_{reg} characterization and functional abilities in order to explain thereafter their diverse influence in the pathogenesis of GvHD which is mainly studied in preclinical models and conclude with a review over completed and current clinical trials.

F. M. Uhl · R. Zeiser (✉)
Department of Hematology and Oncology, Albert Ludwig University Freiburg, Freiburg, Germany
e-mail: franziska.uhl@uniklinik-freiburg.de; robert.zeiser@uniklinik-freiburg.de

M.-A. Perales et al. (eds.), *Cell and Gene Therapies*, Advances and Controversies in Hematopoietic Transplantation and Cell Therapy, https://doi.org/10.1007/978-3-319-54368-0_9

9.2 Characterization of T_{reg}

In 1995, Sakaguchi and colleagues observed a population of cluster of differentiation 4 positive ($CD4^+$) T cells which even in homeostatic conditions expressed high levels of CD25, the interleukin-2 receptor (IL-2R) α-chain (Sakaguchi et al. 1995). A further characterization by depletion experiments revealed their suppressive function to prevent autoimmune symptoms. Two decades later, this suppressive T cell population became known as regulatory T cells (T_{reg}). The cells are characterized by the expression of the transcription factor Forkhead-Box-Protein P3 (FoxP3), which is not only important for the development yet also for continued suppressive functionality of T_{reg} (Fontenot et al. 2005). Mutations within the FoxP3 locus lead to severe autoimmunity, and the genetic dysfunction of the transcription factor is associated with the fatal IPEX (immunodysregulation polyendocrinopathy enteropathy X-linked) syndrome (Bennett et al. 2001; Brunkow et al. 2001; Wildin et al. 2001). Furthermore, they strongly express the high-affinity IL-2R α-chain which developed to be a well-established T_{reg} marker indicating the importance of IL-2. Indeed, this cytokine is essential for T_{reg} homeostasis, survival, and function (Malek 2008; Setoguchi et al. 2005) also shown by the phenotype of CD25 deficiency in human disease (Sharfe et al. 1997). Naturally occurring T_{reg} (nT_{reg}) undergo the same developmental path like conventional T cells (T_{con}) migrating from the bone marrow into the thymus where the lineage commitment occurs. nT_{reg} recognize self-antigens but are not undergoing negative selection. Instead they upregulate FoxP3 and form a suppressive T cell population guarding the lymphatics and tissues from excessive immune responses (Sakaguchi et al. 2006). Nevertheless, $CD4^+$ naïve T cells are able to develop to so-called induced T_{reg} (iT_{reg}) in the periphery when they are activated in a suppressive environment with the presence of transforming growth factor β (TGF-β) and IL-2 (Fantini et al. 2004; Bluestone and Abbas 2003). iT_{reg} can also be developed in vitro by T cell receptor (TCR) stimulation together with TGF-β and IL-2 which leaves them as an attractive tool in clinical use to suppress unwanted immune responses (Fantini et al. 2004; Chen et al. 2003). Additionally, T_{reg} can be divided depending on their location and homeostatic signaling requirements into two subsets, central and effector T_{reg} (Smigiel et al. 2014).

Moreover, besides the classic $CD4^+$ T_{reg}, also the $CD8^+$ counterpart which proves to partake in immune modulation of GvHD (Hahn et al. 2005; Beres et al. 2012) is characterized as well as several subpopulations of T_{reg} such as Tr1 (Roncarolo et al. 2014) or Th3 (Weiner 2001) cells. Recent studies suggest that the initial bias of an immune response shapes the developing T_{reg} which are armed with the proper features such as homing receptors to suppress Th1-, Th2-, or Th17-specific immune reactions (Koch et al. 2009; Zheng et al. 2009; Chaudhry et al. 2009). Yet, a recent study could show that this represents no stable commitment to one lineage but rather a dynamic process in order to maintain homeostatic conditions (Yu et al. 2015).

In order to fulfil their function in suppression of excessive immune responses or aid in the contraction phase after elimination of an infection, T_{reg} have to be able to enter various tissues including lymphoid and nonlymphoid tissues. Highly functional T_{reg} are characterized by expression of CD62L, a lymph node homing molecule which enables them to reach the secondary lymphoid organs where the T cell priming takes place (Venturi et al. 2007). Tissue-specific homing receptors such as C-C chemokine receptor type 5 (CCR5) (Yurchenko et al. 2006), CCR8 (Soler et al. 2006), or CCR9 (Guo et al. 2008) lead the way to the target organs since they are specific for the location of inflammation which needs to be suppressed and are imprinted on the T_{reg} during their activation.

The specific mechanisms in which T_{reg} suppress immune responses are versatile and will be discussed further on with a focus on the suppression of acute GvHD.

9.3 Immunmodulation by T_{reg} in Preclinical Models of GvHD

A study from 2007 could prove that the progressive loss of T_{reg} in the course of GvHD leads to continued disease pathology and conversion of acute to chronic GvHD (Chen et al. 2007). Early T_{reg} depletion studies during allo-HCT indicated an essential role of these cells for tolerance to alloantigen and a highly deteriorated GvHD when T_{reg} were lost (Taylor et al. 2001). Sawamukai et al. further investigated the donor T_{reg} composition and found that nT_{reg} as well as iT_{reg} and both T cell subsets, $CD8^+$ and $CD4^+$ T_{reg}, partake in the protection from GvHD (Sawamukai et al. 2012). Nevertheless, not only donor T_{reg} contained in the graft attenuate alloimmune responses, but also recipient-type T_{reg} which survive the conditioning regimen were able to dampen disease development (Anderson et al. 2004; Bayer et al. 2009).

Based on the finding that donor T_{reg} play a major role in the regulation of alloimmunity, in the following years, several murine adoptive transfer studies were performed in parallel in order to fathom the possibility of improving GvHD by cellular therapy (Cohen et al. 2002; Hoffmann et al. 2002; Taylor et al. 2002; Edinger et al. 2003; Jones et al. 2003; Trenado et al. 2003).

By adding T_{reg} to the transplant, either freshly isolated from a donor (Hoffmann et al. 2002) or expanded ex vivo before transplantation (Taylor et al. 2002), the development of acute GvHD could be prevented. In addition, Jones et al. proved the efficacy of T_{reg} co-transplantation also in a minor mismatch model since in the clinical setting major mismatch transplantations are virtually never performed any more (Jones et al. 2003). Furthermore, first approaches were conducted with the selection and expansion of allo-specific T_{reg} by coculture with recipient antigen-presenting cells (APCs) (Trenado et al. 2003). Despite the unsatisfactory results compared to unspecific T_{reg}, this approach is further evaluated in order to generate T_{reg} specific against major and minor histocompatibility antigens without diminishing the GvL effect (Veerapathran et al. 2011).

Studying the kinetics of allogeneic T cell activation, expansion, and effector phase, T_{reg} were proven to be essential in the early phases after bone marrow transplantation (BMT) in order to efficiently suppress T cell expansion and GvHD development (Edinger et al. 2003). Transplantation of T_{reg} at later time points severely diminished their efficacy to prevent GvHD (Nguyen et al. 2007). Moreover, the transplantation of T_{reg} prior to T_{con} allowed for a transfer of smaller numbers since T_{reg} strongly expand after BMT in vivo. T_{reg} only represent 5–10% of all peripheral

$CD4^+$ T cells which leaves isolation of large numbers of this cell subset challenging (Sakaguchi et al. 2006). One way to increase the number of transplantable cells is ex vivo expansion with a classic protocol of IL-2 administration together with CD3/CD28 stimulation (Taylor et al. 2002; Hoffmann et al. 2004; Earle et al. 2005). Nevertheless, the contamination of the starting cell pool with T_{con} has to be kept in mind since it could lead to an unpreferential expansion of effector T cells (Battaglia et al. 2005).

Another possibility to overcome low T_{reg} numbers is the in vitro induction and expansion of iT_{reg} by generation from T_{con} as mentioned above. Initial studies demonstrated a serious problem emerging when using in vitro generated T_{reg} (Fantini et al. 2004; Beres et al. 2011). The T_{reg} quickly lost FoxP3 expression and adopted an inflammatory T cell phenotype failing to prevent GvHD. FoxP3 expression is epigenetically controlled by hypomethylation of a conserved region in the *foxp3* promoter. In contrast to nT_{reg}, iT_{reg} remain only partially demethylated leading to a progressive loss of FoxP3 expression upon restimulation and absence of suppressive TGF-β (Floess et al. 2007). Novel approaches including hypomethylating agents such as decitabine in the protocol show promising results concerning a sustained FoxP3 expression (Choi et al. 2010).

Nevertheless, clinical approaches which include in vitro handling of human cells always require elaborate cell culture techniques to ensure safety which leaves them at substantial costs. An alternative is provided by studies attempting the in vivo expansion of nT_{reg}. Blockade of the IL-6 signaling pathway increased T_{reg} frequency with simultaneous reduction of effector T cells in a murine allo-HCT model (Chen et al. 2009). Furthermore, studies with CD28 antibody (Kitazawa et al. 2009) as well as CD1d ligand (Duramad et al. 2011) show promising results for the in vivo expansion of T_{reg} and the resulting attenuation of GvHD in preclinical models which yields hope for possible implementation in the clinic. A recent publication shows that administration of an anti-CD45RB monoclonal antibody resulted in increased T_{reg}-APC interaction which led to enhanced T_{reg} proliferation (Camirand et al. 2014).

Several groups reported that rapamycin in combination with IL-2 application was efficient in the expansion of T cells with a regulatory phenotype (Shin et al. 2011; Zhang et al. 2013) which led to extensive research investigating the practical range and the mechanism behind these observations. Since rapamycin exclusively expands T_{reg} by simultaneously inhibiting other T cell subsets (Battaglia et al. 2005, 2006; Tresoldi et al. 2011), the drug represents a powerful tool to expand T_{reg} for further use for adoptive transfer (Battaglia et al. 2012). In a murine model of acute GvHD, the transplantation of T_{reg} and rapamycin treatment showed a synergistic effect by improving disease outcome and preserving long-term tolerance by highly active T_{reg} (Zeiser et al. 2008). Furthermore, the authors could show that, in response to IL-2 and alloantigen stimulation, T_{reg} upregulated signal transducer and activator of transcription 5 (STAT5) by simultaneous high expression of phosphatase and tensin homolog (PTEN), a negative regulator of the phosphatidylinositol-3-kinase/protein kinase B/mammalian target of rapamycin (PI3K/Akt/mTOR) pathway. In order to understand the mechanism behind the differential responses of T_{reg} and T_{con} to rapamycin treatment, Sauer et al. brought evidence for the antagonizing cross talk of TCR signaling and subsequent activation of the PI3K/Akt/mTOR cascade and FoxP3 expression (Sauer et al. 2008). This leads to the conclusion that T_{reg} are not impacted by immune modulation by rapamycin since their signal for survival and function passes through the IL-2R without activating the PI3K/Akt/mTOR pathway (Malek and Castro 2010). In this T cell subset, the signaling cascade is interrupted through high expression of the phosphatase PTEN (Bensinger et al. 2004). The block leaves signaling through the JAK-STAT pathway intact leading to the known hypoproliferative phenotype because of the impaired response to IL-2 signaling compared to T_{con} (Walsh et al. 2006).

9.4 Mechanism of Immunosuppression by T_{reg}

The pathogenesis of acute GvHD is classically divided into three phases in which the innate immune system establishes the inflammatory environment triggered by the conditioning regimen, whereupon APCs build the link between innate and adaptive immune system by activating alloreactive T cells (Fig. 9.1) which ultimately execute the destruction of target organs (Jenq and van den Brink 2010). T_{reg} are able to modulate an immune response at its initiation in the secondary lymphoid organs where APCs prime naïve T cells, as well as during the progression and termination in the inflamed or infected nonlymphoid tissues such as the skin or gastrointestinal tract in case of GvHD (Campbell and Koch 2011). Nevertheless, studies by Nguyen et al. suggested an essential role of T_{reg} particularly during the early phases of disease induction in which T_{reg} colocalize with T_{con} in the lymphoid organs and continue to provide efficient long-term protection since T_{reg} transfer at later time points after BMT decreased GvHD attenuation (Nguyen et al. 2007). In an established full-blown inflammation, T_{reg} are numerically and functionally probably overrun by allogeneic effector T cells and the storm of inflammatory cytokines which is characteristic for acute GvHD.

Generally, T_{reg} are anergic, therefore do not proliferate upon antigen stimulation, yet need TCR stimulation for activation. Since T_{reg} are selected in the thymus by their increased autoreactive potential, they are prone for self-recognition (Hsieh et al. 2004) and only a small stimulus suffices for activation (Takahashi et al. 1998). Thereupon, T_{reg} exhibit suppressive activity regardless of antigen specificity which gives reason for hope in treatment of allo-HCT as T_{reg}/T_{con} histocompatibility seems not to be essential for suppression (Thornton and Shevach 2000). Nevertheless, recent findings indicate that sustained TCR signaling is required for T_{reg} suppressive function (Levine et al. 2014).

In the initial phase of acute GvHD, when the conditioning regimen, irradiation or chemotherapy, leads to local tissue damage, pathogens and so-called pathogen-associated molecular patterns (PAMPs) cross the damaged epithelial barriers of the skin and gastrointestinal tract (Fig. 9.1). Cytokines, chemokines, adhesion molecules, and danger signals (danger-associated molecular patterns, DAMPs) are expressed which ultimately induce the maturation of host dendritic cells (DCs) and the priming of alloreactive T cells (Zeiser et al. 2011; Hill and Ferrara 2000). In

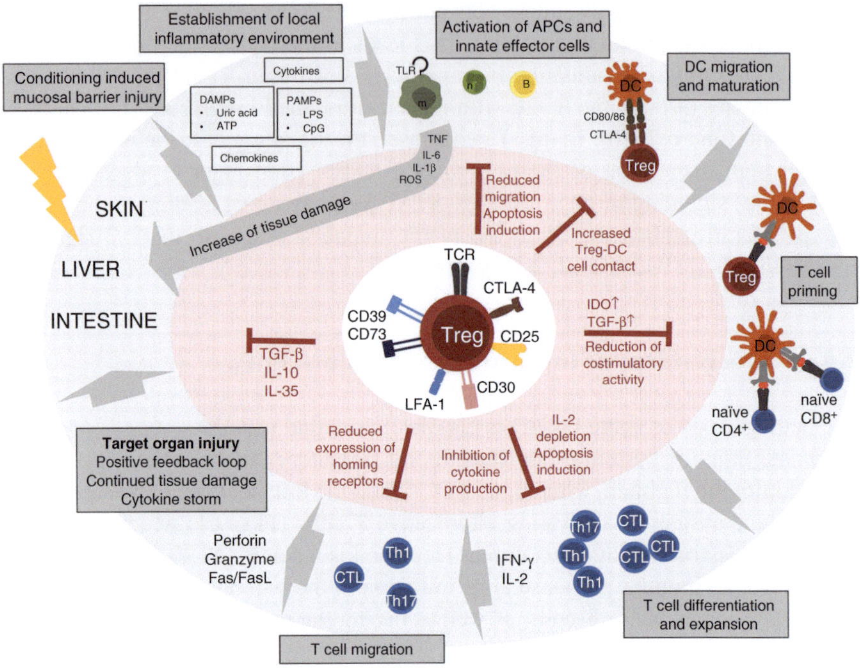

Fig. 9.1 The conditioning regimen such as irradiation or chemotherapy which is necessary in the recipient of allo-HCT to create space for the new immune system and eliminate the malignant cells, the underlying disease, or previous infections leads to host tissue damage in particular in the gut. The resulting release of DAMPs and PAMPs as well as cytokines and chemokines by the local cells leads to an establishment of the inflammatory environment and the activation of local immune cells by their pattern recognition receptors (PRRs). Macrophages and neutrophils in turn secrete inflammatory cytokines such as TNF or IL-6 which enhance the immune activation and aggravate the existing tissue damage. DCs maturing in the periphery migrate to the secondary lymphoid organs where they present host-specific antigens and prime naïve allogeneic T cells which represents the central reaction in GvHD pathogenesis. The activated T cells proliferate and secrete cytokines such as interferon γ (IFN-γ) and IL-2 which contribute to the development of a Th1-biased response. Ultimately, T cells migrate to the target tissues where they destroy cells from the liver, skin, and gastrointestinal tract by mechanisms involving perforin, granzymes, and Fas/FasL. The resulting cell death leads to the continued release of danger signals which perpetuates the GvHD reaction and induces the characteristic cytokine storm. T_{reg} cells are able to interfere at multiple levels within this process in order to attenuate GvHD (references are cited in the main text). (1) Maturation and AG presentation of APC: T_{reg} are able to impair the maturation, migration, and effector function of innate immune cells. Furthermore, they induce apoptosis in B cells and neutrophils. T_{reg} reduce the costimulatory activity of DCs by means of CTLA-4 binding and destabilize the contact of effector T cells with DCs. (2) Inhibition of effector T cells: T_{reg} constrain proliferation by means of IL-2 depletion. Moreover they limit cytokine production and survival by inducing a cytokine-deprived milieu and decrease the expression of homing receptors leading to impaired migration of the effector cells. (3) Effects on local inflamed tissue: T_{reg} secrete a variety of anti-inflammatory cytokines including TGF-β, IL-10, and IL-35 which dampen inflammation

order for the T_{reg} to prevent APC and T_{con} activation, they have to enter the draining lymph nodes by means of CD62L expression since it has been proven that GvHD is only efficiently suppressed by $CD62L^{hi}$ T_{reg} (Taylor et al. 2004; Ermann et al. 2005). Furthermore, expression of homing receptors such as CCR5 mentioned above is essential for the migration in the target tissues in the later stages of GvHD.

Reducing the costimulatory activity and ability of APCs represents the first level of suppression of T cell activation managed by T_{reg}. Already early after T_{reg} discovery, Cederbom and colleagues could show decreased CD80 and CD86 expression on DCs (Cederbom et al. 2000). In 2006, two groups could prove with two-photon microscopy that T_{reg} have long sustained contact with DCs while inhibiting prolonged binding of T_{con} with their APCs in the secondary lymphoid organs (Tadokoro et al. 2006; Tang et al. 2006). One major receptor responsible for inhibition of immune activation by T_{reg} is cytotoxic T-lymphocyte-associated protein 4 (CTLA-4), a high-affinity receptor for CD80 and CD86. Its essential role became apparent in receptor-deficient mice developing severe lymphoproliferative disorders (Tivol et al. 1995). Since a direct inhibitory signaling pathway emanating from CTLA-4 engagement remains still controversial, common hypotheses include that one mechanism of DC inhibition originates from competitive binding of CD80/86 by means of higher affinity of CLTA-4 compared to CD28 (Salomon and Bluestone 2001). This theory is supported by data that show an upregulation of lymphocyte function-associated antigen 1 (LFA-1) by CTLA-4 which may result in even increased sustained cell-cell contact between T_{reg} and APC (Schneider et al. 2005). Recent findings suggest a second mechanism in which by a process called trans-endocytosis CTLA-4 binds and removes CD80/86 from the DC surface by internalization and degradation within the T_{reg} leading to a profound and sustained DC suppression (Qureshi et al. 2011). Moreover, CTLA-4 induces indoleamine dioxygenase (IDO) production in DCs thereby initiating tryptophan metabolism (Grohmann et al. 2002). Tryptophan depletion strongly inhibits T cell proliferation and cytokine production (Fallarino et al. 2003), and IDO expression may also lead to a tolerogenic phenotype of the IDO-expressing cells themselves (Mellor and Munn 2004). IDO represents a major suppression-inducing molecule since it also stimulates the new development of T_{reg} by high TGF-β production of DCs as well as the strong activation of existing T_{reg} and the inhibition of reprogramming of T_{reg} into inflammatory T cells (Chung et al. 2009; Yan et al. 2010; Munn 2011).

Lymphocyte-activation gene 3 (LAG-3) represents another T_{reg} receptor which binds major histocompatibility complex (MHC) class II and may mediate suppression of T_{con} and APC activation (Huang et al. 2004; Liang et al. 2008). Moreover, LAG-3 is also expressed by T_{con} which leaves these cells more susceptible to regulation by T_{reg} (Durham et al. 2014). Further inhibitory surface molecules of T_{reg} include CD30 which has been shown to be essential during early T_{reg} protection from GvHD (Zeiser et al. 2007), as well as CD39 and CD73 which degrade the danger signal extracellular adenosine triphosphate (ATP) to the immunomodulatory molecule adenosine leading to metabolic inhibition of effector T cells (Deaglio et al. 2007; Han et al. 2013).

Besides the receptors involved in T_{reg} activation and enhancement of suppressor function, multiple publications describe glucocorticoid-induced tumor necrosis factor-related protein (GITR) expressed on T_{reg} as a negative regulator which upon stimulation diminishes T_{reg} suppression (Shimizu et al. 2002), while the role of Toll-like receptors (TLRs) such as TLR8 or TLR4 in dampening or inducing T_{reg} responses seems to depend on the type of TLR (Peng et al. 2005; Caramalho et al. 2003).

Nevertheless, T_{reg} also exhibit direct killing mechanisms by means of perforin release for DC killing (Boissonnas et al. 2010) as well as granzyme A and B in order to induce apoptosis in target cells such as $CD4^+$ and $CD8^+$ T cells, monocytes, and DCs (Zeiser et al. 2007; Grossman et al. 2004a, b).

Besides inhibition of DCs, several groups investigated T_{reg}-suppressive capability of B cells regarding the interference with activation, class switch, and antibody production as well as apoptosis induction by perforin and granzymes, the programmed cell death protein 1 (PD-1)/PD-L1 interaction, or the Fas/FasL pathway (Zhao et al. 2006; Lim et al. 2005; Gotot et al. 2012; Xu et al. 2016; Janssens et al. 2003). B cell inhibition is worth consideration in the context of GvHD since B cells are able to act as APCs for effector cells and play a major role in chronic GvHD.

Recent data prove the importance of early neutrophil activation and migration into target organs for the pathogenesis of acute GvHD (Schwab et al. 2014) which leaves inhibition of this cell compartment by T_{reg} during GvHD of serious interest. T_{reg} cells are not only able to reduce migratory potential and induce apoptosis in neutrophils (Richards et al. 2010; Lewkowicz et al. 2006), yet a recent study found that T_{reg} could even promote immunosuppressive features in neutrophils resulting in their contribution to immune modulation (Lewkowicz et al. 2013). Regarding other innate immune cell compartments, T_{reg} are also able to inhibit the cytotoxic capacity of natural killer (NK) cells in a cell-cell contact-dependent mechanism (Trzonkowski et al. 2004). Moreover, T_{reg} were shown to directly downregulate monocyte and macrophage activation leading to reduced cytokine secretion and stimulatory molecule expression (Taams et al. 2005) as well as induce apoptosis in monocytes by means of Fas/FasL interaction (Venet et al. 2006).

Besides the vast possibilities of constraining APC activation by T_{reg}, several studies describe mechanisms of T_{con} inhibition including the impaired expression of homing receptors, adhesion molecules, and chemokine receptors leading to reduced migration (Mavin et al. 2012; Sarween et al. 2004) as well as impaired proliferation (Edinger et al. 2003; Trenado et al. 2003) and cytokine production (Bergerot et al. 1999). The consistent expression of the high-affinity IL-2 receptor chain CD25 is not only required for T_{reg} survival and function, yet is also thought to deplete IL-2 access to T_{con} resulting in apoptosis induction by means of cytokine deprivation (Pandiyan et al. 2007). Furthermore, T_{reg} can not only interact with DCs via CTLA-4 but also with T_{con} thereby inhibiting T cell priming (Fig. 9.1) (Matheu et al. 2015). Several studies show the interference of T_{reg} with $CD8^+$ cytotoxic activity, which is either cell contact mediated or originates from a TGF-β-dependent mechanism (Trzonkowski et al. 2004; Mempel et al. 2006).

TGF-β represents a major factor of tolerance induction since its presence without further inflammatory stimuli such as IL-6 leads to FoxP3 expression and the generation of iT_{reg} in the periphery (Chen et al. 2003). Moreover, TGF-β enhances the expansion and suppressive activity of T_{reg} (Huber et al. 2004) while simultaneously suppressing effector T cell proliferation and function and immunoglobulin production of B cells (Chen et al. 2005; Green et al. 2003; Nakamura et al. 2001). Lastly, T_{reg} interfere with DC maturation in a TGF-β-dependent manner (Misra et al. 2004).

IL-10 represents another important effector molecule of T_{reg} during GvHD since IL-10 mediates immunosuppression particularly at epithelial barriers with contact to the environment such as the lungs or the skin representing target organs in GvHD (Rubtsov et al. 2008). Several studies indicate the important role of IL-10 secretion likely by donor T_{reg} in the regulation of GvHD induction (Hoffmann et al. 2002; Tawara et al. 2012). These data are supported by a study which found a correlation between polymorphisms in the *IL10* promoter and GvHD (Lin et al. 2003).

Investigations by the group around Dario Vignali revealed IL-35 as an important suppressive cytokine produced and secreted by T_{reg} (Collison et al. 2007). On the one hand IL-35 suppresses proliferation of effector T cells which is partly contact dependent since the secretion of IL-35 is increased upon T_{reg}-T_{con} cell contact (Collison et al. 2009). Furthermore, IL-35 drives the conversion of T_{con} to induced T_{reg} (iTr35) whose regulatory activity is mainly driven by IL-35 (Collison et al. 2010).

Altogether, the data presented here draw a complex picture of T_{reg} cell inhibition at multiple levels of an immune response including direct cell contact-mediated effects as well as indirect mechanisms of soluble factor secretion and metabolic inhibition of the target cells.

9.5 Impact of T_{reg} on Antitumor Immunity

Multiple studies particularly in solid tumors delineate the role of T_{reg} in the establishment of tumor tolerance and escape from immune surveillance with T_{reg} infiltrating the tumor tissue and inhibiting an effective T cell response against the cancer cells. Curiel et al. could show in ovarian cancer patients that human T_{reg} specifically inhibit antitumor activity of T cells and contribute to tumor progression. Their accumulation in the tumor mass was supported by CCL22 production by the cancer cells themselves inducing an immune-privileged site; therefore the authors suggest the modulation of T_{reg} function in order to tackle cancer immune escape (Curiel et al. 2004). Besides direct inhibition of T cell immunity, T_{reg} are able to condition intratumoral APCs which could then contribute to tumor tolerance (Bauer et al. 2014). Similar findings were made for gastrointestinal malignancies (Sasada et al. 2003); metastatic melanoma (Vence et al. 2007); breast (Gobert et al. 2009), lung (Tao et al. 2012), and pancreatic cancer (Hiraoka et al. 2006); hepatocellular carcinoma (Fu et al. 2007); classic Hodgkin lymphoma (Schreck et al. 2009); and B cell non-Hodgkin lymphoma (Yang et al. 2006) as well as acute myelogenous leukemia (Szczepanski et al. 2009). These observations led to intensive studies of interrupting

T_{reg} tolerance to increase antitumor immunity by using CTLA-4 blockade (Phan et al. 2003), anti-GITR monoclonal antibody (Ko et al. 2005), or antiangiogenic treatment (Adotevi et al. 2010).

Since an expansion of T_{reg} during allo-HCT represents an interesting option in order to prevent GvHD, the urgent question emerged if increased T_{reg} counts result in diminishment of the greatly appreciated (GvT/GvL) effect. Already early publications showed that engraftment and long-term tolerance were facilitated in the presence of donor T_{reg} (Hanash and Levy 2005; Joffre et al. 2004) while preserving GvL mechanisms (Edinger et al. 2003; Jones et al. 2003; Trenado et al. 2003).

Reasons for the different outcomes of T_{reg} expansion after allo-HCT regarding relapse lie in the unique setting after BMT concerning alloreactivity and tumor cell counts. The number of tumor cells is greatly reduced after the conditioning regimen facilitating their elimination by the transplanted immune system. The diverse mechanisms of T_{reg} suppression of allogeneic immune responses discussed in the chapter above mostly limit the extent of T cell activation, their proliferation, and migration yet without impairing their individual cytotoxic capacity (Edinger et al. 2003). Since the count of tumor cells after BMT is rather low, the transplanted T_{con} are able to eliminate the minimal cancer residue without an excessive allogeneic immune response. Furthermore, novel approaches reach to induce alloantigen-specific T_{reg} which efficiently prevent GvHD without a possible impairment of GvL effects (Veerapathran et al. 2011; Semple et al. 2011; Li et al. 2015).

Moreover, the immune reactivity of the cancer cells is not limited to specific tumor antigens which may be already downregulated in later stages of disease but include classic self-antigens which are recognized by the alloreactive T cells of the graft leaving them more immunogenic (Kloosterman et al. 1995; Reddy et al. 2005). Donor lymphocyte infusions in case of a relapse utilize this effect.

Furthermore, the T_{reg} efficacy is a space-limited process where T_{reg} have to enter similar tissues as effector T cells such as the epithelial GvHD target organs. At later time points after BMT, T_{reg} migrate to the target organs in order to suppress GvHD. Emerging leukemic cells reside in the secondary lymphoid organs or the bone marrow which hosts low T_{reg} numbers (Booth et al. 2010) where they can be eliminated by effector T cells (Nguyen et al. 2007). Supporting this hypothesis, Kim et al. restrained T cells within the secondary lymphoid organs resulting in efficient GvL without GvHD development (Kim et al. 2003).

9.6 Clinical Application of T_{reg} Transfer

The transfer of a tolerogenic cell population such as T_{reg}, mesenchymal stroma cells, or Tr1 cells which persist in the body could ideally lead to long-term tolerance without the need for additional pharmacological interventions. This concept has been recently applied when T_{reg} were transferred in the prophylactic setting to patients that had undergone allo-HCT.

The first study on T_{reg} transfer was performed in 28 patients with high-risk hematologic malignancies who underwent human leukocyte antigen (HLA)-haploidentical HCT and showed that T_{reg} prevented GvHD and promoted immune reconstitution (Di Ianni et al. 2011). The authors reported that T_{reg} prevented GvHD in the absence of any posttransplantation immunosuppression and enhanced lymphoid reconstitution compared to historical controls without any evidence for an increased relapse rate (Di Ianni et al. 2011). Another group studied the safety profile of umbilical cord blood (UCB)-derived T_{reg} in 23 patients (Brunstein et al. 2011). After infusion, UCB T_{reg} could be detected for 14 days, indicating that the infused cells survived the pro-inflammatory cytokine milieu in patients post-HCT. The authors compared their patients with identically treated 108 historical controls without T_{reg} and found a reduced incidence of grade II–IV acute GvHD (43% vs 61%, $P = 0.05$) with no deleterious effect on risks of infection (Brunstein et al. 2011). The same group reported later on the transfer of UCB-derived T_{reg} that had been expanded in cultures stimulated with K562 cells modified to express the high-affinity Fc receptor (CD64) and CD86. The authors reported that the incidence of grade II–IV acute GvHD at 100 days was 9% in the UCB-T_{reg} group compared to 45% in control patients (Brunstein et al. 2016).

Besides those preemptive T_{reg} transfer studies, more evidence indicates a central role for T_{reg} in prevention of GvHD post allo-HCT. Patients who received the antibody mogamulizumab for their adult T cell acute lymphoblastic leukemia (T-ALL) experienced prolonged suppression of normal T_{reg} (Ishida et al. 2012). Importantly, pretransplant use of mogamulizumab in those T-ALL patients that later underwent allo-HCT was connected to severe acute GvHD, which is consistent with a suppressive role of T_{reg} against GvHD (Inoue et al. 2016).

Since it was shown that T_{reg} require IL-2 post allo-HCT to expand and survive (Zeiser et al. 2006), multiple studies later investigated the effects of IL-2 on T_{reg} expansion in patients and GvHD (Koreth et al. 2011, 2016). In a recent phase 2 study, 35 adult patients with steroid-refractory chronic GvHD received daily IL-2 (1×10^6 IU/m^2/d) for 12 weeks (Koreth et al. 2016). The authors reported that 20/33 evaluable patients (61%) had clinical responses at multiple chronic GvHD sites such as the liver, skin, and gastrointestinal tract (Koreth et al. 2016). An important predictor of response seemed to be initiation of IL-2 early after transplantation, suggesting that later established chronic GvHD is harder to modify by IL-2 treatment.

Furthermore, investigators used human donor T_{reg} that were cultivated for 7–12 days and then given to patients suffering from chronic GvHD (Nishimori et al. 2012). The authors reported that two of five patients showed a clinical response with improvement of chronic GvHD symptoms and three patients showed stable symptoms for up to 21 months (Theil et al. 2015). Further clinical trials are in progress and planned to extend these studies also to the treatment of acute GvHD by adoptive T_{reg} transfer.

Summarized, the findings support the attractive option of T_{reg} expansion in patients undergoing allo-HCT in order to suppress the development of GvHD with simultaneous preservation of the appreciated anti-infectious immunity and GvL effect which in turn allows for reduced intensity conditioning regimens. First clinical trials are promising but need confirmation in larger prospective randomized trials.

9.7 Expert Point of View and Future Directions

Since their discovery, T_{reg} have risen rapidly to a well investigated cell population with various possibilities of application. Profound characterization of T_{reg} markers enables the specific enrichment of this regulatory cell compartment which makes them an interesting tool for clinical application. Furthermore, due to their unique signaling pathways such as their specific response to IL-2 treatment and rapamycin, protocols for the efficient expansion have been developed and are already applied successfully. Since classic standard prophylaxis and treatment options for GvHD do not interfere and even possibly enhance T_{reg} function, including rapamycin, glucocorticosteroids, and FTY720, the combined therapy could even provide a synergistic effect, while recent studies indicate that therapy with calcineurin inhibitors has an adverse effect on T_{reg} concerning proliferation and function and MMF application is still discussed controversially (Wu et al. 2012; Scotta et al. 2016; Demirkiran et al. 2009; Lim et al. 2010). First clinical trials show promising results concerning acute as well as chronic GvHD disease outcome both by in vivo as well as in vitro expansion of T_{reg}. Nevertheless, intense research has to be continued in order to further improve the experimental protocols such as the optimal time point of adoptive transfer and investigate the best option for T_{reg} expansion regarding efficacy and safety. Furthermore, the various mechanisms of T_{reg} suppression have to be delineated to better understand their role in the clinical picture of GvHD.

A clinically valuable approach may be the use of third-party T_{reg} and was investigated by Pierini et al. (2015). The researchers suggested this method as more practical since the availability and access of T_{reg} in certain allo-HCT settings such as grafts from cord blood or an unrelated donor may be limited. Furthermore, the T_{reg} could be easily stored and readily applied when most needed. Yet, due to the observed reduced survival of third-party T_{reg}, this technique needs more profound studies. Another urgent question to be clarified is the characterization of common antigens inducing a GvHD reaction. With this knowledge, allo-specific T_{reg} could be generated which would limit their suppressive activity to alloreactive T_{con}. Lastly, certain patient cohorts may be more susceptible to T_{reg} application, and in these, adoptive T_{reg} transfer may be found to be favorable depending on their type of disease pathology.

Concluding, clinical application of T_{reg} for prophylaxis and treatment of GvHD is an upcoming treatment option which not only prevents GvHD by simultaneously preserving the GvL effect but leads to profound long-term immunotolerance instead of medically induced immunosuppression which ceases upon discontinuation of treatment.

References

Adotevi O et al (2010) A decrease of regulatory T cells correlates with overall survival after sunitinib-based antiangiogenic therapy in metastatic renal cancer patients. J Immunother 33:991–998

Anderson BE et al (2004) Recipient CD4+ T cells that survive irradiation regulate chronic graft-versus-host disease. Blood 104:1565–1573

Battaglia M, Stabilini A, Roncarolo MG (2005) Rapamycin selectively expands CD4+CD25+FoxP3+ regulatory T cells. Blood 105:4743–4748
Battaglia M et al (2006) Rapamycin promotes expansion of functional CD4+CD25+FOXP3+ regulatory T cells of both healthy subjects and type 1 diabetic patients. J Immunol 177:8338–8347
Battaglia M, Stabilini A, Tresoldi E (2012) Expanding human T regulatory cells with the mTOR-inhibitor rapamycin. Methods Mol Biol 821:279–293
Bauer CA et al (2014) Dynamic Treg interactions with intratumoral APCs promote local CTL dysfunction. J Clin Invest 124:2425–2440
Bayer AL et al (2009) Host CD4+CD25+ T cells can expand and comprise a major component of the Treg compartment after experimental HCT. Blood 113:733–743
Bennett CL et al (2001) The immune dysregulation, polyendocrinopathy, enteropathy, X-linked syndrome (IPEX) is caused by mutations of FOXP3. Nat Genet 27:20–21
Bensinger SJ et al (2004) Distinct IL-2 receptor signaling pattern in CD4+CD25+ regulatory T cells. J Immunol 172:5287–5296
Beres A, Komorowski R, Mihara M, Drobyski WR (2011) Instability of Foxp3 expression limits the ability of induced regulatory T cells to mitigate graft versus host disease. Clin Cancer Res 17:3969–3983
Beres AJ et al (2012) CD8+ Foxp3+ regulatory T cells are induced during graft-versus-host disease and mitigate disease severity. J Immunol 189:464–474
Bergerot I et al (1999) Insulin B-chain reactive CD4+ regulatory T-cells induced by oral insulin treatment protect from type 1 diabetes by blocking the cytokine secretion and pancreatic infiltration of diabetogenic effector T-cells. Diabetes 48:1720–1729
Bluestone JA, Abbas AK (2003) Natural versus adaptive regulatory T cells. Nat Rev Immunol 3:253–257
Boissonnas A et al (2010) Foxp3+ T cells induce perforin-dependent dendritic cell death in tumor-draining lymph nodes. Immunity 32:266–278
Booth NJ et al (2010) Different proliferative potential and migratory characteristics of human CD4+ regulatory T cells that express either CD45RA or CD45RO. J Immunol 184:4317–4326
Brunkow ME et al (2001) Disruption of a new forkhead/winged-helix protein, scurfin, results in the fatal lymphoproliferative disorder of the scurfy mouse. Nat Genet 27:68–73
Brunstein CG, Miller JS, Cao Q, McKenna DH, Hippen KL, Curtsinger J et al (2011) Infusion of ex vivo expanded T regulatory cells in adults transplanted with umbilical cord blood: safety profile and detection kinetics. Blood 117:1061–1070
Brunstein CG, Miller JS, McKenna DH, Hippen KL, DeFor TE, Sumstad D et al (2016) Umbilical cord blood-derived T regulatory cells to prevent GVHD: kinetics, toxicity profile and clinical effect. Blood 127:1044–1051
Camirand G et al (2014) CD45 ligation expands Tregs by promoting interactions with DCs. J Clin Invest 124:4603–4613
Campbell DJ, Koch MA (2011) Phenotypical and functional specialization of FOXP3+ regulatory T cells. Nat Rev Immunol 11:119–130
Caramalho I et al (2003) Regulatory T cells selectively express toll-like receptors and are activated by lipopolysaccharide. J Exp Med 197:403–411
Cederbom L, Hall H, Ivars F (2000) CD4+CD25+ regulatory T cells down-regulate co-stimulatory molecules on antigen-presenting cells. Eur J Immunol 30:1538–1543
Chaudhry A et al (2009) CD4+ regulatory T cells control TH17 responses in a Stat3-dependent manner. Science 326:986–991
Chen W et al (2003) Conversion of peripheral CD4+CD25- naive T cells to CD4+CD25+ regulatory T cells by TGF-beta induction of transcription factor Foxp3. J Exp Med 198:1875–1886
Chen ML et al (2005) Regulatory T cells suppress tumor-specific CD8 T cell cytotoxicity through TGF-beta signals in vivo. Proc Natl Acad Sci U S A 102:419–424
Chen X et al (2007) Absence of regulatory T-cell control of TH1 and TH17 cells is responsible for the autoimmune-mediated pathology in chronic graft-versus-host disease. Blood 110:3804–3813

Chen X et al (2009) Blockade of interleukin-6 signaling augments regulatory T-cell reconstitution and attenuates the severity of graft-versus-host disease. Blood 114:891–900
Choi J et al (2010) In vivo administration of hypomethylating agents mitigate graft-versus-host disease without sacrificing graft-versus-leukemia. Blood 116:129–139
Chung DJ et al (2009) Indoleamine 2,3-dioxygenase-expressing mature human monocyte-derived dendritic cells expand potent autologous regulatory T cells. Blood 114:555–563
Cohen JL, Trenado A, Vasey D, Klatzmann D, Salomon BL (2002) CD4(+)CD25(+) immunoregulatory T cells: new therapeutics for graft-versus-host disease. J Exp Med 196:401–406
Collison LW et al (2007) The inhibitory cytokine IL-35 contributes to regulatory T-cell function. Nature 450:566–569
Collison LW, Pillai MR, Chaturvedi V, Vignali DA (2009) Regulatory T cell suppression is potentiated by target T cells in a cell contact, IL-35- and IL-10-dependent manner. J Immunol 182:6121–6128
Collison LW et al (2010) IL-35-mediated induction of a potent regulatory T cell population. Nat Immunol 11:1093–1101
Curiel TJ et al (2004) Specific recruitment of regulatory T cells in ovarian carcinoma fosters immune privilege and predicts reduced survival. Nat Med 10:942–949
Deaglio S et al (2007) Adenosine generation catalyzed by CD39 and CD73 expressed on regulatory T cells mediates immune suppression. J Exp Med 204:1257–1265
Demirkiran A et al (2009) Conversion from calcineurin inhibitor to mycophenolate mofetil-based immunosuppression changes the frequency and phenotype of CD4+FOXP3+ regulatory T cells. Transplantation 87:1062–1068
Di Ianni M, Falzetti F, Carotti A, Terenzi A, Castellino F, Bonifacio E et al (2011) Tregs prevent GVHD and promote immune reconstitution in HLA-haploidentical transplantation. Blood 117:3921–3928
Duramad O, Laysang A, Li J, Ishii Y, Namikawa R (2011) Pharmacologic expansion of donor-derived, naturally occurring CD4(+)Foxp3(+) regulatory T cells reduces acute graft-versus-host disease lethality without abrogating the graft-versus-leukemia effect in murine models. Biol Blood Marrow Transplant 17:1154–1168
Durham NM et al (2014) Lymphocyte Activation Gene 3 (LAG-3) modulates the ability of CD4 T-cells to be suppressed in vivo. PLoS One 9:e109080
Earle KE et al (2005) In vitro expanded human CD4+CD25+ regulatory T cells suppress effector T cell proliferation. Clin Immunol 115:3–9
Edinger M et al (2003) CD4+CD25+ regulatory T cells preserve graft-versus-tumor activity while inhibiting graft-versus-host disease after bone marrow transplantation. Nat Med 9:1144–1150
Ermann J et al (2005) Only the CD62L+ subpopulation of CD4+CD25+ regulatory T cells protects from lethal acute GVHD. Blood 105:2220–2226
Fallarino F et al (2003) Modulation of tryptophan catabolism by regulatory T cells. Nat Immunol 4:1206–1212
Fantini MC et al (2004) Cutting edge: TGF-beta induces a regulatory phenotype in CD4+CD25- T cells through Foxp3 induction and down-regulation of Smad7. J Immunol 172:5149–5153
Ferrara JL, Levine JE, Reddy P, Holler E (2009) Graft-versus-host disease. Lancet 373:1550–1561
Floess S et al (2007) Epigenetic control of the foxp3 locus in regulatory T cells. PLoS Biol 5:e38
Fontenot JD et al (2005) Regulatory T cell lineage specification by the forkhead transcription factor foxp3. Immunity 22:329–341
Fu J et al (2007) Increased regulatory T cells correlate with CD8 T-cell impairment and poor survival in hepatocellular carcinoma patients. Gastroenterology 132:2328–2339
Gobert M et al (2009) Regulatory T cells recruited through CCL22/CCR4 are selectively activated in lymphoid infiltrates surrounding primary breast tumors and lead to an adverse clinical outcome. Cancer Res 69:2000–2009
Gotot J et al (2012) Regulatory T cells use programmed death 1 ligands to directly suppress autoreactive B cells in vivo. Proc Natl Acad Sci U S A 109:10468–10473

Green EA, Gorelik L, McGregor CM, Tran EH, Flavell RA (2003) CD4+CD25+ T regulatory cells control anti-islet CD8+ T cells through TGF-beta-TGF-beta receptor interactions in type 1 diabetes. Proc Natl Acad Sci U S A 100:10878–10883

Grohmann U et al (2002) CTLA-4-Ig regulates tryptophan catabolism in vivo. Nat Immunol 3:1097–1101

Grossman WJ et al (2004a) Differential expression of granzymes A and B in human cytotoxic lymphocyte subsets and T regulatory cells. Blood 104:2840–2848

Grossman WJ et al (2004b) Human T regulatory cells can use the perforin pathway to cause autologous target cell death. Immunity 21:589–601

Guo Z et al (2008) CD4+CD25+ regulatory T cells in the small intestinal lamina propria show an effector/memory phenotype. Int Immunol 20:307–315

Hahn BH, Singh RP, La Cava A, Ebling FM (2005) Tolerogenic treatment of lupus mice with consensus peptide induces Foxp3-expressing, apoptosis-resistant, TGFbeta-secreting CD8+ T cell suppressors. J Immunol 175:7728–7737

Han KL et al (2013) Adenosine A(2)A receptor agonist-mediated increase in donor-derived regulatory T cells suppresses development of graft-versus-host disease. J Immunol 190:458–468

Hanash AM, Levy RB (2005) Donor CD4+CD25+ T cells promote engraftment and tolerance following MHC-mismatched hematopoietic cell transplantation. Blood 105:1828–1836

Hill GR, Ferrara JL (2000) The primacy of the gastrointestinal tract as a target organ of acute graft-versus-host disease: rationale for the use of cytokine shields in allogeneic bone marrow transplantation. Blood 95:2754–2759

Hiraoka N, Onozato K, Kosuge T, Hirohashi S (2006) Prevalence of FOXP3+ regulatory T cells increases during the progression of pancreatic ductal adenocarcinoma and its premalignant lesions. Clin Cancer Res 12:5423–5434

Hoffmann P, Ermann J, Edinger M, Fathman CG, Strober S (2002) Donor-type CD4(+)CD25(+) regulatory T cells suppress lethal acute graft-versus-host disease after allogeneic bone marrow transplantation. J Exp Med 196:389–399

Hoffmann P, Eder R, Kunz-Schughart LA, Andreesen R, Edinger M (2004) Large-scale in vitro expansion of polyclonal human CD4(+)CD25 high regulatory T cells. Blood 104:895–903

Hsieh CS et al (2004) Recognition of the peripheral self by naturally arising CD25+ CD4+ T cell receptors. Immunity 21:267–277

Huang CT et al (2004) Role of LAG-3 in regulatory T cells. Immunity 21:503–513

Huber S et al (2004) Cutting edge: TGF-beta signaling is required for the in vivo expansion and immunosuppressive capacity of regulatory CD4+CD25+ T cells. J Immunol 173:6526–6531

Inoue Y, Fuji S, Tanosaki R, Fukuda T (2016) Pretransplant mogamulizumab against ATLL might increase the risk of acute GVHD and non-relapse mortality. Bone Marrow Transplant 51:725–727. https://doi.org/10.1038/bmt.2015.315

Ishida T, Joh T, Uike N, Yamamoto K, Utsunomiya A, Yoshida S et al (2012) Defucosylated anti-CCR4 monoclonal antibody (KW-0761) for relapsed adult T-cell leukemia-lymphoma: a multicenter phase II study. J Clin Oncol 30:837–842

Janssens W et al (2003) CD4+CD25+ T cells lyse antigen-presenting B cells by Fas-Fas ligand interaction in an epitope-specific manner. J Immunol 171:4604–4612

Jenq RR, van den Brink MR (2010) Allogeneic haematopoietic stem cell transplantation: individualized stem cell and immune therapy of cancer. Nat Rev Cancer 10:213–221

Joffre O, Gorsse N, Romagnoli P, Hudrisier D, van Meerwijk JP (2004) Induction of antigen-specific tolerance to bone marrow allografts with CD4+CD25+ T lymphocytes. Blood 103:4216–4221

Jones SC, Murphy GF, Korngold R (2003) Post-hematopoietic cell transplantation control of graft-versus-host disease by donor CD425 T cells to allow an effective graft-versus-leukemia response. Biol Blood Marrow Transplant 9:243–256

Kim YM, Sachs T, Asavaroengchai W, Bronson R, Sykes M (2003) Graft-versus-host disease can be separated from graft-versus-lymphoma effects by control of lymphocyte trafficking with FTY720. J Clin Invest 111:659–669

Kitazawa Y et al (2009) Superagonist CD28 antibody preferentially expanded Foxp3-expressing nTreg cells and prevented graft-versus-host diseases. Cell Transplant 18:627–637
Kloosterman TC, Martens AC, van Bekkum DW, Hagenbeek A (1995) Graft-versus-leukemia in rat MHC-mismatched bone marrow transplantation is merely an allogeneic effect. Bone Marrow Transplant 15:583–590
Ko K et al (2005) Treatment of advanced tumors with agonistic anti-GITR mAb and its effects on tumor-infiltrating Foxp3+CD25+CD4+ regulatory T cells. J Exp Med 202:885–891
Koch MA et al (2009) The transcription factor T-bet controls regulatory T cell homeostasis and function during type 1 inflammation. Nat Immunol 10:595–602
Koreth J, Matsuoka K, Kim HT, McDonough SM, Bindra B, Alyea EP et al (2011) Interleukin-2 and regulatory T cells in graft-versus-host disease. N Engl J Med 365:2055–2066
Koreth J, Kim HT, Jones KT, Lange PB, Reynolds CG, Chammas MJ et al (2016) Efficacy, durability, and response predictors of low-dose interleukin-2 therapy for chronic graft vs. host disease. Blood 128:130–137. pii: blood-2016-02-702852
Levine AG, Arvey A, Jin W, Rudensky AY (2014) Continuous requirement for the TCR in regulatory T cell function. Nat Immunol 15:1070–1078
Lewkowicz P, Lewkowicz N, Sasiak A, Tchorzewski H (2006) Lipopolysaccharide-activated CD4+CD25+ T regulatory cells inhibit neutrophil function and promote their apoptosis and death. J Immunol 177:7155–7163
Lewkowicz N, Klink M, Mycko MP, Lewkowicz P (2013) Neutrophil--CD4+CD25+ T regulatory cell interactions: a possible new mechanism of infectious tolerance. Immunobiology 218:455–464
Li J et al (2015) HY-specific induced regulatory T cells display high specificity and efficacy in the prevention of acute graft-versus-host disease. J Immunol 195:717–725
Liang B et al (2008) Regulatory T cells inhibit dendritic cells by lymphocyte activation gene-3 engagement of MHC class II. J Immunol 180:5916–5926
Lim HW, Hillsamer P, Banham AH, Kim CH (2005) Cutting edge: direct suppression of B cells by CD4+ CD25+ regulatory T cells. J Immunol 175:4180–4183
Lim DG et al (2010) Impact of immunosuppressants on the therapeutic efficacy of in vitro-expanded CD4+CD25+Foxp3+ regulatory T cells in allotransplantation. Transplantation 89:928–936
Lin MT et al (2003) Relation of an interleukin-10 promoter polymorphism to graft-versus-host disease and survival after hematopoietic-cell transplantation. N Engl J Med 349:2201–2210
Malek TR (2008) The biology of interleukin-2. Annu Rev Immunol 26:453–479
Malek TR, Castro I (2010) Interleukin-2 receptor signaling: at the interface between tolerance and immunity. Immunity 33:153–165
Matheu MP et al (2015) Imaging regulatory T cell dynamics and CTLA4-mediated suppression of T cell priming. Nat Commun 6:6219
Mavin E et al (2012) Regulatory T cells inhibit CD8(+) T-cell tissue invasion in human skin graft-versus-host reactions. Transplantation 94:456–464
Mellor AL, Munn DH (2004) IDO expression by dendritic cells: tolerance and tryptophan catabolism. Nat Rev Immunol 4:762–774
Mempel TR et al (2006) Regulatory T cells reversibly suppress cytotoxic T cell function independent of effector differentiation. Immunity 25:129–141
Misra N, Bayry J, Lacroix-Desmazes S, Kazatchkine MD, Kaveri SV (2004) Cutting edge: human CD4+CD25+ T cells restrain the maturation and antigen-presenting function of dendritic cells. J Immunol 172:4676–4680
Munn DH (2011) Indoleamine 2,3-dioxygenase, Tregs and cancer. Curr Med Chem 18:2240–2246
Nakamura K, Kitani A, Strober W (2001) Cell contact-dependent immunosuppression by CD4(+) CD25(+) regulatory T cells is mediated by cell surface-bound transforming growth factor beta. J Exp Med 194:629–644
Nguyen VH et al (2007) In vivo dynamics of regulatory T-cell trafficking and survival predict effective strategies to control graft-versus-host disease following allogeneic transplantation. Blood 109:2649–2656

Nishimori H, Maeda Y, Teshima T, Sugiyama H, Kobayashi K, Yamasuji Y et al (2012) Synthetic retinoid Am80 ameliorates chronic graft-versus-host disease by down-regulating Th1 and Th17. Blood 119:285–295
Pandiyan P, Zheng L, Ishihara S, Reed J, Lenardo MJ (2007) CD4+CD25+Foxp3+ regulatory T cells induce cytokine deprivation-mediated apoptosis of effector CD4+ T cells. Nat Immunol 8:1353–1362
Peng G et al (2005) Toll-like receptor 8-mediated reversal of CD4+ regulatory T cell function. Science 309:1380–1384
Phan GQ et al (2003) Cancer regression and autoimmunity induced by cytotoxic T lymphocyte-associated antigen 4 blockade in patients with metastatic melanoma. Proc Natl Acad Sci U S A 100:8372–8377
Pierini A et al (2015) Donor requirements for regulatory T cell suppression of murine graft-versus-host disease. J Immunol 195:347–355
Qureshi OS et al (2011) Trans-endocytosis of CD80 and CD86: a molecular basis for the cell-extrinsic function of CTLA-4. Science 332:600–603
Reddy P et al (2005) A crucial role for antigen-presenting cells and alloantigen expression in graft-versus-leukemia responses. Nat Med 11:1244–1249
Richards H et al (2010) Novel role of regulatory T cells in limiting early neutrophil responses in skin. Immunology 131:583–592
Roncarolo MG, Gregori S, Bacchetta R, Battaglia M (2014) Tr1 cells and the counter-regulation of immunity: natural mechanisms and therapeutic applications. Curr Top Microbiol Immunol 380:39–68
Rubtsov YP et al (2008) Regulatory T cell-derived interleukin-10 limits inflammation at environmental interfaces. Immunity 28:546–558
Sakaguchi S, Sakaguchi N, Asano M, Itoh M, Toda M (1995) Immunologic self-tolerance maintained by activated T cells expressing IL-2 receptor alpha-chains (CD25). Breakdown of a single mechanism of self-tolerance causes various autoimmune diseases. J Immunol 155:1151–1164
Sakaguchi S et al (2006) Foxp3+ CD25+ CD4+ natural regulatory T cells in dominant self-tolerance and autoimmune disease. Immunol Rev 212:8–27
Salomon B, Bluestone JA (2001) Complexities of CD28/B7: CTLA-4 costimulatory pathways in autoimmunity and transplantation. Annu Rev Immunol 19:225–252
Sarween N et al (2004) CD4+CD25+ cells controlling a pathogenic CD4 response inhibit cytokine differentiation, CXCR-3 expression, and tissue invasion. J Immunol 173:2942–2951
Sasada T, Kimura M, Yoshida Y, Kanai M, Takabayashi A (2003) CD4+CD25+ regulatory T cells in patients with gastrointestinal malignancies: possible involvement of regulatory T cells in disease progression. Cancer 98:1089–1099
Sauer S et al (2008) T cell receptor signaling controls Foxp3 expression via PI3K, Akt, and mTOR. Proc Natl Acad Sci U S A 105:7797–7802
Sawamukai N et al (2012) Cell-autonomous role of TGFbeta and IL-2 receptors in CD4+ and CD8+ inducible regulatory T-cell generation during GVHD. Blood 119:5575–5583
Schneidawind D, Pierini A, Negrin RS (2013) Regulatory T cells and natural killer T cells for modulation of GVHD following allogeneic hematopoietic cell transplantation. Blood 122:3116–3121
Schneider H, Valk E, da Rocha Dias S, Wei B, Rudd CE (2005) CTLA-4 up-regulation of lymphocyte function-associated antigen 1 adhesion and clustering as an alternate basis for coreceptor function. Proc Natl Acad Sci U S A 102:12861–12866
Schreck S et al (2009) Prognostic impact of tumour-infiltrating Th2 and regulatory T cells in classical Hodgkin lymphoma. Hematol Oncol 27:31–39
Schwab L et al (2014) Neutrophil granulocytes recruited upon translocation of intestinal bacteria enhance graft-versus-host disease via tissue damage. Nat Med 20:648–654
Scotta C et al (2016) Impact of immunosuppressive drugs on the therapeutic efficacy of ex vivo expanded human regulatory T cells. Haematologica 101:91–100

Semple K, Yu Y, Wang D, Anasetti C, Yu XZ (2011) Efficient and selective prevention of GVHD by antigen-specific induced Tregs via linked-suppression in mice. Biol Blood Marrow Transplant 17:309–318

Setoguchi R, Hori S, Takahashi T, Sakaguchi S (2005) Homeostatic maintenance of natural Foxp3(+) CD25(+) CD4(+) regulatory T cells by interleukin (IL)-2 and induction of autoimmune disease by IL-2 neutralization. J Exp Med 201:723–735

Sharfe N, Dadi HK, Shahar M, Roifman CM (1997) Human immune disorder arising from mutation of the alpha chain of the interleukin-2 receptor. Proc Natl Acad Sci U S A 94:3168–3171

Shimizu J, Yamazaki S, Takahashi T, Ishida Y, Sakaguchi S (2002) Stimulation of CD25(+)CD4(+) regulatory T cells through GITR breaks immunological self-tolerance. Nat Immunol 3:135–142

Shin HJ et al (2011) Rapamycin and IL-2 reduce lethal acute graft-versus-host disease associated with increased expansion of donor type CD4+CD25+Foxp3+ regulatory T cells. Blood 118:2342–2350

Smigiel KS et al (2014) CCR7 provides localized access to IL-2 and defines homeostatically distinct regulatory T cell subsets. J Exp Med 211:121–136

Soler D et al (2006) CCR8 expression identifies CD4 memory T cells enriched for FOXP3+ regulatory and Th2 effector lymphocytes. J Immunol 177:6940–6951

Szczepanski MJ et al (2009) Increased frequency and suppression by regulatory T cells in patients with acute myelogenous leukemia. Clin Cancer Res 15:3325–3332

Taams LS et al (2005) Modulation of monocyte/macrophage function by human CD4+CD25+ regulatory T cells. Hum Immunol 66:222–230

Tadokoro CE et al (2006) Regulatory T cells inhibit stable contacts between CD4+ T cells and dendritic cells in vivo. J Exp Med 203:505–511

Takahashi T et al (1998) Immunologic self-tolerance maintained by CD25+CD4+ naturally anergic and suppressive T cells: induction of autoimmune disease by breaking their anergic/suppressive state. Int Immunol 10:1969–1980

Tang Q et al (2006) Visualizing regulatory T cell control of autoimmune responses in nonobese diabetic mice. Nat Immunol 7:83–92

Tao H et al (2012) Prognostic potential of FOXP3 expression in non-small cell lung cancer cells combined with tumor-infiltrating regulatory T cells. Lung Cancer 75:95–101

Tawara I et al (2012) Donor- but not host-derived interleukin-10 contributes to the regulation of experimental graft-versus-host disease. J Leukoc Biol 91:667–675

Taylor PA, Noelle RJ, Blazar BR (2001) CD4(+)CD25(+) immune regulatory cells are required for induction of tolerance to alloantigen via costimulatory blockade. J Exp Med 193:1311–1318

Taylor PA, Lees CJ, Blazar BR (2002) The infusion of ex vivo activated and expanded CD4(+) CD25(+) immune regulatory cells inhibits graft-versus-host disease lethality. Blood 99:3493–3499

Taylor PA et al (2004) L-Selectin(hi) but not the L-selectin(lo) CD4+25+ T-regulatory cells are potent inhibitors of GVHD and BM graft rejection. Blood 104:3804–3812

Theil A, Tuve S, Oelschlägel U, Maiwald A, Döhler D, Oßmann D et al (2015) Adoptive transfer of allogeneic regulatory T cells into patients with chronic graft-versus-host disease. Cytotherapy 17:473–486

Thornton AM, Shevach EM (2000) Suppressor effector function of CD4+CD25+ immunoregulatory T cells is antigen nonspecific. J Immunol 164:183–190

Tivol EA et al (1995) Loss of CTLA-4 leads to massive lymphoproliferation and fatal multiorgan tissue destruction, revealing a critical negative regulatory role of CTLA-4. Immunity 3:541–547

Trenado A et al (2003) Recipient-type specific CD4+CD25+ regulatory T cells favor immune reconstitution and control graft-versus-host disease while maintaining graft-versus-leukemia. J Clin Invest 112:1688–1696

Tresoldi E et al (2011) Stability of human rapamycin-expanded CD4+CD25+ T regulatory cells. Haematologica 96:1357–1365

Trzonkowski P, Szmit E, Mysliwska J, Dobyszuk A, Mysliwski A (2004) CD4+CD25+ T regulatory cells inhibit cytotoxic activity of T CD8+ and NK lymphocytes in the direct cell-to-cell interaction. Clin Immunol 112:258–267

Veerapathran A, Pidala J, Beato F, Yu XZ, Anasetti C (2011) Ex vivo expansion of human Tregs specific for alloantigens presented directly or indirectly. Blood 118:5671–5680

Vence L et al (2007) Circulating tumor antigen-specific regulatory T cells in patients with metastatic melanoma. Proc Natl Acad Sci U S A 104:20884–20889

Venet F et al (2006) Human CD4+CD25+ regulatory T lymphocytes inhibit lipopolysaccharide-induced monocyte survival through a Fas/Fas ligand-dependent mechanism. J Immunol 177:6540–6547

Venturi GM, Conway RM, Steeber DA, Tedder TF (2007) CD25+CD4+ regulatory T cell migration requires L-selectin expression: L-selectin transcriptional regulation balances constitutive receptor turnover. J Immunol 178:291–300

Walsh PT et al (2006) PTEN inhibits IL-2 receptor-mediated expansion of CD4+ CD25+ Tregs. J Clin Invest 116:2521–2531

Weiner HL (2001) Induction and mechanism of action of transforming growth factor-beta-secreting Th3 regulatory cells. Immunol Rev 182:207–214

Wildin RS et al (2001) X-linked neonatal diabetes mellitus, enteropathy and endocrinopathy syndrome is the human equivalent of mouse scurfy. Nat Genet 27:18–20

Wu T et al (2012) Immunosuppressive drugs on inducing Ag-specific CD4(+)CD25(+)Foxp3(+) Treg cells during immune response in vivo. Transpl Immunol 27:30–38

Xu A et al (2016) TGF-beta-induced regulatory T cells directly suppress B cell responses through a noncytotoxic mechanism. J Immunol 196(9):3631–3641

Yan Y et al (2010) IDO upregulates regulatory T cells via tryptophan catabolite and suppresses encephalitogenic T cell responses in experimental autoimmune encephalomyelitis. J Immunol 185:5953–5961

Yang ZZ, Novak AJ, Ziesmer SC, Witzig TE, Ansell SM (2006) Attenuation of CD8(+) T-cell function by CD4(+)CD25(+) regulatory T cells in B-cell non-Hodgkin's lymphoma. Cancer Res 66:10145–10152

Yu F, Sharma S, Edwards J, Feigenbaum L, Zhu J (2015) Dynamic expression of transcription factors T-bet and GATA-3 by regulatory T cells maintains immunotolerance. Nat Immunol 16:197–206

Yurchenko E et al (2006) CCR5-dependent homing of naturally occurring CD4+ regulatory T cells to sites of Leishmania major infection favors pathogen persistence. J Exp Med 203:2451–2460

Zeiser R, Nguyen VH, Beilhack A, Buess M, Schulz S, Baker J, Contag CH, Negrin RS (2006) Inhibition of CD4+CD25+ regulatory T cell function by calcineurin dependent interleukin-2 production. Blood 108:390–399

Zeiser R et al (2007) Early CD30 signaling is critical for adoptively transferred CD4+CD25+ regulatory T cells in prevention of acute graft-versus-host disease. Blood 109:2225–2233

Zeiser R et al (2008) Differential impact of mammalian target of rapamycin inhibition on CD4+CD25+Foxp3+ regulatory T cells compared with conventional CD4+ T cells. Blood 111:453–462

Zeiser R, Penack O, Holler E, Idzko M (2011) Danger signals activating innate immunity in graft-versus-host disease. J Mol Med (Berl) 89:833–845

Zhang P et al (2013) Induced regulatory T cells promote tolerance when stabilized by rapamycin and IL-2 in vivo. J Immunol 191:5291–5303

Zhao DM, Thornton AM, DiPaolo RJ, Shevach EM (2006) Activated CD4+CD25+ T cells selectively kill B lymphocytes. Blood 107:3925–3932

Zheng Y et al (2009) Regulatory T-cell suppressor program co-opts transcription factor IRF4 to control T(H)2 responses. Nature 458:351–356

Part III

Beyond T-Cells

Natural Killer Cells: What Have We Learned?

10

Dhifaf Sarhan and Jeffery S. Miller

10.1 Introduction

Before their discovery in the 1970s, NK cells were originally interpreted as an artifact. Subsequently, they were recognized as essential immune effectors capable of fighting viral infections and cancer. Studies in transgenic mouse models established that NK cells play an important role in immune surveillance against tumors. Many approaches using NK cells as cancer immunotherapy have since been proposed. NK cell antitumor activity is best demonstrated in patients with myeloid leukemia. Many challenges persist when considering NK cell therapy for more common solid tumors. Our group hypothesizes that inhibitory checkpoints in the tumor microenvironment may explain some of the barriers to successful treatment in such patients using NK cells.

NK cells are components of the innate immune system. Their functional behavior is classically described as a result of a balance between inhibitory and activating receptor signaling. Unlike T cells and B cells, NK cells do not express germ-line rearranged antigen-specific receptors. NK cells comprise 15% of peripheral blood mononuclear cells (PBMC). The majority of circulating blood NK cells are $CD56^{dim}$. These cells express the potent activation receptor FcRγIII (CD16) and exhibit potent cytotoxicity without activation or prior exposure (Fig. 10.1, left panel). A second major NK cell subset is defined by high-density CD56 ($CD56^{bright}$), lack of CD16,

D. Sarhan
Department of Microbiology, Tumour and Cell Biology, Karolinska Institutet, Stockholm, Sweden
e-mail: dhifaf.sarhan@ki.se

J. S. Miller (✉)
Adult and Pediatric Blood and Marrow Transplant Program, University of Minnesota Cancer Center, Minneapolis, MN, USA
e-mail: mille011@umn.edu

M.-A. Perales et al. (eds.), *Cell and Gene Therapies*, Advances and Controversies in Hematopoietic Transplantation and Cell Therapy,
https://doi.org/10.1007/978-3-319-54368-0_10

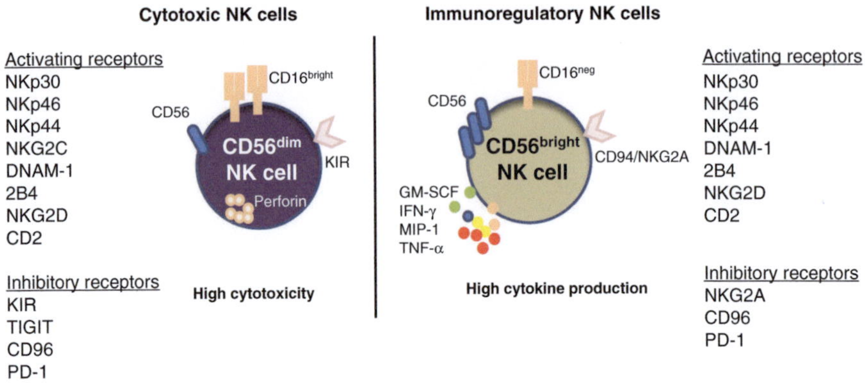

Fig. 10.1 Two major subsets of NK cells found in human blood have different functional properties and receptor expression (printed with permission)

and high proliferative potential with unique regulatory function to produce cytokines (Fig. 10.1, right panel). NK cell recognition is defined by "missing-self" human leukocyte antigen (HLA) that is downregulated after viral infection or malignant transformation as well as a collection of activation receptor interactions that differ between tumor types. Therefore, the final determinant of NK cell attack is the net sum of these activation and inhibitory interactions.

10.2 NK Cell Biology and Function

10.2.1 MHC I-Dependent Regulation of NK Cells

NK cell function is regulated by the interaction between killer-cell immunoglobulin-like receptors (KIRs) and class I MHC molecules on target cells. Killing by lack of MHC recognition is referred to as the "missing-self hypothesis" (Fig. 10.2a, b) (Karre et al. 1986; Ljunggren and Karre 1985). All resting blood NK cells are presumed to express at least one inhibitory receptor that is ligated by self-MHC class I in order to mediate tolerance (Valiante et al. 1997). Greater tolerance in NK cells was shown to correlate with expression of all inhibitory KIR. These receptors are expressed on human chromosome 19 independent of cognate HLA ligands expressed on human chromosome 6. This makes KIR expression stochastic (Andersson et al. 2009). Inhibitory KIR bind to HLA-A, HLA-B, or HLA-C to initiate a cascade of signals through their long cytoplasmic tails, containing tyrosine-based inhibitory motifs that are phosphorylated upon crosslinking and deliver inhibitory signals to NK cells (Thielens et al. 2012; Binstadt et al. 1996). Some activating KIR (e.g., KIR2DS1) can also ligate MHC I molecules, but many of the activating KIR ligands remain unknown. These receptors are characterized by having a short cytoplasmic tail with ITAM-bearing subunits linked to DAP12 signaling molecules associated with the recruitment of SYK and ZAP70 protein tyrosine kinases resulting in NK

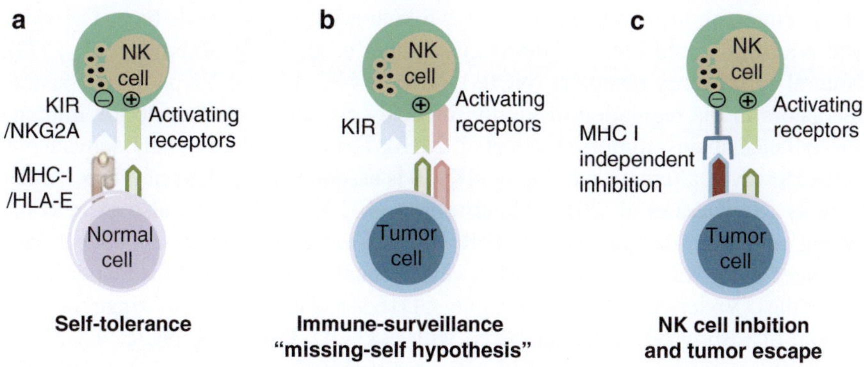

Fig. 10.2 NK cell function is regulated by the interaction between the killer-cell immunoglobulin-like receptors (KIRs) and class I MHC molecules on target cells. Alternatively, self-tolerance is regulated by the interaction of NKG2A and HLA-E. Killing by lack of MHC recognition is referred to as the "missing-self hypothesis." However, NK cells are still inhibited by incomplete or variable HLA downregulation in tumor cells and other potent NK cell inhibitory checkpoint pathways (e.g., PD-1 and CD96/TIGIT) (printed with permission)

cell activation (Lanier et al. 1998). Besides KIR, there are other receptors binding to MHC I molecules. These include the inhibitory receptor NKG2A that binds HLA-E and the activating receptor NKG2C that binds HLA-E with lower affinity (Tomasec et al. 2000; Wada et al. 2004). NKG2A is downregulated on NK cells in adults compared to newborns (Manser and Uhrberg 2016). It is also less expressed in terminal differentiated NK cells (Beziat et al. 2010). NK cells that lack the expression of all inhibitory receptors are hyporesponsive with poor cytotoxicity and reduced IFNγ production (Cooley et al. 2007). NKG2A expression contributes to NK cell tolerance when cells express low levels of KIR to maintain mature function (Bjorklund et al. 2010). Therefore, NK cells require inhibitory receptor ligation for tolerance and to acquire and maintain their normal function.

10.2.2 MHC I-Independent Regulation of NK Cells

NK cells encode a variety of activating and inhibitory receptors that regulate their function independent of HLA interactions. NKG2D is expressed on the surface of NK cells and binds the stress-induced nonclassical MHC molecules MICA/B and ULBP1–6 to induce NK cell cytolytic activity (Lanier 2005). DNAM-1, CD96, and the inhibitory receptors T cell immunoreceptor with immunoglobulin and ITIM domains (TIGIT) are also regulatory receptors that play a role in controlling killing and adhesion. All three receptors ligate the poliovirus receptor (PVR [CD155]) and Nectins and nectin-like proteins (nectin-2 [CD112]). CD96 and TIGIT compete with DNAM-1 for binding to CD155 resulting in NK cell inhibition (Chan et al. 2014). While many activating receptors including NKG2D, DNAM-1, CD2, and 2B4 are unable to induce NK cell cytotoxicity in resting NK cells when triggered alone, engaging the same receptors in cytokine-activated NK cells (e.g., DNAM-1 and NKG2D) could induce cytotoxicity (Bauer et al. 1999; Shibuya et al. 1998). Natural cytotoxicity receptors (NCRs), NKp30, NKp44, and NKp46, are essential mediators in the regulation of virally infected cells and contribute to the immune surveillance against tumors (Koch et al. 2013). These receptors usually activate NK cells. However, alternate splicing of NKp30 is associated with loss of NK cell cytotoxicity (Siewiera et al. 2015; Mantovani et al. 2015). NK cells also express the potent activating receptor CD16 (FcRγIII) that controls antibody-dependent cell-mediated cytotoxicity (ADCC) by NK cells through recognition of the Fc portion of antibodies (Vivier et al. 1991). Engaging CD16 alone is sufficient to trigger degranulation of resting NK cells compared with NKG2D, DNAM-1, NCRs, CD2, and 2B4 that have to be combined with other activating signals (Bryceson et al. 2006, 2009). These discoveries explain why monoclonal antibodies targeting specific tumor antigens with good Fc binding have changed the practice of cancer therapy.

10.2.3 NK Cell Education and Tolerance

NK cells undergo education to tolerate self and avoid autoaggression. The process by which NK cells acquire function by ligation of inhibitory KIR interactions with class I MHC ligands is termed education (or licensing). Expressing KIR throughout NK cell development is critical for functional maturation (Elliott and Yokoyama 2011). Several hypotheses have been proposed for NK cell education, the first suggesting that NK cells are initially uneducated and KIR engagement with self-MHC I by different affinities during development results in competent effector cells (Kim et al. 2005). Alternatively, NK cells are initially active during development through in vivo stimulation as a result of constitutive expression of an activating ligand, but their activity gets downregulated after ligating cognate class I MHC. This process is referred to as the "disarming model." Thus, NK cells are rendered anergic in the absence of inhibitory receptor ligation (Gasser and Raulet 2006; Tripathy et al. 2008). In vivo studies show that NK cells developed in class I MHC-deficient mice are unable to reject tumor cells lacking the class I MHC expression and are hyporesponsive (Liao et al. 1991). In addition, NK cells that developed in a class I MHC-deficient environment acquire function and become quickly educated after infusion into mice that expressed normal class I MHC, thus demonstrating the considerable flexibility of NK cells to respond to their environment (Elliott et al. 2010; Belanger et al. 2012). However, the exact function of uneducated NK cells in the blood remains unknown. Those cells may simply be precursors awaiting a response from their environment or they may have specialized function. A study by Orr and colleagues suggests that depleting unlicensed NK cells in a CMV mouse model may diminish control of viral titers (Orr et al. 2010). A second study by Alvarez et al. showed that depleting host-licensed NK cells may result in increased donor engraftment, while donor engraftment is reduced after depletion of all NK cells (licensed and unlicensed), which suggests that unlicensed NK cells promote donor allogeneic engraftment by production of GM-CSF (Alvarez et al. 2016).

10.2.4 NK Cell Regulation by Cytokines

In the early 1980s, López-Botet's group demonstrated that interleukin-2 (IL-2)-containing supernatant induces strong proliferation of NK cells (Toribio et al. 1983). Subsequently, Brenner's group showed that IL-2-activated NK cells have augmented cytotoxicity against NK cell-resistant hairy cell leukemia targets (Cordingley et al. 1988). A decade later, the Caligiuri laboratory showed that IL-15 binds to the shared βγ subunits of the IL-2 receptor and induces proliferation, cytotoxicity, and cytokine production of NK cells (Carson et al. 1994). It is now established that IL-15Rα is expressed on dendritic cells (DC) to trans-present IL-15 to NK cells to promote proliferation, survival, and antitumoral activity (Ferlazzo et al. 2004; Van den Bergh et al. 2015). This physiologic signaling by IL-15 also regulates the homeostasis of NK cells. Recently, IL-15 was shown to induce activation of mTOR (mammalian target of rapamycin) to maintain NK cell metabolism. In addition, mTOR activation was shown to be specific to IL-15 stimulation and unresponsive to other cytokines including IL-18, IL-12, IFNβ, IL-7, and TGFβ (Marcais et al. 2014). However, Viel et al. showed that TGFβ suppressed NK cell function through an inhibition of mTOR signaling to a similar level as when inhibited with the mTOR-specific inhibitor rapamycin. Blocking TGFβ restored mTOR activity in response to IL-15 and IL-2 stimulation in NK cells (Viel et al. 2016). When use in cancer patients is contemplated, rapamycin treatment should be carefully assessed to avoid NK cell inhibition. Other cytokines like IL-12 and IL-18 are potent inducers of IFNγ production in NK cells by stabilization of IFN-gamma mRNA (Mavropoulos et al. 2005). These cytokines, when combined with IL-15 for 16 h, induce a unique activation signal for NK cells to survive and mediate an antitumor response (Ni et al. 2012; Leong et al. 2014).

10.2.5 NK Cell Memory and Adaptive Features

Although NK cells were felt to be short lived, emerging data in mice and humans suggests that NK cells possess characteristics of adaptive immunity and immunological memory. NK cell memory was first observed in a murine study showing that liver-resident NK cells could recall a secondary response against haptens independent of T and B cell responses. These Ly49C-I(+) NK cells (the Ly49 family in mice is analogous to KIR in humans) persisted for at least 4 weeks upon hapten restimulation (O'Leary et al. 2006). In 2009, Sun et al. demonstrated that a subpopulation of NK cells expressing the activating receptor Ly49H undergoes an antigen-specific expansion against the murine cytomegalovirus (MCMV) antigen m157, followed by contraction and then long-lived memory NK cells that persist over time. These NK cells exhibited enhanced effector function following rechallenge with MCMV (Sun et al. 2009). NK cells are important in controlling viral infections such as human cytomegalovirus (HCMV), Epstein-Barr virus (EBV), and human papillomavirus (HPV) (Orange 2002). Human NK cells do not express Ly49. Instead, a HCMV-responsive human NK cell subset has been characterized by the expression of the activating receptor NKG2C and the maturation marker CD57 (Guma et al. 2004). These NK cells are defined by epigenetic silencing of one or more of the signaling molecules SYK, EAT-2, and FcεRγ along with silencing of the transcription factor PLZF and are referred to as "adaptive NK cells." Adaptive NK cells exhibit a whole-genome methylation signature that is similar to effector $CD8^+$ T cells (Schlums et al. 2015; Wiencke et al. 2016). The expansion of the $NKG2C^+$ NK cells is not limited to autologous settings as these cells are found to expand after allogeneic transplantation in cancer patients who reactivate CMV (Foley et al. 2012). Current knowledge suggests that $NKG2C^+$ NK cells may be specific to CMV exposure as these cells do not expand in response to other viral antigens such as herpes simplex virus type 2 (HSV-2) or EBV (Bjorkstrom et al. 2011a; Hendricks et al. 2014). Mechanistically, NKG2C has not yet been shown to specifically bind CMV. Although a small percentage (4%) of all humans carry a homozygous deletion of the gene that encodes for NKG2C (NKG2C(−/−)), cells from these individuals still exhibit characteristics of adaptive NK cells functionally and by epigenetic remodeling (Liu et al. 2016). This suggests that NKG2C is either redundant or may not be directly involved with HCMV recognition. While the frequency of NK cells expressing NKG2C is reduced in correlation with a drop in anti-HCMV IgG titers (Goodier et al. 2014), other studies show that $NKG2C^+$ NK cells can expand in patients infected during an outbreak of hantavirus infection (Bjorkstrom et al. 2011b). In this Swedish cohort, almost all were CMV seropositive, making interactions unclear. Therefore, while adaptive NK cell responses are seen in the context of prior CMV exposure, they have not been shown to be CMV antigen-specific. Rather, they appear to be broadly primed for function when challenged with targets or ADCC when antibody-coated targets are involved.

10.3 Adoptive Cell Therapies

10.3.1 NK Cell Therapies in Hematological Malignancies

An abundance of clinical studies has been performed with the goal of stimulating autologous NK cells to target a variety of cancers. However, NK cells remain tolerant after autologous transplantation or adoptive transfer based on the premise that all NK cells contain at least one inhibitory KIR for MHC ligands expressed on residual tumor cells. In haploidentical transplantation, where the donor and recipient are matched for one HLA haplotype, 2/3 of patients would have at least one KIR ligand missing on the host cells, resulting in a reduced inhibition of donor NK cells and greater tumor kill. Donor selection for KIR-ligand incompatibility or KIR/KIR-ligand mismatch can result in superior disease-free survival for patients with myeloid malignancies after transplantation. Moreover, missing one or more KIR ligands, compared to the presence of all ligands, protected against relapse in patients with early myeloid leukemia (Miller et al. 2007). In 92 acute myeloid leukemia (AML) patients receiving haploidentical hematopoietic cell transplantation (HCT), donor KIR-ligand mismatching was the only independent predictor of survival

(Ruggeri et al. 2002). However, no beneficial effect of KIR-ligand mismatching was observed in acute lymphoblastic leukemia (ALL) (Ruggeri et al. 1999). Possible explanations include lack of class I-independent activating receptor ligands or differences in MHC expression levels on the blasts (Verheyden et al. 2009). In addition to the KIR incompatibility models in allogeneic HCT, other factors might play a role including donor KIR immunogenetics where different KIR gene clusters may predict clinical outcomes. KIR genes are divided into two haplotypes including haplotype A that consists mostly of inhibitory KIRs (KIR3DL3, KIR2DL3, KIR2DL1, KIR3DL1, and KIR2DL2) and one activating KIR (KIR2DS4). Alternatively, haplotype B involves up to five activating KIRs. Several studies have evaluated the impact of KIR haplotypes on clinical outcome, concluding that in AML but not in adult ALL patients, combinations of different KIR genes within the B haplotype including KIR2DS1, KIR2DS2, KIR2DS3, KIR2DS5, KIR3DS1, and KIR2DL5A are associated with relapse protection (McQueen et al. 2007; Stringaris et al. 2010; Cooley et al. 2009). While KIR-ligand incompatibility/mismatch and donor KIR immunogenetics clearly play a role in transplantation outcome, there is no data supporting this paradigm for NK cell adoptive transfer. A possible explanation may be activation and maturation differences between NK cells that reconstitute from stem cells versus the transient persistence of blood NK cells after infusion. Studies with bigger cohorts are required to re-examine these parameters and their association with clinical outcome using NK cell-based strategies.

For allogeneic adoptive transfer, lymphodepletion is used both to create space and to compete with endogenous cytokines for the donor cells to proliferate in vivo (Boni et al. 2008; Dudley et al. 2002). Adoptively transferred NK cells are expected to be transient without permanent engraftment and to require the need for cytokines like IL-2 or IL-15 to maintain their persistence, proliferation, and function. We have developed a clinical protocol that enables transferred haploidentical NK cells to expand in patients and persist for up to 1 month using high-dose cyclophosphamide and fludarabine (Hi-Cy/Flu). The persistence of adoptive transferred NK cells was believed to be a result of a surge in endogenous IL-15 found in the serum of AML patients in combination with low-dose IL-2 administered during the first 2 weeks after adoptive transfer (Miller et al. 2005). AML patients with advanced AML failing standard therapy were treated with haploidentical NK cell adoptive transfer ($n = 19$). Twenty-six percent ($n = 5$) demonstrated a complete remission (CR). This response correlated with persistence and in in vivo expansion. Additional patients were treated with this strategy ($n = 42$) and an update has been published (Bachanova et al. 2014).

10.3.2 NK Cell Therapies in Solid Tumors

Driven by the promise of NK cell therapy in AML, allogeneic NK cell adoptive transfer and IL-2 administration were tested with or without total-body irradiation (TBI) in recurrent metastatic breast and ovarian cancer. Although the lymphodepletion and IL-2 administration were the same as used in patients with AML, NK cells did not persist or expand in these patients. However, regulatory T cells (T_{reg}) were increased following 14 days of IL-2 infusion, possibly explaining the inhibition of NK cell expansion (Geller et al. 2011). A follow-up study in AML patients using IL-2 diphtheria toxin fusion protein (Ontak) to eliminate T_{reg} supports this interpretation. Compared to therapy without Ontak, T_{reg} numbers and T_{reg}-produced IL-35 were decreased and resulted in overall improved complete remission rates (53% vs 21%; $P = 0.02$) and disease-free survival (33% vs 5%; $P < 0.01$). This clinical response correlated with lower T_{reg} and a higher frequency of patients with NK cell persistence and in vivo expansion (Bachanova et al. 2014). These observations support the suppressive role of T_{reg} on adoptive transferred NK cells. In a small metastatic melanoma and renal cell carcinoma trial, autologous NK cells infusions and IL-2 appeared to persist transiently but could not induce tumor regression. These NK cells could not lyse tumor cells and had lower expression of the activation receptor NKG2D, unless reactivated with exogenous IL-2. Nevertheless, evaluation of NK cells after infusion could still mediate antibody-dependent cell-mediated cytotoxicity (ADCC) without exogenous IL-2 suggesting that NK cell adoptive transfer could be more effective against solid tumors in a combination with antibody treatment (Parkhurst et al. 2011).

Using a different strategy, the NK-92 cell line has also been tested in a phase I clinical trial in patients with advanced solid tumors. Outcomes showed that even with the highest dose of infusion, 12 of 15 tested patients demonstrated disease progression. However, one patient with non-small cell lung cancer had a stable disease and two with small cell lung cancer experienced mixed response (Tonn et al. 2013). Genetic engineering of NK-92 to express ErbB2-chimeric antigen receptor (CAR) has been developed and tested in a preclinical glioblastoma model with good antitumor effects (Zhang et al. 2016). Despite these encouraging results, clinical testing of NK cells in solid tumors remains limited. Preclinical studies suggest that limitations such as immune-suppressive cells, immune-suppressive cytokines, and inhibitory checkpoints on NK cells need to be considered to achieve efficacy in solid tumors with NK cell-based therapies (Fig. 10.2c).

10.3.3 Other Approaches for Cell Therapies

Allogeneic adoptive transfer studies conclude that persistence and expansion of NK cells correlate with clinical efficacy. One way to better promote in vivo expansion and persistence is to use better cytokines such as IL-15 or trans-presented superagonist IL-15 complexes, an approach that is under study at the University of Minnesota (ClinicalTrials.gov identifier: NCT01885897 and NCT02395822). Another approach is to develop protocols for ex vivo expansion of NK cells. While PBMC is a convenient source for this approach, hematopoietic stem cells (HSC, $CD34^{+}$) from placenta or umbilical cord blood and even unlimited human-induced pluripotent stem cells (iPSC) are being considered.

While technically more challenging, these approaches are under development for clinical implementation. NK cells are known to best expand with accessory cells. In the early 1990s, we demonstrated the importance of contact with accessory cell monocytes for NK cell expansion from PBMC (Miller et al. 1992). Several other expansion protocols were tested utilizing different irradiated feeder cells including K562-IL-15/4-1BBL (Shah et al. 2015), K562-IL-21/4-1BBL (Liu et al. 2013), or Epstein-Barr virus-transformed lymphoblastoid cells (Berg et al. 2009) to expand blood-derived NK cells. Spanholtz and Dolstra's group have been developing a stroma-free clinical grade NK cell product form UCB $CD34^+$ in the presence of IL-15 and IL-12 resulting in highly pure, mature functional NK cells in high numbers (Spanholtz et al. 2011; Cany et al. 2015), which still needs definitive clinical testing.

10.4 NK Cell Dysfunction in Cancer

Tumor cells have multiple mechanisms to escape the immune system. One of the well-known tumor escape mechanisms for NK cells is the shedding of the NKG2D ligands on tumor cells that may result in impaired cytotoxicity (Salih et al. 2002). NKG2D ligand shedding has been explained by the high proteolytic and hypoxic activities of the tumor cells and the tumor microenvironment (Waldhauer and Steinle 2006; Siemens et al. 2008). Tumor stroma cells are a major source to support tumor growth and metastasis. In fact, NK cell function is frequently suppressed in the tumor microenvironment not only by tumor cells but also by the suppression of a complex system that is orchestrated by immune-suppressive compartments like myeloid-derived suppressor cells (MDSCs), T_{reg}, and stromal cells such as mesenchymal stem cells (Li et al. 2009; Wolf et al. 2003; Vasold et al. 2015). The tumor microenvironment generates a solid pressure on the immune effector cells, resulting in their hypofunction and ineffective responses against tumors. For example, MDSCs are increased in patients with different types of cancer and associated with poor prognosis (Poschke et al. 2010; Xu et al. 2016; Chen et al. 2014). In addition, sustained suppression by MDSC on T cells and NK cells was explained by MDSC secretion of immune-regulatory factors like TGFβ and nitric oxygen (NO) (Sevko et al. 2013; Mao et al. 2014). T_{reg} are identified as $CD3^+CD4^+CD127^-CD25^{high}FOXP3^+$ and could suppress NK cell responses by IL-2 deprivation and also through TGFβ secretion (Wang et al. 2010; Ghiringhelli et al. 2006). T_{reg} expansion and increased activities in patients with cancer correlate with poor prognosis (Wolf et al. 2005; Shenghui et al. 2011). Adding to all the suppressive factors in the tumor microenvironment, both tumor cells and immune-suppressive cells express several inhibitory ligands for the immune effector checkpoints including programmed death ligand 1 (PD-L1) and CTLA-4 (Curran et al. 2010). In summary, the tumor microenvironment plays a critical role in NK cell antitumor responses that could explain their dysfunction in patients with cancer (Fig. 10.3).

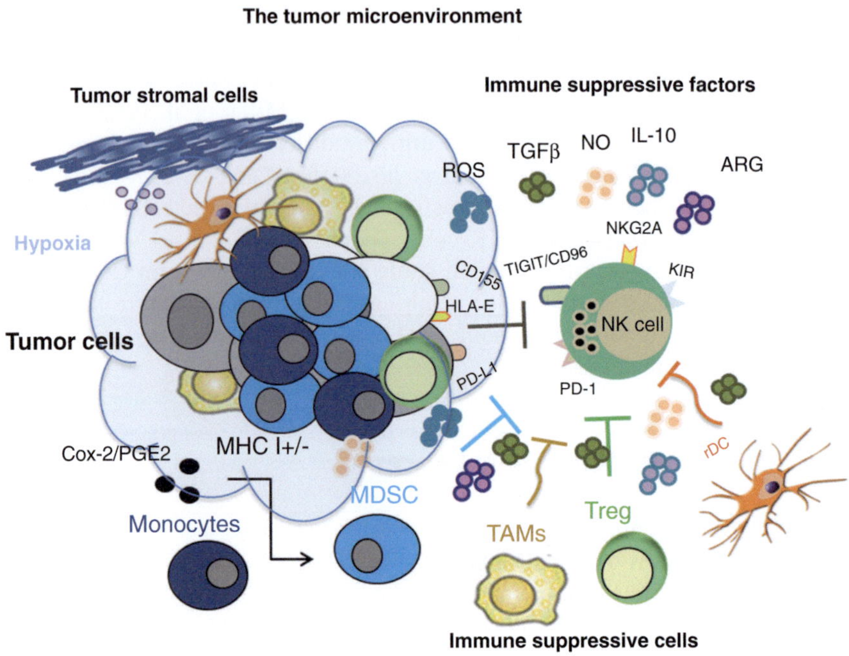

Fig. 10.3 The tumor microenvironment is a complex system associated with suppressed NK cell function. This system is tightly regulated by immune-suppressive compartments that inhibit NK cell function through suppressive cytokines and through contact-dependent mechanisms. The immune-suppressive compartments include myeloid-derived suppressor cells (MDSCs), tumor-associated macrophages (TAMs), regulatory dendritic cells (rDC), regulatory T cells (T_{reg}), killer-cell immunoglobulin-like receptor (KIR), T-cell immunoglobulin and ITIM domain (TIGIT), and contact-independent factors such as IL-10, TGFβ, nitric oxide (NO), reactive oxygen species (ROS), arginase (ARG), and the general hypoxic tumor milieu (printed with permission)

10.5 NK Cell Preclinical Therapies

10.5.1 Innovative Antibody Therapies Targeting NK Cell Activation

Many preclinical NK cell studies show promising results worthy of clinical testing. Besides NK cell adoptive transfer, few therapies targeting NK cell activation have been tested in clinical trials, and no NK cell therapy approach is Food and Drug Administration (FDA) approved. However, in the past decade, antibody therapies for cancer have changed the practice of cancer care, and many of these approaches work in part through NK cells. New antibody treatments targeting different T cell inhibitory checkpoints have shown remarkable clinical success. Unfortunately, very little is known how these influence NK cell responses. Specific checkpoint inhibitors and other antibody therapies have been manufactured and investigated. Examples include targeting inhibitory KIR to prevent tolerance of

NK cells to patient tumor. Preclinical and clinical studies in AML and multiple myeloma show that the monoclonal anti-KIR restores NK cell function when tested ex vivo and that the treatment is safe and does not induce autoimmunity. However, no objective responses have yet been seen after infusion of anti-KIR antibodies alone (Vey et al. 2012; Benson et al. 2012; Korde et al. 2014). Similarly, NKG2A blocking antibodies have been developed and may prove useful in the clinic if supporting data emerges.

In our laboratory, we have developed bi- or tri-specific killer engagers (BiKEs or TriKEs) as a non-gene therapy approach to make NK cells antigen-specific. These specific engagers are constructed by DNA fragments from two fully humanized single-chain fragment variable (scFv) antibodies recognizing CD16 on NK cells and also a tumor target antigen like CD33, CD19, CD133, and CD22 to facilitate an immunological synapse. One advantage of BiKEs and TriKEs is that they bind CD16 with high-affinity compared to low-affinity Fc binding of whole antibodies. Gleason et al. showed that healthy PBMC and CD33xCD16 BiKE augmented the ability to kill cytokine-induced MDSCs and the $CD33^+$ human acute promyelocytic leukemia cell line HL-60 (Gleason et al. 2014). In the TriKE, we have added IL-15 to maintain NK cell proliferation and persistence (Gleason et al. 2012, 2014; Vallera et al. 2016; Schmohl et al. 2015). CD16xIL-15xCD33 TriKE proved to be more potent than CD16xCD33 BiKE. NK cells targeted with TriKE produced significantly more pro-inflammatory cytokines IFNγ, TNFα, and GM-CSF and the chemokine MIP1α when cultured with $CD33^+$ targets. These NK cells proliferated, had better survival, and had greater cytolytic activity against primary AML blasts than NK cells and BiKE. In an in vivo xenograft model of AML (HL-60), NK cells infused together with the CD16xIL-15xCD33 TriKE were best at controlling AML growth after 21 days. This response correlated the in vivo function of the modified IL-15 linker that promoted the persistence, expansion, and function of NK cells (Vallera et al. 2016). Thus, TriKE have the potential to be an effective cancer treatment by increasing the specificity of NK cell antitumor activity and enhancing in vivo persistence and in vivo expansion of NK cells. However, it is still unknown whether TriKE can activate heavily suppressed NK cells in cancer patients or whether adoptive transfer will still be needed.

10.5.2 Targeting Adaptive NK Cells for Immunotherapy in Cancer

CMV past exposure is associated with the presence of a population of $NKG2C^+CD57^+$ NK cells in CMV seropositive individuals. Following CMV reactivation in patients with hematological malignancies ($n = 674$) that underwent allogeneic hematopoietic cell transplantation (HCT), higher absolute numbers of $CD56^{dim}NKG2C^+CD57^+$ NK cells were found to correlate with lower disease relapse (26% [17–35%], $p = 0.05$) and greater disease-free survival (DFS) (55% [45–65%] $p = 0.04$) (Cichocki et al. 2016). Collectively, CMV has a powerful effect on shaping the NK cell repertoire to enhance persistence, survival, and function. This knowledge provides the motivation to develop strategies to expand adaptive NK cells for clinical therapy. Investigations are in progress. These adaptive NK cells will be particularly useful with the CD16-targeted approaches discussed above with whole antibodies, BiKEs and TriKEs. In another approach, specific cytokine stimulation cocktails could induce NK cells that also have memory-like properties. Compared to IL-15 activation alone, IL-15, IL-18, and IL-12 overnight activation resulted in long-term production of IFNγ by NK cells (more than 4 weeks but less than 12 months) after adoptive transfer in mice (Leong et al. 2014; Cooper et al. 2009). A clinical trial in humans is ongoing with cytokine-induced memory-like NK cells in advanced AML and myelodysplastic syndrome patients (ClinicalTrials.gov identifier: NCT01898793).

10.5.3 Targeting NK Cell Checkpoint Inhibitors

Other strategies to improve NK cell antitumor activity have been proposed including blocking novel inhibitory checkpoints involving NK cells. Blake et al. demonstrated that $CD96^{-/-}$ transgenic mice had significantly fewer lung metastases in three different tumor models including lung, prostate carcinoma, and melanoma. A dose-dependent beneficial effect of blockade between the inhibitory receptor CD96 and its ligand CD155 was also observed. Additionally, their data showed that combining anti-PD1 blockade together with anti-CD96 is more powerful in reducing lung metastases than either alone, resulting in enhanced NK cell IFNγ production (Blake et al. 2016). The FDA has approved two cancer immunotherapy checkpoints for patients with advanced melanoma: ipilimumab against CTLA-4 in 2011 and nivolumab and pembrolizumab against programmed death 1 (PD-1) in 2014. Other PD-1 and PD-L1 antibodies are also being developed. Interestingly, anti-PD-L1 may also have a dual role by mediating ADCC against $PD\text{-}L1^{+}$ targets (Boyerinas et al. 2015). A study showed that NK cells derived from multiple myeloma (MM) patients have increased PD-1 expression on NK cells compared to healthy controls and blocking the PD-1/PD-L1 axis enhanced NK cell cytotoxicity against autologous MM cells (Benson et al. 2010). These findings suggest that blocking the inhibitory checkpoints of NK cells may improve their antitumor activity. Clinical trials are needed to corroborate this possibility.

10.6 Expert Point of View

A balance between activating and inhibitory receptors tightly regulates NK cells. However, inhibition of NK cell responses needs to be controlled to promote efficacious responses against established tumors. Through extensive research we have learned that adoptive NK cell transfer in AML patients can generate complete remission and prolonged survival but also that their clinical effect is diminished by the suppression of T_{reg} increased in the blood of cancer patients. We have also learned that adoptive transfer of NK cells may be different in patients with solid tumors. Barriers to therapeutic efficacy may be explained by the suppressive tumor microenvironment on NK cells. It is possible that adaptive/memory-like NK cells will better persist in vivo, making them therapeutically useful, especially in combination with enhanced specificity through the Fc receptor CD16. However, these strategies alone may be insufficient as a result of the complex immune-suppressive tumor microenvironment. The best IL-15 strategy to enhance adoptive transfer or facilitate endogenous NK cells in cancer patients remains undetermined. Lastly, known and newly recognized checkpoint inhibitors specifically targeting the inhibitory receptors CD96 and PD-1 on NK cells may strengthen many of the approaches discussed in this chapter.

10.7 Future Directions

Although NK cells are "natural" in targeting tumor cells and play an important role in the immune surveillance against tumors, the probability of NK cells eliminating well-established tumors is low without strategies to increase their activity. The tumor suppression mechanisms of the immune system are complex. Targeting only one suppressive pathway of NK cells may be inadequate. Currently, immunotherapy is focused on targeting individual immune checkpoints. However we expect that future immunotherapies will combine therapies to target more than one suppressive factor and more than one tumor-specific antigen to enhance tumor recognition. As our healthy immune cells have many regulatory elements to avoid autoaggression, malignantly transformed cells adapt to these mechanisms. Combinatorial approaches hold promise to overcome these problems.

References

Alvarez M, Sun K, Murphy WJ (2016) Mouse host unlicensed NK cells promote donor allogeneic bone marrow engraftment. Blood 127(9):1202–1205. https://doi.org/10.1182/blood-2015-08-665570

Andersson S, Fauriat C, Malmberg JA, Ljunggren HG, Malmberg KJ (2009) KIR acquisition probabilities are independent of self-HLA class I ligands and increase with cellular KIR expression. Blood 114(1):95–104. https://doi.org/10.1182/blood-2008-10-184549

Bachanova V, Cooley S, Defor TE, Verneris MR, Zhang B, McKenna DH, Curtsinger J, Panoskaltsis-Mortari A, Lewis D, Hippen K, McGlave P, Weisdorf DJ, Blazar BR, Miller JS (2014) Clearance of acute myeloid leukemia by haploidentical natural killer cells is improved using IL-2 diphtheria toxin fusion protein. Blood 123(25):3855–3863. https://doi.org/10.1182/blood-2013-10-532531

Bauer S, Groh V, Wu J, Steinle A, Phillips JH, Lanier LL, Spies T (1999) Activation of NK cells and T cells by NKG2D, a receptor for stress-inducible MICA. Science 285(5428):727–729

Belanger S, Tu MM, Rahim MM, Mahmoud AB, Patel R, Tai LH, Troke AD, Wilhelm BT, Landry JR, Zhu Q, Tung KS, Raulet DH, Makrigiannis AP (2012) Impaired natural killer cell self-education and "missing-self" responses in Ly49-deficient mice. Blood 120(3):592–602. https://doi.org/10.1182/blood-2012-02-408732

Benson DM Jr, Bakan CE, Mishra A, Hofmeister CC, Efebera Y, Becknell B, Baiocchi RA, Zhang J, Yu J, Smith MK, Greenfield CN, Porcu P, Devine SM, Rotem-Yehudar R, Lozanski G, Byrd JC, Caligiuri MA (2010) The PD-1/PD-L1 axis modulates the natural killer cell versus multiple myeloma effect: a therapeutic target for CT-011, a novel monoclonal anti-PD-1 antibody. Blood 116(13):2286–2294. https://doi.org/10.1182/blood-2010-02-271874

Benson DM Jr, Hofmeister CC, Padmanabhan S, Suvannasankha A, Jagannath S, Abonour R, Bakan C, Andre P, Efebera Y, Tiollier J, Caligiuri MA, Farag SS (2012) A phase 1 trial of the anti-KIR antibody IPH2101 in patients with relapsed/refractory multiple myeloma. Blood 120(22):4324–4333. https://doi.org/10.1182/blood-2012-06-438028

Berg M, Lundqvist A, McCoy P Jr, Samsel L, Fan Y, Tawab A, Childs R (2009) Clinical-grade ex vivo-expanded human natural killer cells up-regulate activating receptors and death receptor ligands and have enhanced cytolytic activity against tumor cells. Cytotherapy 11(3):341–355. https://doi.org/10.1080/14653240902807034

Beziat V, Descours B, Parizot C, Debre P, Vieillard V (2010) NK cell terminal differentiation: correlated stepwise decrease of NKG2A and acquisition of KIRs. PLoS One 5(8):e11966. https://doi.org/10.1371/journal.pone.0011966

Binstadt BA, Brumbaugh KM, Dick CJ, Scharenberg AM, Williams BL, Colonna M, Lanier LL, Kinet JP, Abraham RT, Leibson PJ (1996) Sequential involvement of Lck and SHP-1 with MHC-recognizing receptors on NK cells inhibits FcR-initiated tyrosine kinase activation. Immunity 5(6):629–638

Bjorklund AT, Schaffer M, Fauriat C, Ringden O, Remberger M, Hammarstedt C, Barrett AJ, Ljungman P, Ljunggren HG, Malmberg KJ (2010) NK cells expressing inhibitory KIR for non-self-ligands remain tolerant in HLA-matched sibling stem cell transplantation. Blood 115(13):2686–2694. https://doi.org/10.1182/blood-2009-07-229740

Bjorkstrom NK, Svensson A, Malmberg KJ, Eriksson K, Ljunggren HG (2011a) Characterization of natural killer cell phenotype and function during recurrent human HSV-2 infection. PLoS One 6(11):e27664. https://doi.org/10.1371/journal.pone.0027664

Bjorkstrom NK, Lindgren T, Stoltz M, Fauriat C, Braun M, Evander M, Michaelsson J, Malmberg KJ, Klingstrom J, Ahlm C, Ljunggren HG (2011b) Rapid expansion and long-term persistence of elevated NK cell numbers in humans infected with hantavirus. J Exp Med 208(1):13–21. https://doi.org/10.1084/jem.20100762

Blake SJ, Stannard K, Liu J, Allen S, Yong MC, Mittal D, Roman Aguilera A, Miles JJ, Lutzky VP, Ferrari de Andrade L, Martinet L, Colonna M, Takeda K, Kuhnel F, Gurlevik E, Bernhardt G, Teng MW, Smyth MJ (2016) Suppression of metastases using a new lymphocyte checkpoint target for cancer immunotherapy. Cancer Discov 6(4):446–459. https://doi.org/10.1158/2159-8290.CD-15-0944

Boni A, Muranski P, Cassard L, Wrzesinski C, Paulos CM, Palmer DC, Gattinoni L, Hinrichs CS, Chan CC, Rosenberg SA, Restifo NP (2008) Adoptive transfer of allogeneic tumor-specific T cells mediates effective regression of large tumors across major histocompatibility barriers. Blood 112(12):4746–4754. https://doi.org/10.1182/blood-2008-07-169797

Boyerinas B, Jochems C, Fantini M, Heery CR, Gulley JL, Tsang KY, Schlom J (2015) Antibody-dependent cellular cytotoxicity activity of a novel Anti-PD-L1 antibody Avelumab (MSB0010718C) on human tumor cells. Cancer Immunol Res 3(10):1148–1157. https://doi.org/10.1158/2326-6066.CIR-15-0059

Bryceson YT, March ME, Ljunggren HG, Long EO (2006) Synergy among receptors on resting NK cells for the activation of natural cytotoxicity and cytokine secretion. Blood 107(1):159–166. https://doi.org/10.1182/blood-2005-04-1351

Bryceson YT, Ljunggren HG, Long EO (2009) Minimal requirement for induction of natural cytotoxicity and intersection of activation signals by inhibitory receptors. Blood 114(13):2657–2666. https://doi.org/10.1182/blood-2009-01-201632

Cany J, van der Waart AB, Spanholtz J, Tordoir M, Jansen JH, van der Voort R, Schaap NM, Dolstra H (2015) Combined IL-15 and IL-12 drives the generation of CD34-derived natural killer cells with superior maturation and alloreactivity potential following adoptive transfer. Oncoimmunology 4(7):e1017701. https://doi.org/10.1080/2162402X.2015.1017701

Carson WE, Giri JG, Lindemann MJ, Linett ML, Ahdieh M, Paxton R, Anderson D, Eisenmann J, Grabstein K, Caligiuri MA (1994) Interleukin (IL) 15 is a novel cytokine that activates human natural killer cells via components of the IL-2 receptor. J Exp Med 180(4):1395–1403. https://doi.org/10.1084/jem.180.4.1395

Chan CJ, Martinet L, Gilfillan S, Souza-Fonseca-Guimaraes F, Chow MT, Town L, Ritchie DS, Colonna M, Andrews DM, Smyth MJ (2014) The receptors CD96 and CD226 oppose each other in the regulation of natural killer cell functions. Nat Immunol 15(5):431–438. https://doi.org/10.1038/ni.2850

Chen MF, Kuan FC, Yen TC, Lu MS, Lin PY, Chung YH, Chen WC, Lee KD (2014) IL-6-stimulated CD11b+ CD14+ HLA-DR- myeloid-derived suppressor cells, are associated with progression and poor prognosis in squamous cell carcinoma of the esophagus. Oncotarget 5(18):8716–8728. https://doi.org/10.18632/oncotarget.2368

Cichocki F, Cooley S, Davis Z, DeFor TE, Schlums H, Zhang B, Brunstein CG, Blazar BR, Wagner J, Diamond DJ, Verneris MR, Bryceson YT, Weisdorf DJ, Miller JS (2016) CD56(dim) CD57(+)NKG2C(+) NK cell expansion is associated with reduced leukemia relapse after reduced intensity HCT. Leukemia 30(2):456–463. https://doi.org/10.1038/leu.2015.260

Cooley S, Xiao F, Pitt M, Gleason M, McCullar V, Bergemann TL, McQueen KL, Guethlein LA, Parham P, Miller JS (2007) A subpopulation of human peripheral blood NK cells that lacks inhibitory receptors for self-MHC is developmentally immature. Blood 110(2):578–586. https://doi.org/10.1182/blood-2006-07-036228

Cooley S, Trachtenberg E, Bergemann TL, Saeteurn K, Klein J, Le CT, Marsh SG, Guethlein LA, Parham P, Miller JS, Weisdorf DJ (2009) Donors with group B KIR haplotypes improve relapse-free survival after unrelated hematopoietic cell transplantation for acute myelogenous leukemia. Blood 113(3):726–732. https://doi.org/10.1182/blood-2008-07-171926

Cooper MA, Elliott JM, Keyel PA, Yang L, Carrero JA, Yokoyama WM (2009) Cytokine-induced memory-like natural killer cells. Proc Natl Acad Sci U S A 106(6):1915–1919. https://doi.org/10.1073/pnas.0813192106

Cordingley FT, Hoffbrand AV, Brenner MK (1988) Cytokine-induced enhancement of the susceptibility of hairy cell leukaemia lymphocytes to natural killer cell lysis. Br J Haematol 70(1):37–41

Curran MA, Montalvo W, Yagita H, Allison JP (2010) PD-1 and CTLA-4 combination blockade expands infiltrating T cells and reduces regulatory T and myeloid cells within B16 melanoma tumors. Proc Natl Acad Sci U S A 107(9):4275–4280. https://doi.org/10.1073/pnas.0915174107

Dudley ME, Wunderlich JR, Robbins PF, Yang JC, Hwu P, Schwartzentruber DJ, Topalian SL, Sherry R, Restifo NP, Hubicki AM, Robinson MR, Raffeld M, Duray P, Seipp CA, Rogers-Freezer L, Morton KE, Mavroukakis SA, White DE, Rosenberg SA (2002) Cancer regression and autoimmunity in patients after clonal repopulation with antitumor lymphocytes. Science 298(5594):850–854. https://doi.org/10.1126/science.1076514

Elliott JM, Yokoyama WM (2011) Unifying concepts of MHC-dependent natural killer cell education. Trends Immunol 32(8):364–372. https://doi.org/10.1016/j.it.2011.06.001

Elliott JM, Wahle JA, Yokoyama WM (2010) MHC class I-deficient natural killer cells acquire a licensed phenotype after transfer into an MHC class I-sufficient environment. J Exp Med 207(10):2073–2079. https://doi.org/10.1084/jem.20100986

Ferlazzo G, Pack M, Thomas D, Paludan C, Schmid D, Strowig T, Bougras G, Muller WA, Moretta L, Münz C (2004) Distinct roles of IL-12 and IL-15 in human natural killer cell activation by dendritic cells from secondary lymphoid organs. Proc Natl Acad Sci U S A 101(47):16606–16611. https://doi.org/10.1073/pnas.0407522101

Foley B, Cooley S, Verneris MR, Curtsinger J, Luo X, Waller EK, Anasetti C, Weisdorf D, Miller JS (2012) Human cytomegalovirus (CMV)-induced memory-like NKG2C(+) NK cells are transplantable and expand in vivo in response to recipient CMV antigen. J Immunol 189(10):5082–5088. https://doi.org/10.4049/jimmunol.1201964

Gasser S, Raulet DH (2006) Activation and self-tolerance of natural killer cells. Immunol Rev 214:130–142. https://doi.org/10.1111/j.1600-065X.2006.00460.x

Geller MA, Cooley S, Judson PL, Ghebre R, Carson LF, Argenta PA, Jonson AL, Panoskaltsis-Mortari A, Curtsinger J, McKenna D, Dusenbery K, Bliss R, Downs LS, Miller JS (2011) A phase II study of allogeneic natural killer cell therapy to treat patients with recurrent ovarian and breast cancer. Cytotherapy 13(1):98–107. https://doi.org/10.3109/14653249.2010.515582

Ghiringhelli F, Menard C, Martin F, Zitvogel L (2006) The role of regulatory T cells in the control of natural killer cells: relevance during tumor progression. Immunol Rev 214:229–238. https://doi.org/10.1111/j.1600-065X.2006.00445.x

Gleason MK, Verneris MR, Todhunter DA, Zhang B, McCullar V, Zhou SX, Panoskaltsis-Mortari A, Weiner LM, Vallera DA, Miller JS (2012) Bispecific and trispecific killer cell engagers directly activate human NK cells through CD16 signaling and induce cytotoxicity and cytokine production. Mol Cancer Ther 11(12):2674–2684. https://doi.org/10.1158/1535-7163.MCT-12-0692

Gleason MK, Ross JA, Warlick ED, Lund TC, Verneris MR, Wiernik A, Spellman S, Haagenson MD, Lenvik AJ, Litzow MR, Epling-Burnette PK, Blazar BR, Weiner LM, Weisdorf DJ, Vallera DA, Miller JS (2014) CD16xCD33 bispecific killer cell engager (BiKE) activates NK cells against primary MDS and MDSC CD33+ targets. Blood 123(19):3016–3026. https://doi.org/10.1182/blood-2013-10-533398

Goodier MR, White MJ, Darboe A, Nielsen CM, Goncalves A, Bottomley C, Moore SE, Riley EM (2014) Rapid NK cell differentiation in a population with near-universal human cytomegalovirus infection is attenuated by NKG2C deletions. Blood 124(14):2213–2222. https://doi.org/10.1182/blood-2014-05-576124

Guma M, Angulo A, Vilches C, Gomez-Lozano N, Malats N, Lopez-Botet M (2004) Imprint of human cytomegalovirus infection on the NK cell receptor repertoire. Blood 104(12):3664–3671. https://doi.org/10.1182/blood-2004-05-2058

Hendricks DW, Balfour HH Jr, Dunmire SK, Schmeling DO, Hogquist KA, Lanier LL (2014) Cutting edge: NKG2C(hi)CD57+ NK cells respond specifically to acute infection with cytomegalovirus and not Epstein-Barr virus. J Immunol 192(10):4492–4496. https://doi.org/10.4049/jimmunol.1303211

Karre K, Ljunggren HG, Piontek G, Kiessling R (1986) Selective rejection of H-2-deficient lymphoma variants suggests alternative immune defence strategy. Nature 319(6055):675–678. https://doi.org/10.1038/319675a0

Kim S, Poursine-Laurent J, Truscott SM, Lybarger L, Song YJ, Yang L, French AR, Sunwoo JB, Lemieux S, Hansen TH, Yokoyama WM (2005) Licensing of natural killer cells by host major histocompatibility complex class I molecules. Nature 436(7051):709–713. https://doi.org/10.1038/nature03847

Koch J, Steinle A, Watzl C, Mandelboim O (2013) Activating natural cytotoxicity receptors of natural killer cells in cancer and infection. Trends Immunol 34(4):182–191. https://doi.org/10.1016/j.it.2013.01.003

Korde N, Carlsten M, Lee MJ, Minter A, Tan E, Kwok M, Manasanch E, Bhutani M, Tageja N, Roschewski M, Zingone A, Costello R, Mulquin M, Zuchlinski D, Maric I, Calvo KR, Braylan R, Tembhare P, Yuan C, Stetler-Stevenson M, Trepel J, Childs R, Landgren O (2014) A phase II trial of pan-KIR2D blockade with IPH2101 in smoldering multiple myeloma. Haematologica 99(6):e81–e83. https://doi.org/10.3324/haematol.2013.103085

Lanier LL (2005) NK cell recognition. Annu Rev Immunol 23:225–274. https://doi.org/10.1146/annurev.immunol.23.021704.115526

Lanier LL, Corliss BC, Wu J, Leong C, Phillips JH (1998) Immunoreceptor DAP12 bearing a tyrosine-based activation motif is involved in activating NK cells. Nature 391(6668):703–707. https://doi.org/10.1038/35642

Leong JW, Chase JM, Romee R, Schneider SE, Sullivan RP, Cooper MA, Fehniger TA (2014) Preactivation with IL-12, IL-15, and IL-18 induces CD25 and a functional high-affinity IL-2 receptor on human cytokine-induced memory-like natural killer cells. Biol Blood Marrow Transplant 20(4):463–473. https://doi.org/10.1016/j.bbmt.2014.01.006

Li H, Han Y, Guo Q, Zhang M, Cao X (2009) Cancer-expanded myeloid-derived suppressor cells induce anergy of NK cells through membrane-bound TGF-beta 1. J Immunol 182(1):240–249

Liao NS, Bix M, Zijlstra M, Jaenisch R, Raulet D (1991) MHC class I deficiency: susceptibility to natural killer (NK) cells and impaired NK activity. Science 253(5016):199–202

Liu Y, Wu HW, Sheard MA, Sposto R, Somanchi SS, Cooper LJ, Lee DA, Seeger RC (2013) Growth and activation of natural killer cells ex vivo from children with neuroblastoma for adoptive cell therapy. Clin Cancer Res 19(8):2132–2143. https://doi.org/10.1158/1078-0432.CCR-12-1243

Liu LL, Landskron J, Ask EH, Enqvist M, Sohlberg E, Traherne JA, Hammer Q, Goodridge JP, Larsson S, Jayaraman J, Oei VY, Schaffer M, Tasken K, Ljunggren HG, Romagnani C, Trowsdale J, Malmberg KJ, Beziat V (2016) Critical Role of CD2 Co-stimulation in Adaptive Natural Killer Cell Responses Revealed in NKG2C-Deficient Humans. Cell Rep 15(5):1088–1099. https://doi.org/10.1016/j.celrep.2016.04.005

Ljunggren HG, Karre K (1985) Host resistance directed selectively against H-2-deficient lymphoma variants. Analysis of the mechanism. J Exp Med 162(6):1745–1759

Manser AR, Uhrberg M (2016) Age-related changes in natural killer cell repertoires: impact on NK cell function and immune surveillance. Cancer Immunol Immunother 65(4):417–426. https://doi.org/10.1007/s00262-015-1750-0

Mantovani S, Mele D, Oliviero B, Barbarini G, Varchetta S, Mondelli MU (2015) NKp30 isoforms in patients with chronic hepatitis C virus infection. Immunology 146(2):234–242. https://doi.org/10.1111/imm.12495

Mao Y, Sarhan D, Steven A, Seliger B, Kiessling R, Lundqvist A (2014) Inhibition of tumor-derived prostaglandin-e2 blocks the induction of myeloid-derived suppressor cells and recovers natural killer cell activity. Clin Cancer Res 20(15):4096–4106. https://doi.org/10.1158/1078-0432.CCR-14-0635

Marcais A, Cherfils-Vicini J, Viant C, Degouve S, Viel S, Fenis A, Rabilloud J, Mayol K, Tavares A, Bienvenu J, Gangloff YG, Gilson E, Vivier E, Walzer T (2014) The metabolic checkpoint kinase mTOR is essential for IL-15 signaling during the development and activation of NK cells. Nat Immunol 15(8):749–757. https://doi.org/10.1038/ni.2936

Mavropoulos A, Sully G, Cope AP, Clark AR (2005) Stabilization of IFN-gamma mRNA by MAPK p38 in IL-12- and IL-18-stimulated human NK cells. Blood 105(1):282–288. https://doi.org/10.1182/blood-2004-07-2782

McQueen KL, Dorighi KM, Guethlein LA, Wong R, Sanjanwala B, Parham P (2007) Donor-recipient combinations of group A and B KIR haplotypes and HLA class I ligand affect the outcome of HLA-matched, sibling donor hematopoietic cell transplantation. Hum Immunol 68(5):309–323. https://doi.org/10.1016/j.humimm.2007.01.019

Miller JS, Oelkers S, Verfaillie C, McGlave P (1992) Role of monocytes in the expansion of human activated natural killer cells. Blood 80(9):2221–2229

Miller JS, Soignier Y, Panoskaltsis-Mortari A, McNearney SA, Yun GH, Fautsch SK, McKenna D, Le C, Defor TE, Burns LJ, Orchard PJ, Blazar BR, Wagner JE, Slungaard A, Weisdorf DJ, Okazaki IJ, McGlave PB (2005) Successful adoptive transfer and in vivo expansion of human haploidentical NK cells in patients with cancer. Blood 105(8):3051–3057. https://doi.org/10.1182/blood-2004-07-2974

Miller JS, Cooley S, Parham P, Farag SS, Verneris MR, McQueen KL, Guethlein LA, Trachtenberg EA, Haagenson M, Horowitz MM, Klein JP, Weisdorf DJ (2007) Missing KIR ligands are associated with less relapse and increased graft-versus-host disease (GVHD) following unrelated donor allogeneic HCT. Blood 109(11):5058–5061. https://doi.org/10.1182/blood-2007-01-065383

Ni J, Miller M, Stojanovic A, Garbi N, Cerwenka A (2012) Sustained effector function of IL-12/15/18-preactivated NK cells against established tumors. J Exp Med 209(13):2351–2365. https://doi.org/10.1084/jem.20120944

O'Leary JG, Goodarzi M, Drayton DL, von Andrian UH (2006) T cell- and B cell-independent adaptive immunity mediated by natural killer cells. Nat Immunol 7(5):507–516. https://doi.org/10.1038/ni1332

Orange JS (2002) Human natural killer cell deficiencies and susceptibility to infection. Microbes Infect 4(15):1545–1558

Orr MT, Murphy WJ, Lanier LL (2010) 'Unlicensed' natural killer cells dominate the response to cytomegalovirus infection. Nat Immunol 11(4):321–327. https://doi.org/10.1038/ni.1849

Parkhurst MR, Riley JP, Dudley ME, Rosenberg SA (2011) Adoptive transfer of autologous natural killer cells leads to high levels of circulating natural killer cells but does not mediate tumor regression. Clin Cancer Res 17(19):6287–6297. https://doi.org/10.1158/1078-0432.CCR-11-1347

Poschke I, Mougiakakos D, Hansson J, Masucci GV, Kiessling R (2010) Immature immunosuppressive CD14+HLA-DR−/low cells in melanoma patients are Stat3hi and overexpress CD80, CD83, and DC-sign. Cancer Res 70(11):4335–4345. https://doi.org/10.1158/0008-5472.CAN-09-3767

Ruggeri L, Capanni M, Casucci M, Volpi I, Tosti A, Perruccio K, Urbani E, Negrin RS, Martelli MF, Velardi A (1999) Role of natural killer cell alloreactivity in HLA-mismatched hematopoietic stem cell transplantation. Blood 94(1):333–339

Ruggeri L, Capanni M, Urbani E, Perruccio K, Shlomchik WD, Tosti A, Posati S, Rogaia D, Frassoni F, Aversa F, Martelli MF, Velardi A (2002) Effectiveness of donor natural killer cell alloreactivity in mismatched hematopoietic transplants. Science 295(5562):2097–2100. https://doi.org/10.1126/science.1068440

Salih HR, Rammensee HG, Steinle A (2002) Cutting edge: down-regulation of MICA on human tumors by proteolytic shedding. J Immunol 169(8):4098–4102

Schlums H, Cichocki F, Tesi B, Theorell J, Beziat V, Holmes TD, Han H, Chiang SC, Foley B, Mattsson K, Larsson S, Schaffer M, Malmberg KJ, Ljunggren HG, Miller JS, Bryceson YT (2015) Cytomegalovirus infection drives adaptive epigenetic diversification of NK cells with altered signaling and effector function. Immunity 42(3):443–456. https://doi.org/10.1016/j.immuni.2015.02.008

Schmohl JU, Gleason MK, Dougherty PR, Miller JS, Vallera DA (2015) Heterodimeric Bispecific Single Chain Variable Fragments (scFv) Killer Engagers (BiKEs) Enhance NK-cell Activity Against CD133+ Colorectal Cancer Cells. Target Oncol 11(3):353–361. https://doi.org/10.1007/s11523-015-0391-8

Sevko A, Sade-Feldman M, Kanterman J, Michels T, Falk CS, Umansky L, Ramacher M, Kato M, Schadendorf D, Baniyash M, Umansky V (2013) Cyclophosphamide promotes chronic inflammation-dependent immunosuppression and prevents antitumor response in melanoma. J Investig Dermatol 133(6):1610–1619. https://doi.org/10.1038/jid.2012.444

Shah NN, Baird K, Delbrook CP, Fleisher TA, Kohler ME, Rampertaap S, Lemberg K, Hurley CK, Kleiner DE, Merchant MS, Pittaluga S, Sabatino M, Stroncek DF, Wayne AS, Zhang H, Fry TJ, Mackall CL (2015) Acute GVHD in patients receiving IL-15/4-1BBL activated NK cells following T-cell-depleted stem cell transplantation. Blood 125(5):784–792. https://doi.org/10.1182/blood-2014-07-592881

Shenghui Z, Yixiang H, Jianbo W, Kang Y, Laixi B, Yan Z, Xi X (2011) Elevated frequencies of CD4(+) CD25(+) CD127lo regulatory T cells is associated to poor prognosis in patients with acute myeloid leukemia. Int J Cancer 129(6):1373–1381. https://doi.org/10.1002/ijc.25791

Shibuya A, Lanier LL, Phillips JH (1998) Protein kinase C is involved in the regulation of both signaling and adhesion mediated by DNAX accessory molecule-1 receptor. J Immunol 161(4):1671–1676

Siemens DR, Hu N, Sheikhi AK, Chung E, Frederiksen LJ, Pross H, Graham CH (2008) Hypoxia increases tumor cell shedding of MHC class I chain-related molecule: role of nitric oxide. Cancer Res 68(12):4746–4753. https://doi.org/10.1158/0008-5472.CAN-08-0054

Siewiera J, Gouilly J, Hocine HR, Cartron G, Levy C, Al-Daccak R, Jabrane-Ferrat N (2015) Natural cytotoxicity receptor splice variants orchestrate the distinct functions of human natural killer cell subtypes. Nat Commun 6:10183. https://doi.org/10.1038/ncomms10183

Spanholtz J, Preijers F, Tordoir M, Trilsbeek C, Paardekooper J, de Witte T, Schaap N, Dolstra H (2011) Clinical-grade generation of active NK cells from cord blood hematopoietic progenitor cells for immunotherapy using a closed-system culture process. PLoS One 6(6):e20740. https://doi.org/10.1371/journal.pone.0020740

Stringaris K, Adams S, Uribe M, Eniafe R, Wu CO, Savani BN, Barrett AJ (2010) Donor KIR Genes 2DL5A, 2DS1 and 3DS1 are associated with a reduced rate of leukemia relapse after HLA-identical sibling stem cell transplantation for acute myeloid leukemia but not other hematologic malignancies. Biol Blood Marrow Transplant. 16(9):1257–1264. https://doi.org/10.1016/j.bbmt.2010.03.004

Sun JC, Beilke JN, Lanier LL (2009) Adaptive immune features of natural killer cells. Nature 457(7229):557–561. https://doi.org/10.1038/nature07665

Thielens A, Vivier E, Romagne F (2012) NK cell MHC class I specific receptors (KIR): from biology to clinical intervention. Curr Opin Immunol 24(2):239–245. https://doi.org/10.1016/j.coi.2012.01.001

Tomasec P, Braud VM, Rickards C, Powell MB, McSharry BP, Gadola S, Cerundolo V, Borysiewicz LK, McMichael AJ, Wilkinson GW (2000) Surface expression of HLA-E, an inhibitor of natural killer cells, enhanced by human cytomegalovirus gpUL40. Science 287(5455):1031

Tonn T, Schwabe D, Klingemann HG, Becker S, Esser R, Koehl U, Suttorp M, Seifried E, Ottmann OG, Bug G (2013) Treatment of patients with advanced cancer with the natural killer cell line NK-92. Cytotherapy 15(12):1563–1570. https://doi.org/10.1016/j.jcyt.2013.06.017

Toribio ML, De Landazuri MO, Lopez-Botet M (1983) Induction of natural killer-like cytotoxicity in cultured human thymocytes. Eur J Immunol 13(12):964–969. https://doi.org/10.1002/eji.1830131203

Tripathy SK, Keyel PA, Yang L, Pingel JT, Cheng TP, Schneeberger A, Yokoyama WM (2008) Continuous engagement of a self-specific activation receptor induces NK cell tolerance. J Exp Med 205(8):1829–1841. https://doi.org/10.1084/jem.20072446

Valiante NM, Uhrberg M, Shilling HG, Lienert-Weidenbach K, Arnett KL, D'Andrea A, Phillips JH, Lanier LL, Parham P (1997) Functionally and structurally distinct NK cell receptor repertoires in the peripheral blood of two human donors. Immunity 7(6):739–751

Vallera DA, Felices M, McElmurry RT, McCullar V, Zhou X, Schmohl J, Zhang B, Lenvik A, Panoskaltsis-Mortari A, Verneris MR, Tolar J, Cooley S, Weisdorf D, Blazar BR, Miller JS (2016) IL-15 Trispecific Killer Engagers (TriKEs) Make Natural Killer Cells Specific to CD33+ Targets While Also Inducing In Vivo Expansion, and Enhanced Function. Clin Cancer Res 22(14):3440–3450. https://doi.org/10.1158/1078-0432.CCR-15-2710

Van den Bergh J, Willemen Y, Lion E, Acker HV, De Reu H, Anguille S, Goossens H, Berneman Z, Van Tendeloo V, Smits E (2015) Transpresentation of interleukin-15 by IL-15/IL-15Rα mRNA-engineered human dendritic cells boosts antitumoral natural killer cell activity. Oncotarget 6(42):44123–44133

Vasold J, Wagner M, Drolle H, Deniffel C, Kutt A, Oostendorp R, Sironi S, Rieger C, Fiegl M (2015) The bone marrow microenvironment is a critical player in the NK cell response against acute myeloid leukaemia in vitro. Leuk Res 39(2):257–262. https://doi.org/10.1016/j.leukres.2014.12.001

Verheyden S, Ferrone S, Mulder A, Claas FH, Schots R, De Moerloose B, Benoit Y, Demanet C (2009) Role of the inhibitory KIR ligand HLA-Bw4 and HLA-C expression levels in the recognition of leukemic cells by Natural Killer cells. Cancer ImmunolImmunother 58(6):855–865. https://doi.org/10.1007/s00262-008-0601-7

Vey N, Bourhis JH, Boissel N, Bordessoule D, Prebet T, Charbonnier A, Etienne A, Andre P, Romagne F, Benson D, Dombret H, Olive D (2012) A phase 1 trial of the anti-inhibitory KIR mAb IPH2101 for AML in complete remission. Blood 120(22):4317–4323. https://doi.org/10.1182/blood-2012-06-437558

Viel S, Marcais A, Guimaraes FS, Loftus R, Rabilloud J, Grau M, Degouve S, Djebali S, Sanlaville A, Charrier E, Bienvenu J, Marie JC, Caux C, Marvel J, Town L, Huntington ND, Bartholin L, Finlay D, Smyth MJ, Walzer T (2016) TGF-beta inhibits the activation and functions of NK cells by repressing the mTOR pathway. Sci Signal 9(415):ra19. https://doi.org/10.1126/scisignal.aad1884

Vivier E, Morin P, O'Brien C, Druker B, Schlossman SF, Anderson P (1991) Tyrosine phosphorylation of the Fc gamma RIII(CD16): zeta complex in human natural killer cells. Induction by antibody-dependent cytotoxicity but not by natural killing. J Immunol 146(1):206–210

Wada H, Matsumoto N, Maenaka K, Suzuki K, Yamamoto K (2004) The inhibitory NK cell receptor CD94/NKG2A and the activating receptor CD94/NKG2C bind the top of HLA-E through mostly shared but partly distinct sets of HLA-E residues. Eur J Immunol 34(1):81–90. https://doi.org/10.1002/eji.200324432

Waldhauer I, Steinle A (2006) Proteolytic release of soluble UL16-binding protein 2 from tumor cells. Cancer Res 66(5):2520–2526. https://doi.org/10.1158/0008-5472.CAN-05-2520

Wang G, Khattar M, Guo Z, Miyahara Y, Linkes SP, Sun Z, He X, Stepkowski SM, Chen W (2010) IL-2-deprivation and TGF-beta are two non-redundant suppressor mechanisms of CD4+CD25+ regulatory T cell which jointly restrain CD4+CD25- cell activation. Immunol Lett 132(1–2):61–68. https://doi.org/10.1016/j.imlet.2010.06.001

Wiencke JK, Butler R, Hsuang G, Eliot M, Kim S, Sepulveda MA, Siegel D, Andres Houseman E, Kelsey KT (2016) The dna methylation profile of activated human natural killer cells. Epigenetics 11(5):363–380. https://doi.org/10.1080/15592294.2016.1163454

Wolf AM, Wolf D, Steurer M, Gastl G, Gunsilius E, Grubeck-Loebenstein B (2003) Increase of regulatory T cells in the peripheral blood of cancer patients. Clin Cancer Res 9(2):606–612

Wolf D, Wolf AM, Rumpold H, Fiegl H, Zeimet AG, Muller-Holzner E, Deibl M, Gastl G, Gunsilius E, Marth C (2005) The expression of the regulatory T cell-specific forkhead box transcription factor FoxP3 is associated with poor prognosis in ovarian cancer. Clin Cancer Res 11(23):8326–8331. https://doi.org/10.1158/1078-0432.CCR-05-1244

Xu XD, Hu J, Wang M, Peng F, Tian R, Guo XJ, Xie Y, Qin RY (2016) Circulating myeloid-derived suppressor cells in patients with pancreatic cancer. Hepatobiliary Pancreat Dis Int 15(1):99–105

Zhang C, Burger MC, Jennewein L, Genssler S, Schonfeld K, Zeiner P, Hattingen E, Harter PN, Mittelbronn M, Tonn T, Steinbach JP, Wels WS (2016) ErbB2/HER2-Specific NK Cells for Targeted Therapy of Glioblastoma. J Natl Cancer Inst 108(5):djv375. https://doi.org/10.1093/jnci/djv375

Dendritic Cells in Hematopoietic Cell Transplantation

11

David J. Chung

11.1 Human Dendritic Cells

11.1.1 Dendritic Cells: Critical Regulators of Immunity

Dendritic cells (DCs) are specialized bone marrow-derived leukocytes that orchestrate both innate and adaptive immunity. DCs reside in all tissues where they continuously survey the local environment and inform cells of the immune system to modulate their responses (Banchereau and Steinman 1998; Steinman and Banchereau 2007; Steinman 2012). Under physiologic steady-state conditions, DCs are predominantly immature or semi-mature and efficiently process self-antigens to induce and maintain self-tolerance (Hawiger et al. 2001; Bonifaz et al. 2002; Lutz and Schuler 2002). Under inflammatory conditions, DCs undergo terminal maturation and activation to become fully immunogenic. DC heterogeneity and differential activation states ultimately determine the type and quality of immune responses.

DCs initiate an immune response by capturing and presenting antigen in the form of peptide–major histocompatibility complex (MHC) molecule complexes to naive T cells in lymphoid tissues (Banchereau and Steinman 1998; Steinman and Banchereau 2007; Steinman 2012). DCs share most features of antigen-processing cells and class I and II MHC-restricted presentation with other antigen-presenting cells (APCs). DCs, however, are endowed with the capacity to cross-present exogenous antigens on their own class I MHC molecules to autologous T cells regardless of the MHC alleles expressed by the antigen source (Albert et al. 1998; Guermonprez et al. 2003; Ackerman et al. 2005). When compared with other APCs, like macrophages, DCs are much more efficient and can elicit responses from very low numbers of T cells (Steinman 2012).

D. J. Chung
Memorial Sloan Kettering Cancer Center, New York, NY, USA
e-mail: chungd1@mskcc.org

M.-A. Perales et al. (eds.), *Cell and Gene Therapies*, Advances and Controversies in Hematopoietic Transplantation and Cell Therapy,
https://doi.org/10.1007/978-3-319-54368-0_11

In peripheral tissues, DCs capture antigens by different complementary mechanisms (Trombetta and Mellman 2005) and then migrate through the afferent lymphatics to draining lymph nodes. DCs process proteins into peptides that bind to both MHC class I and class II molecules. Lipid antigens are processed differently through nonclassical MHC molecules of the CD1 family (Banchereau et al. 2000). Antigens also reach lymph node-resident DCs directly through the lymph (Itano and Jenkins 2003). On interaction with DCs, naive $CD4^+$ and $CD8^+$ T cells differentiate into antigen-specific effector cells with diverse functions. $CD4^+$ T cells can become T helper 1 (T_H1) cells, T_H2 cells, T_H17 cells, or T follicular helper (T_{FH}) cells, as well as regulatory T (T_{Reg}) cells that suppress the function of other lymphocytes. Naive $CD8^+$ T cells can give rise to effector cytotoxic T lymphocytes (CTLs). The type of $CD4^+$ or $CD8^+$ T-cell response is at least in part dependent on the DC subset presenting the antigen (Banchereau and Steinman 1998). DCs also interact with cells of the innate immune system, including natural killer (NK) cells and mast cells (Banchereau and Steinman 1998; Steinman and Banchereau 2007; Steinman 2012). DCs control humoral immunity, directly by interacting with B cells and indirectly by inducing $CD4^+$ helper T-cell expansion and differentiation (Jego et al. 2005; Qi et al. 2006).

11.1.2 DC Maturation and Activation

DC maturation and activation is pivotal to the control of immune responses. Immature or non-activated DCs in peripheral tissues induce immune tolerance either through T-cell deletion or T_{Reg} expansion (Steinman et al. 2003). Immature DCs efficiently capture antigens, accumulate MHC class II molecules in the late endosome–lysosomal compartment, express low levels of co-stimulatory molecules, and have a limited capacity for cytokine secretion (Trombetta and Mellman 2005). In response to environmental signals, immature DCs differentiate into mature forms that efficiently induce immune responses. Maturation is associated with decreased antigen-capture activity, increased expression of surface MHC class II and co-stimulatory molecules, increased cytokine secretion (Trombetta and Mellman 2005), increased CCR7 expression to enable migration to draining lymph nodes (Trombetta and Mellman 2005), and upregulation of CD83, the prototypical marker of DC maturation (Zhou and Tedder 1995). DCs also upregulate the immune-modulatory enzyme, indoleamine 2,3-dioxygenase, with maturation to induce T_{Regs}, thus providing an intrinsic brake to counter otherwise unrestrained immune responses (Munn et al. 2002; Chung et al. 2009).

Microbial products provide a physiologic activation stimulus to DCs via pathogen-associated molecular patterns (PAMPs), including toll-like receptors. Although most microbes activate DCs, a few can block DC maturation (Steinman and Banchereau 2007; Pulendran et al. 2001; Palucka and Banchereau 2002). Tissue-localized DCs can also be polarized into distinct phenotypes by products released from neighboring immune cells responding to injury, including interferon (IFN)-γ from γδ-T cells and NK cells, preformed interleukin (IL)-4 and TNF from mast cells, IFNα from pDCs, and IL-15 and thymic stromal lymphopoietin (TSLP) from stromal cells (Ueno et al. 2010; Cheng et al. 2010). A combination of pro-inflammatory cytokines that include IL-1-β, IL-6, prostaglandin E2, and tumor necrosis factor (TNF)-α (Jonuleit et al. 1997) simulates physiologic stimulation and is often used to mature DCs for study in vitro and use in clinical vaccine trials. In addition, adjuvant components of many vaccines trigger DC activation through distinct molecular pathways, resulting in varied T-cell responses (Maldonado-Lopez et al. 1999; Pulendran et al. 1999).

11.1.3 Human DC Subsets

Comparative phenotypic and functional studies have identified distinct DC subsets present in all mammals. Human DCs express MHC class II (HLA-DR) at high levels but lack T cell (CD3), B cell (CD19/CD20), and NK cell (CD56) lineage markers. The classical descriptions of DCs as HLA-DR$^+$ lineage$^-$ cells have been refined to include additional positive DC lineage markers that categorize DCs as either "myeloid" (or "conventional") or "plasmacytoid" (Ziegler-Heitbrock et al. 2010). Human DC subsets in the blood can be distinguished by the differential expression of the cell-surface molecules CD303 (BDCA2 and CLEC4C), CD1C (BDCA1), and CD141 (BDCA3 and thrombomodulin) (Dzionek et al. 2000).

Myeloid DCs (mDCs) express the myeloid antigens CD11c, CD13, CD33, and CD11b, corresponding to mouse CD11c$^+$ "classical" or "conventional" DCs. In humans, both monocytes and mDCs express CD11c, but DCs lack CD14 or CD16 and can be subclassified into two populations by the reciprocal expression of CD1c and CD141. These two subpopulations share homology with mouse classical DCs expressing either CD11b (CD1c$^+$ DCs) or CD8/CD103 (CD141$^+$ DCs). Human CD141$^+$ mDCs are adept at taking up dead or necrotic cells via CLEC9A, sensing viral nucleic acids via TLR3 and TLR8, and cross-presenting antigen to CD8$^+$ T cells in vitro (Collin et al. 2013). Thus, human CD141$^+$ DCs are well equipped to stimulate CD8$^+$ T-cell-mediated immune responses. It is important to note that other human DCs, such as epidermal Langerhans cells (Klechevsky et al. 2008), also cross-present antigens effectively. Whether CD141$^+$ blood mDCs are related to DC subsets in peripheral tissues is unknown. CD1c$^+$ mDCs are the major population of human mDCs in blood, tissues, and lymphoid organs, and defining their unique function(s) remains an area of active research. Overall, the division of labor between CD141$^+$ DCs and other myeloid DCs in humans appears less sharply demarcated than in the mouse, underscoring the imprecise nature of cross-species comparisons.

Langerhans cells (LCs) and dermal interstitial DCs (dermal DCs) are the two primary subsets of mDCs present in the skin. LCs express high levels of langerin, a C-type lectin, and CD1a, a non-polymorphic class I MHC molecule, and are superior stimulators of cytotoxic T lymphocytes (CTLs) in vitro, at least against recall viral antigen and cross-presented tumor antigen (Ratzinger et al. 2004). Dermal DCs can be further subdivided into CD1a$^+$ DCs and CD14$^+$ DCs (Valladeau and Saeland 2005; Nestle et al. 1993). CD14$^+$ DCs appear to be specialized participants in humoral responses (Klechevsky et al. 2008; Ueno et al. 2007), as they can directly help activated B cells and induce naive T cells to differentiate into cells with T_{FH} cell-like properties (Klechevsky et al. 2008; Caux et al. 1997).

Plasmacytoid DCs (pDCs) secrete copious amounts of type I interferon (IFN--α/β) in response to foreign nucleic acids and thereby mediate antiviral immunity (Siegal et al. 1999). pDCs are distinguished by the absence of myeloid antigens and expression of CD123 (IL-3R), CD303, and CD304. Freshly isolated plasmacytoid DCs express much lower levels of MHC and co-stimulatory molecules than their conventional DC counterparts (Grouard et al. 1997). Non-activated pDCs capture, process, and load antigens onto MHC molecules less effectively and are therefore relatively poor stimulators of T cells. In their resting state, pDCs participate in immune tolerance, including oral tolerance (Reizis et al. 2011). IL-3, in combination with CD40L or microbial products, leads to full pDC activation, abundant type I IFN secretion, and more potent lymphocyte stimulation (Siegal et al. 1999; Cella et al. 1999; Fonteneau et al. 2003). Activated pDCs also induce the maturation of activated B cells into plasma cells through cytokines and surface signaling (Jego et al. 2003; Shaw et al. 2010).

11.1.4 DC Receptors

DCs sense the environment with a diverse repertoire of surface and intracellular receptors, including toll-like receptors (TLRs), C-type lectins (CLRs), and helicases. TLRs recognize specific components conserved among microorganisms, and ligand binding to TLRs on DCs initiates the entire range of innate and acquired immunity (Takeda et al. 2003). TLR ligands include peptidoglycan (TLR2), viral dsRNA (TLR3), LPS (TLR4), viral ssRNA (TLR7), and unmethylated bacterial CpG DNA motif (TLR9). Myeloid DCs express various combinations of TLR1–TLR6 and TLR8, depending on the subset and activation state (Kadowaki et al. 2001; Jarrossay et al. 2001). pDCs are the only human DC subtype with TLR7 and TLR9 expression (Kadowaki et al. 2001; Jarrossay et al. 2001). CLRs bind carbohydrate moieties of glycoprotein self-antigens and pathogens, as well as many non-carbohydrate ligands such as lipids and proteins, by mechanisms that are not yet fully understood, to variably trigger pro-inflammatory or anti-inflammatory reactions (Reis e Sousa 2006). CLRs can synergize with, antagonize, or regulate signals from other receptors, thereby fine-tuning responses to infection or damage. CLR expression by DCs varies with activation status (Valladeau et al. 2000; Ebner et al. 2004; Bonifaz et al. 2004) and includes DEC-205 (CD205), DC-SIGN (CD209), BDCA-2, Dectin-1, Langerin (CD207), and CLEC9A. Helicases are members of a large family of molecules, including retinoic acid-inducible gene I (RIGI), which recognize nucleic acids. Activation of helicases can differentially affect DC function to yield distinct immune responses (Takeuchi and Akira 2010; Zhang et al. 2011). DCs also express a combination of activating (CD16, CD32a, and CD64) and inhibitory (CD32b) Fc-γ receptors that influence processing and presentation of antigens in the steady state and during inflammation (Guilliams et al. 2014).

11.2 Human DCs in Clinical Hematopoietic Cell Transplantation

11.2.1 DC Antigen Presentation and Chimerism After Allogeneic Hematopoietic Cell Transplantation

DCs initiate T-cell responses to MHC and minor histocompatibility antigens (miHAs) and are both initiators and targets of graft–host interactions in hematopoietic cell transplantation (HCT). Specifically, DCs participate in the induction of graft-versus-tumor (GVT) activity and graft-versus-host disease (GvHD), two distinct but overlapping syndromes. The cytokine storm associated with pretransplantation conditioning and the early peri-transplant period can activate DCs to present MHC and miHAs through two separate pathways in an immunogenic manner (Hill and Ferrara 2000). Persistent host DCs present antigen by direct ligation of the donor T-cell receptor (TCR) by MHC molecules on recipient DCs. Engrafting donor DCs use an indirect pathway to cross-present host antigens. In both cases, antigens are presented to engrafting donor T cells. Polymorphic residues in the MHC binding groove, which themselves are not accessible to TCRs, affect binding of peptides recognized by allogeneic T cells. This intensifies the antigenic effect of MHC polymorphisms and explains the much higher frequency of T cells (1–10%) reactive with allogeneic MHC compared with those that react with miHAs presented by MHC-identical individuals (Sherman and Chattopadhyay 1993). Donor T cells use an indirect pathway to recognize miHAs, which are peptides derived from polymorphic genes unique to the host but recognized because they are presented by shared MHC molecules in matched allogeneic HCT (allo-HCT) (Bleakley and Riddell 2004). The ultimate goal in clinical transplantation is to stimulate T cells against miHAs unique to a malignancy that are absent from normal tissues, thus achieving GVT activity without GvHD.

DCs are terminally differentiated and, due to their nonproliferating state, are resistant to myeloablative regimens that target dividing cells, including total body irradiation. This results in the persistence of host DCs that coexist with new donor-derived DCs after allo-HCT. Most chimerism studies have evaluated conventional or myeloid DCs, identifying rapid conversion to donor type even though small numbers of residual host DCs may persist for extended periods, especially after reduced-intensity conditioning. In one study, approximately 80% of peripheral blood DCs were of donor origin by day +14 after allo-HCT, increasing to >95% by day +56 (Auffermann-Gretzinger et al. 2002). The kinetics of DC chimerism in peripheral tissues varies by conditioning regimen. A study of epidermal LC chimerism after allo-HCT found an average 97% donor-derived LCs with full-intensity conditioning, but only 36.5% donor-derived LCs with reduced-intensity conditioning 40 days after allo-HCT; at least 90% of LCs were donor-derived by day +100 (Collin et al. 2006). Donor chimerism is delayed in the presence of acute GvHD (Collin et al. 2006; Auffermann-Gretzinger et al. 2006), but the presence of residual host DCs is also seen in the absence of acute GvHD (Andani et al. 2014).

11.2.2 DCs and GvHD

GvHD is a frequent complication of allo-HCT and causes significant morbidity and mortality. At its root, GvHD is an inflammatory process mediated by both the innate and adaptive arms of the immune system (Ball and Egeler 2008; Ferrara et al. 2009). Residual host- and donor-derived DCs participate in GvHD pathogenesis. In murine models, host-derived DCs are essential for the induction of acute GvHD, whereas donor-derived DCs amplify acute GvHD and may be involved in the development of chronic GvHD (Shlomchik et al. 1999; Matte et al. 2004). During the effector phase of GvHD, tissue-resident, host-derived macrophages and DCs control the migration of alloreactive donor T cells into the tissues and subsequent local development of GvHD in mice (Zhang et al. 2002).

Mouse models of GvHD demonstrate that DC homeostasis after transplant influences GvHD outcome. LCs can self-renew in the skin of parabiotic mice from local precursors and remain of host origin for a prolonged period (Merad et al. 2004). LCs and dermal DCs can survive myeloablative radiation and persist for months after transplantation of purified stem cells or T-cell-depleted bone marrow in the absence of GvHD (Merad et al. 2004; Bogunovic et al. 2006). The presence or absence of GvHD is crucial to DC composition. In the absence of GvHD, trace populations of low-level cycling precursors in the skin can replace LCs or dermal DCs that exit to secondary lymphoid tissues, thus maintaining DCs of host origin. In contrast, in the setting of GvHD, the loss of DCs exceeds the capacity of local precursors to replenish host populations, allowing for circulating donor marrow-derived DC precursors to fill the resulting void. Elimination of host LCs and replacement by donor DCs prevent cutaneous GvHD in MHC-mismatched allo-HCT (Merad et al. 2004). In addition, residual allogeneic T cells from donor marrow, once primed against host MHC or miHA, eliminate host DCs from GvHD target organs, with subsequent replacement by donor marrow-derived DCs (Merad et al. 2004). Previous acute GvHD of the skin in humans correlates with complete donor LC chimerism, again supporting a role of allogeneic T cells in promoting donor LC engraftment (Collin et al. 2006).

Resident populations of DCs in peripheral tissues may be more relevant to acute GvHD, as addressed in the murine studies cited above. In humans, host LCs decreased and then recovered with donor LCs more rapidly after myeloablative conditioning than with reduced-intensity conditioning, although the nadirs were comparable between days 14 and 21 (Collin et al. 2006). Donor LC recovery to pretransplant levels was more brisk in the absence of acute GvHD but more complete in the presence of acute GvHD, indicating a role for donor T cells in promoting LC engraftment as in mice (Merad et al. 2002, 2004). Dermal DC reconstitution can exhibit similarly rapid turnover by about day +100 (Auffermann-Gretzinger et al. 2006), although some host dermal DCs persist, especially after reduced-intensity conditioning (Bogunovic et al. 2006). Co-expression of the activation marker, CMRF-44, by conventional or myeloid $CD11c^+$ DCs in peripheral blood precedes the onset of clinically significant acute GvHD (Lau et al. 2007), suggesting the predictive value of monitoring such subsets in the blood.

Prophylactic and therapeutic immunosuppressive agents for GvHD affect DC numbers. During clinically significant acute GvHD, circulating DC levels decline, reflecting the effects of therapy (especially steroids), more rapid turnover and migration into tissues, or both (Reddy et al. 2004). Alemtuzumab rapidly depletes circulating host DCs but does not alter donor DC engraftment or deplete other DCs that lack the CD52 target epitope (LCs or dermal DCs) (Ratzinger et al. 2003; Collin et al. 2005; Klangsinsirikul et al. 2002). Cyclosporin A and tacrolimus can impair antigen processing by DCs (Lee et al. 2005) but, like steroids, are nonselective and also exert broad effects on T cells by calcineurin inhibition. Sirolimus (rapamycin), which blocks the signal transduction resulting from ligation of the IL-2, IL-4, and IL-6 receptors in T cells, also suppresses DC immunogenicity (Hackstein et al. 2003). Thus, drugs that block DC function should modulate immune interactions in allo-HCT. More targeted reagents are still required, however, especially if the goal is to maintain viral immunity and GVT effects while eliminating GvHD and avoiding overly global immune suppression and its attendant complications. The use of tolerogenic recipient DCs to pretreat donor stem cell sources and minimize allogeneic T-cell responses is an alternative consideration.

11.2.3 DCs and GVT Responses

Host DCs presenting tumor antigen(s) either directly or by cross-presentation should induce at least a portion of the GVT response. The precise role of the different human DC subtypes in GVT responses after allo-HCT, however, remains poorly understood. Mouse studies have shown that host DCs may play an important role in GVT effects (Mapara et al. 2002), especially those that are able to cross-present tumor-specific antigen(s) to donor T cells (Toubai et al. 2013). The participation of host DCs in GVT in humans was supported by a study where the combination of donor T cells and mixed chimerism in DC subsets stimulated a potent GVL effect in association with GvHD, whereas donor lymphocyte infusions in patients with donor chimerism in both T cells and DC subsets resulted in GVL reactivity without GvHD (Levenga et al. 2007). Whether DC subtypes separately direct GVH or GVT reactions at the level of antigen presentation to responding T cells is incompletely understood. In the absence of concomitant tissue damage, persistent host LCs migrating from the skin to draining lymph nodes can stimulate potent graft responses against host antigens, thus supporting GVT without GvHD in an MHC-matched murine allo-HCT model (Durakovic et al. 2006). This finding is also relevant to the immunologic effects mediated by donor lymphocyte infusions to treat relapsed/recurrent disease. The ultimate goal is to preferentially target miHAs that are only expressed by tumor cells and not shared with normal tissue to avoid the overlapping development of GvHD (Bleakley and Riddell 2004). Maintaining DCs in an immature or semi-mature state to preserve graft–host tolerance while promoting GVT is an area of ongoing study.

11.2.4 DC Vaccines: General Considerations

Methods for the large-scale generation of human DCs have enabled their clinical evaluation as vaccines. Although early phase I and II trials of DC-based vaccines showed limited success, many studies used immature DCs that were insufficiently immunogenic, suboptimal routes and schedules of vaccination, and patients with advanced disease in whom there was inadequate time to respond. Importantly, numerous other studies have demonstrated the feasibility of DC-based immunization to induce both immune and objective clinical responses against tumors (Palucka and Banchereau 2012), although primarily in the non-transplant setting.

DC precursors can be obtained from several sources, including nondividing peripheral blood monocytes or cycling CD34^{+} progenitors in cord blood, granulocyte colony-stimulating factor-elicited peripheral blood, or bone marrow. Regardless of source, precursor cells require recombinant cytokine support in vitro to generate DCs, with subsequent terminal maturation to ensure optimal stimulation of T-cell immunity. A potential advantage of using CD34^{+}-derived DCs, especially in the setting of cord blood transplantation, is their capacity for expansion prior to DC differentiation to generate larger numbers of DCs from a limited pool of precursor cells. In addition to cytokine-supported methods, preformed circulating DCs can also be isolated from blood by density gradient (Hsu et al. 1996; Timmerman et al. 2002) or direct immunoselection (Dzionek et al. 2000; Lopez et al. 2003).

Almost all previous DC vaccine trials have used monocyte-derived DCs (moDCs), in large part because monocyte precursors are easier to obtain and culture in vitro than CD34^{+}-derived subsets, including LCs. LCs, however, are superior to moDCs and other conventional DC subsets at inducing antigen-specific CTLs against viral and tumor antigens in vitro (Klechevsky et al. 2008; Ratzinger et al. 2004). When compared with moDCs, LCs secrete more IL-15 (Klechevsky et al. 2008; Ratzinger et al. 2004; Munz et al. 2005), which in turn reduces IL-2-induced T-cell apoptosis and decreases T_{Reg} expansion during LC-mediated CTL generation (Romano et al. 2012). LCs can overcome tolerance against tumor-associated antigens by an IL-15Rα/IL-15/pSTAT5-dependent mechanism (Romano et al. 2012). Clinical trial data have shown greater efficacy of DC vaccines that contain LCs (Banchereau et al. 2001), as well as greater tetramer reactivity stimulated by LCs when compared with moDCs (Romano et al. 2011). Thus, selection of DC subtype for use in vaccine formulations is an important consideration.

Optimizing antigen loading is another key parameter of DC vaccine preparation. The simplest and most often used approach is "peptide pulsing," which is the incubation of DCs with synthetic peptides of limited length and defined HLA restrictions, most commonly HLA-A*0201. DNA (Yuan et al. 2006)- or RNA (Gilboa and Vieweg 2004)-based methods of antigen delivery offer the potential advantage of facilitating the processing and presentation of a broad repertoire of multiple class I and II MHC-restricted epitopes from the translated protein (Romano et al. 2011), together with more sustained antigen expression than peptide pulsing. Other approaches have used tumor lysates for uptake and cross-presentation (Ratzinger et al. 2004; Berard et al. 2000; Palucka et al. 2006), DC receptor targeting for antigen delivery in vivo (Bonifaz et al. 2004; Birkholz et al. 2010), and systemic delivery of antigen-encoding RNA lipoplexes to DCs in vivo (Kranz et al. 2016). The majority of DC vaccine studies have been limited to single antigen and restricted epitope targets. Simultaneously targeting more than one antigen, however, offers the potential to improve the breadth of immune responses and clinical response rates (Karan et al. 2011; Walter et al. 2012).

Different routes of immunization have been tested, with subcutaneous administration by far the most common method. Other approaches include intradermal, intravenous, intranodal, and intratumoral injections. Although direct comparisons are generally lacking, intradermal vaccination may be more effective than subcutaneous vaccination due to the rich lymphatics at the epidermal–dermal junction. Intravenous administration does not compare favorably with the intradermal route in animal and limited clinical comparisons. Intranodal vaccination removes considerable uncertainty but cannot be widely implemented. The ideal frequency and duration for vaccination is unknown, but maintaining an ongoing vaccination schedule in responding patients may provide benefit (Palucka et al. 2006).

Early-phase trials often rely on proxy measurements in vitro of responses to vaccines. These include antigen-driven assays for measurement of IFN-γ secretion, intracellular cytokine secretion assays, T-cell reactivity with tetramers/pentamers of defined peptides with known MHC restrictions, CTL assays against antigen-expressing targets, and, more recently, next-generation deep sequencing of the TCR-V-beta CDR3 region to assess changes in T-cell clonal diversity. Clinical responses remain mostly anecdotal in the relatively small numbers of patients among the many treated in the presence of persistent systemic disease.

11.2.5 DC Vaccination After Autologous Stem Cell Transplantation

DC-based vaccination to induce or restore antitumor immunity offers a promising approach to target residual malignancy and to improve clinical outcomes after autologous HCT (auto-HCT). The minimal residual disease state and lymphopenia after auto-HCT afford a unique platform to induce antitumor immune responses by limiting tumor-driven immunosuppression (Kim et al. 2006), eliminating cytokine sinks (Gattinoni et al. 2005), and transiently depleting T_{Regs} (Zhang et al. 2005; Chung et al. 2016). Importantly, $CD8^+$ T cells can respond to autologous DCs presenting tumor antigen in vitro as early as day +12 posttransplant, becoming antigen-specific cytolytic T-lymphocyte effectors and thereby demonstrating preservation of cellular reactivity after transplant (Chung et al. 2016). DC-based vaccination in this setting therefore offers one approach to redirect recovering T cells toward specific MHC-restricted antigen(s).

The feasibility of DC vaccines in the setting of auto-HCT has been demonstrated in multiple myeloma, the most common indication for auto-HCT (Table 11.1). DCs from patients with multiple myeloma are functionally intact, comparable to those from healthy donors, and induce autologous antigen-specific T cells with lytic

Table 11.1 DC vaccine trials after auto-HCT

DC subtype	Cell source	Target	Antigen(s)	Antigen form	Vaccine route	Immune response	Clinical response	SAE	Reference
CD14+	PBMC	MM	Id KLH	Protein	IV/SC	Id 2/12 KLH 11/12	N/A	NR	Reichardt et al. (1999)
CD14+	PBMC	MM	Id	Protein	IV	Not reported	OS benefit	NR	Lacy et al. (2009)
CD14+	PBMC	MM	Autologous tumor	DC–tumor fusion	SC	Expansion of MM-specific T cells 36/36	Increased CR at 1 year	NR	Rosenblatt et al. (2013)
CD14+	PBMC	MM	Autologous tumor	DC–tumor fusion	SC	N/A	N/A	N/A	[a]NCT 02728102
LC	CD34+ HPC	MM	CT7 MAGE-A3 WT1	mRNA	ID	N/A	N/A	N/A	[a]NCT 01995708

ALL acute lymphoblastic leukemia, *AML* acute myeloid leukemia, *CMV* cytomegalovirus, *CR* complete response, *CT7* cancer–testis antigen 7, *DC* dendritic cell, *DTH* delayed-type hypersensitivity, *HPC* hematopoietic progenitor cell, *Id* idiotype, *ID* intradermal, *IV* intravenous, *KLH* keyhole limpet hemocyanin, *LC* Langerhans-type dendritic cell, *MAGE-A3* melanoma-associated antigen 3, *MiHA* minor histocompatibility antigen, *MM* multiple myeloma, *N/A* not applicable, *NHL* non-Hodgkin lymphoma, *NR* none reported, *OS* overall survival, *PBMC* peripheral blood mononuclear cell, *PBSC* peripheral blood stem cell, *RCC* renal cell carcinoma, *SAE* severe adverse events, *SC* subcutaneous, *WT1* Wilms' tumor 1

[a]Trial ongoing

activity in vitro (Chung et al. 2016). Clinical validation of this approach was shown with an idiotype-pulsed autologous DC vaccine for multiple myeloma after auto-HCT that induced idiotype-specific T-cell responses in a subset of patients (Reichardt et al. 1999). Subsequently, posttransplant vaccination with an idiotype-pulsed cellular product containing DCs was associated with improved progression-free survival compared with a historical control cohort (Lacy et al. 2009). More recently, vaccination with a DC–myeloma fusion vaccine following autologous transplant was associated with an increase in myeloma-specific T cells and conversion from partial response to complete response in a subset of patients (Rosenblatt et al. 2013). Vaccination in these three studies was well tolerated without evidence of significant autoimmunity or adverse effect on posttransplant engraftment.

Posttransplant maintenance therapy with lenalidomide improves progression-free and overall survival after auto-HCT (McCarthy et al. 2012; Attal et al. 2012; Palumbo et al. 2014). In addition, lenalidomide has immunostimulatory properties (Benson Jr et al. 2011; Luptakova et al. 2013; Noonan et al. 2012) that could further augment vaccine-induced immunity. This is being assessed in two DC vaccine studies that include lenalidomide maintenance in the treatment regimen. A phase I study is examining early posttransplant vaccination using autologous LCs electroporated with mRNA encoding three MM-associated antigens followed by lenalidomide maintenance (NCT01995708). A phase II, multicenter trial will study posttransplant lenalidomide maintenance alone or in conjunction with serial vaccination with DC–myeloma fusions (NCT02728102).

Immune checkpoint inhibitors enhance vaccine-induced antitumor immune responses in various preclinical models. Both $CD4^+$ and $CD8^+$ T cells from multiple myeloma patients express the negative regulatory molecules, CTLA-4, PD-1, LAG-3, and TIM-3, before and after auto-HCT (Chung et al. 2016). In addition, a subpopulation of hyporesponsive, exhausted/senescent PD-1-expressing $CD8^+$ T cells that characterize immune impairment and relapse after auto-HCT can be revived with PD-1 blockade in vitro (Chung et al. 2016). The combination of DC vaccines with checkpoint blockade to "prime and boost" antitumor immune responses warrants investigation.

11.2.6 DC Vaccination After Allogeneic Stem Cell Transplantation

As in the auto-HCT setting, DC-based vaccination after allo-HCT offers similar advantages in exploiting a minimal residual disease state and the autoreactive potential of recovering T-cell populations, relatively devoid of T_{Regs}. In contrast to auto-HCT, however, allo-HCT regimens often include immunosuppressant agents for GvHD prophylaxis, which could impede responses to vaccines. Nonetheless, DC vaccination after allo-HCT has been well tolerated with evidence of both clinical and immunological antiviral and antitumor responses without increases in adverse events, albeit in a limited number of patients (Table 11.2).

Virus-specific immunity against human cytomegalovirus (CMV) can be induced by DC vaccination after allo-HCT. Patients at high risk for developing CMV

Table 11.2 DC vaccine trials after allo-HCT

DC subtype	Cell source	Target	Antigen(s)	Antigen form	Vaccine route	Immune response	Clinical response	SAE	Reference
CD14+	Donor PBMC	CMV	pp65 pp150	Peptide	SC	Tetramer 7/17	15/17	NR	Grigoleit et al. (2007)
CD14+	Donor PBMC	CMV	pp65	Protein	SC	Protein recall 1/1	1/1	NR	Feuchtinger et al. (2010)
CD14+	Donor PBSC	AML, ALL, NHL	Autologous tumor	Irradiated tumor cells	IV	DTH 3/4	3/4	NR	Fujii et al. (2001)
CD14+	Donor PBSC	RCC	Autologous tumor	Lysate	ID	DTH 0/1	0/1	NR	Tatsugami et al. (2004)
CD14+	Donor PBMC	AML	WT1 KLH	Peptide	ID	WT1 no KLH yes	0/1	NR	Kitawaki et al. (2008)
CD14+	Host PBMC	MM	MiHA	N/A	IV/ID	Protein recall 6/6	0/6	NR	Levenga et al. (2010)

ALL acute lymphoblastic leukemia, *AML* acute myeloid leukemia, *CMV* cytomegalovirus, *CR* complete response, *CT7* cancer–testis antigen 7, *DC* dendritic cell, *DTH* delayed-type hypersensitivity, *HPC* hematopoietic progenitor cell, *Id* idiotype, *ID* intradermal, *IV* intravenous, *KLH* keyhole limpet hemocyanin, *LC* Langerhans-type dendritic cell, *MAGE-A3* melanoma-associated antigen 3, *MiHA* minor histocompatibility antigen, *MM* multiple myeloma, *N/A* not applicable, *NHL* non-Hodgkin lymphoma, *NR* none reported, *OS* overall survival, *PBMC* peripheral blood mononuclear cell, *PBSC* peripheral blood stem cell, *RCC* renal cell carcinoma, *SAE* severe adverse events, *SC* subcutaneous, *WT1* Wilms' tumor 1

disease, defined as a CMV-seropositive patient and a CMV-seronegative donor and/or receipt of a T-cell-depleted graft, received donor CD14-derived peptide-loaded DCs after allo-HCT, with induction of measureable CMV-specific T-cell responses and evidence of clinical benefit, without the stimulation or expansion of allo-reactive T cells (Grigoleit et al. 2007). Vaccination with CMV pp65-pulsed DCs induced antigen-specific CD4 and CD8 cells and sustained CMV viral clearance in a patient with recurrent CMV viremia resistant to standard antiviral therapies (Feuchtinger et al. 2010).

Tumor-specific immunity elicited by donor-derived DCs loaded with irradiated tumor cells was observed in three of four patients with hematologic malignancies relapsed after allo-HCT (Fujii et al. 2001). Additional reports have demonstrated antigen-specific immune responses in patients immunized with DC-based vaccines after allo-HCT (Tatsugami et al. 2004; Kitawaki et al. 2008; Levenga et al. 2010).

Because allo-HCT patients may not be sufficiently immune reconstituted to respond to direct immunization, alternative approaches merit consideration. Donors could be vaccinated with DCs bearing their recipients' tumor antigen(s) before stem cell collection and transplantation. Donor DCs could also be used to stimulate donor lymphocytes ex vivo against specific tumor antigens for adoptive immunotherapy, with less off-target effects that could trigger GvHD.

11.3 Expert Point of View

DCs comprise a complex system of bone marrow-derived leukocytes that are critical to the onset and modulation of immunity. The divisions of labor among distinct human DC subsets maintain an equilibrium between steady-state tolerance and stimulation of antigen-specific immunity against pathogens, tumors, and other insults. Maintenance of tolerance in the steady state is an active process mediated by resting or semi-mature DCs. Under inflammatory conditions, this homeostasis is disrupted, leading to the maturation and activation of DCs and triggering a cascade of events leading to an immune response. In the setting of HCT, the mechanisms that regulate DC homeostasis offer potential targets to fine-tune graft–host interactions. It is not yet known whether a particular subtype of DC is more or less responsible for initiating or being targeted (or both) by GvHD reactions. The precise role of the different DC subtypes in GVT responses after HCT also remains poorly understood. Animal models are providing important data about distinct DC precursors, homeostasis of tissue-resident DCs, and turnover of DCs in response to inflammatory stimuli and pathological conditions like GvHD. Ultimately, therapeutic interventions that use or specifically target defined DC subtypes to selectively induce both the innate and adaptive arms of immunity, either in combination or in a prime-boost sequence, may provide optimal clinical utility by harnessing both effector cell compartments.

11.4 Future Directions

Advancing our knowledge of how different DC subsets are related, their roles in graft–host interactions and disease pathogenesis, and their most favorable therapeutic implementation are among the key issues for future studies. Progress in systems immunology is expected to lend insights into the molecular pathways that determine DC-guided immunity. Thus, an integrated approach combining transcriptional profiling, genetic and small-molecule screening, and proteomics will further our understanding of DC biology and thereby enable the discovery of novel adjuvants and strategies to induce protective immune responses while minimizing the risk of autoimmunity or GvHD. In turn, this will yield more rational and refined clinical applications of DC-based therapies in HCT.

References

Ackerman AL, Kyritsis C, Tampe R, Cresswell P (2005) Access of soluble antigens to the endoplasmic reticulum can explain cross-presentation by dendritic cells. Nat Immunol 6:107–113

Albert ML, Sauter B, Bhardwaj N (1998) Dendritic cells acquire antigen from apoptotic cells and induce class I-restricted CTLs. Nature 392:86–89

Andani R et al (2014) Origin of Langerhans cells in normal skin and chronic GVHD after hematopoietic stem-cell transplantation. Exp Dermatol 23:75–77

Attal M et al (2012) Lenalidomide maintenance after stem-cell transplantation for multiple myeloma. N Engl J Med 366:1782–1791

Auffermann-Gretzinger S et al (2002) Rapid establishment of dendritic cell chimerism in allogeneic hematopoietic cell transplant recipients. Blood 99:1442–1448

Auffermann-Gretzinger S et al (2006) Fast appearance of donor dendritic cells in human skin: dynamics of skin and blood dendritic cells after allogeneic hematopoietic cell transplantation. Transplantation 81:866–873

Ball LM, Egeler RM (2008) Acute GvHD: pathogenesis and classification. Bone Marrow Transplant 41(Suppl 2):S58–S64

Banchereau J, Steinman RM (1998) Dendritic cells and the control of immunity. Nature 392:245–252

Banchereau J et al (2000) Immunobiology of dendritic cells. Annu Rev Immunol 18:767–811

Banchereau J et al (2001) Immune and clinical responses in patients with metastatic melanoma to CD34(+) progenitor-derived dendritic cell vaccine. Cancer Res 61:6451–6458

Benson DM Jr et al (2011) IPH 2101, a novel anti-inhibitory KIR antibody, and lenalidomide combine to enhance the natural killer cell versus multiple myeloma effect. Blood 118:6387–6391

Berard F et al (2000) Cross-priming of naive CD8 T cells against melanoma antigens using dendritic cells loaded with killed allogeneic melanoma cells. J Exp Med 192:1535–1544

Birkholz K et al (2010) Targeting of DEC-205 on human dendritic cells results in efficient MHC class II-restricted antigen presentation. Blood 116:2277–2285

Bleakley M, Riddell SR (2004) Molecules and mechanisms of the graft-versus-leukaemia effect. Nat Rev Cancer 4:371–380

Bogunovic M et al (2006) Identification of a radio-resistant and cycling dermal dendritic cell population in mice and men. J Exp Med 203:2627–2638

Bonifaz L et al (2002) Efficient targeting of protein antigen to the dendritic cell receptor DEC-205 in the steady state leads to antigen presentation on major histocompatibility complex class I products and peripheral CD8+ T cell tolerance. J Exp Med 196:1627–1638

Bonifaz LC et al (2004) In vivo targeting of antigens to maturing dendritic cells via the DEC-205 receptor improves T cell vaccination. J Exp Med 199:815–824

Caux C et al (1997) CD34+ hematopoietic progenitors from human cord blood differentiate along two independent dendritic cell pathways in response to granulocyte-macrophage colony-stimulating factor plus tumor necrosis factor alpha: II. Functional analysis. Blood 90:1458–1470

Cella M et al (1999) Plasmacytoid monocytes migrate to inflamed lymph nodes and produce large amounts of type I interferon. Nat Med 5:919–923

Cheng P, Zhou J, Gabrilovich D (2010) Regulation of dendritic cell differentiation and function by Notch and Wnt pathways. Immunol Rev 234:105–119

Chung DJ et al (2009) Indoleamine 2,3-dioxygenase-expressing mature human monocyte-derived dendritic cells expand potent autologous regulatory T cells. Blood 114:555–563

Chung DJ et al (2016) T-cell exhaustion in multiple myeloma relapse after autotransplant: optimal timing of immunotherapy. Cancer Immunol Res 4:61–71

Collin M, McGovern N, Haniffa M (2013) Human dendritic cell subsets. Immunology 140:22–30

Collin MP et al (2005) In vitro depletion of tissue-derived dendritic cells by CMRF-44 antibody and alemtuzumab: implications for the control of graft-versus-host disease. Transplantation 79:722–725

Collin MP et al (2006) The fate of human Langerhans cells in hematopoietic stem cell transplantation. J Exp Med 203:27–33

Durakovic N et al (2006) Host-derived Langerhans cells persist after MHC-matched allografting independent of donor T cells and critically influence the alloresponses mediated by donor lymphocyte infusions. J Immunol 177:4414–4425

Dzionek A et al (2000) BDCA-2, BDCA-3, and BDCA-4: three markers for distinct subsets of dendritic cells in human peripheral blood. J Immunol 165:6037–6046

Ebner S et al (2004) Expression of C-type lectin receptors by subsets of dendritic cells in human skin. Int Immunol 16:877–887

Ferrara JL, Levine JE, Reddy P, Holler E (2009) Graft-versus-host disease. Lancet 373:1550–1561

Feuchtinger T et al (2010) Dendritic cell vaccination in an allogeneic stem cell recipient receiving a transplant from a human cytomegalovirus (HCMV)-seronegative donor: induction of a HCMV-specific T (helper) cell response. Cytotherapy 12:945–950

Fonteneau JF et al (2003) Activation of influenza virus-specific CD4+ and CD8+ T cells: a new role for plasmacytoid dendritic cells in adaptive immunity. Blood 101:3520–3526

Fujii S et al (2001) Treatment of post-transplanted, relapsed patients with hematological malignancies by infusion of HLA-matched, allogeneic-dendritic cells (DCs) pulsed with irradiated tumor cells and primed T cells. Leuk Lymphoma 42:357–369

Gattinoni L et al (2005) Removal of homeostatic cytokine sinks by lymphodepletion enhances the efficacy of adoptively transferred tumor-specific CD8+ T cells. J Exp Med 202:907–912

Gilboa E, Vieweg J (2004) Cancer immunotherapy with mRNA-transfected dendritic cells. Immunol Rev 199:251–263

Grigoleit GU et al (2007) Dendritic cell vaccination in allogeneic stem cell recipients: induction of human cytomegalovirus (HCMV)-specific cytotoxic T lymphocyte responses even in patients receiving a transplant from an HCMV-seronegative donor. J Infect Dis 196:699–704

Grouard G et al (1997) The enigmatic plasmacytoid T cells develop into dendritic cells with interleukin (IL)-3 and CD40-ligand. J Exp Med 185:1101–1111

Guermonprez P et al (2003) ER-phagosome fusion defines an MHC class I cross-presentation compartment in dendritic cells. Nature 425:397–402

Guilliams M, Bruhns P, Saeys Y, Hammad H, Lambrecht BN (2014) The function of Fcgamma receptors in dendritic cells and macrophages. Nat Rev Immunol 14:94–108

Hackstein H et al (2003) Rapamycin inhibits IL-4--induced dendritic cell maturation in vitro and dendritic cell mobilization and function in vivo. Blood 101:4457–4463

Hawiger D et al (2001) Dendritic cells induce peripheral T cell unresponsiveness under steady state conditions in vivo. J Exp Med 194:769–779

Hill GR, Ferrara JL (2000) The primacy of the gastrointestinal tract as a target organ of acute graft-versus-host disease: rationale for the use of cytokine shields in allogeneic bone marrow transplantation. Blood 95:2754–2759

Hsu FJ et al (1996) Vaccination of patients with B-cell lymphoma using autologous antigen-pulsed dendritic cells. Nat Med 2:52–58

Itano AA, Jenkins MK (2003) Antigen presentation to naive CD4 T cells in the lymph node. Nat Immunol 4:733–739

Jarrossay D, Napolitani G, Colonna M, Sallusto F, Lanzavecchia A (2001) Specialization and complementarity in microbial molecule recognition by human myeloid and plasmacytoid dendritic cells. Eur J Immunol 31:3388–3393

Jego G, Pascual V, Palucka AK, Banchereau J (2005) Dendritic cells control B cell growth and differentiation. Curr Dir Autoimmun 8:124–139

Jego G et al (2003) Plasmacytoid dendritic cells induce plasma cell differentiation through type I interferon and interleukin 6. Immunity 19:225–234

Jonuleit H et al (1997) Pro-inflammatory cytokines and prostaglandins induce maturation of potent immunostimulatory dendritic cells under fetal calf serum-free conditions. Eur J Immunol 27:3135–3142

Kadowaki N et al (2001) Subsets of human dendritic cell precursors express different toll-like receptors and respond to different microbial antigens. J Exp Med 194:863–869

Karan D et al (2011) Dual antigen target-based immunotherapy for prostate cancer eliminates the growth of established tumors in mice. Immunotherapy 3:735–746

Kim R, Emi M, Tanabe K, Arihiro K (2006) Tumor-driven evolution of immunosuppressive networks during malignant progression. Cancer Res 66:5527–5536

Kitawaki T et al (2008) Potential of dendritic-cell immunotherapy for relapse after allogeneic hematopoietic stem cell transplantation, shown by WT1 peptide- and keyhole-limpet-hemocyanin-pulsed, donor-derived dendritic-cell vaccine for acute myeloid leukemia. Am J Hematol 83:315–317

Klangsinsirikul P, Carter GI, Byrne JL, Hale G, Russell NH (2002) Campath-1G causes rapid depletion of circulating host dendritic cells (DCs) before allogeneic transplantation but does not delay donor DC reconstitution. Blood 99:2586–2591

Klechevsky E et al (2008) Functional specializations of human epidermal Langerhans cells and CD14+ dermal dendritic cells. Immunity 29:497–510

Kranz LM et al (2016) Systemic RNA delivery to dendritic cells exploits antiviral defence for cancer immunotherapy. Nature 534:396–401

Lacy MQ et al (2009) Idiotype-pulsed antigen-presenting cells following autologous transplantation for multiple myeloma may be associated with prolonged survival. Am J Hematol 84:799–802

Lau J et al (2007) Activated circulating dendritic cells after hematopoietic stem cell transplantation predict acute graft-versus-host disease. Transplantation 83:839–846

Lee YR et al (2005) Cyclosporin A and tacrolimus, but not rapamycin, inhibit MHC-restricted antigen presentation pathways in dendritic cells. Blood 105:3951–3955

Levenga H et al (2007) Dynamics in chimerism of T cells and dendritic cells in relapsed CML patients and the influence on the induction of alloreactivity following donor lymphocyte infusion. Bone Marrow Transplant 40:585–592

Levenga H et al (2010) Partial T cell-depleted allogeneic stem cell transplantation following reduced-intensity conditioning creates a platform for immunotherapy with donor lymphocyte infusion and recipient dendritic cell vaccination in multiple myeloma. Biol Blood Marrow Transplant 16:320–332

Lopez JA et al (2003) Single step enrichment of blood dendritic cells by positive immunoselection. J Immunol Methods 274:47–61

Luptakova K et al (2013) Lenalidomide enhances anti-myeloma cellular immunity. Cancer Immunol Immunother. 62:39–49

Lutz MB, Schuler G (2002) Immature, semi-mature and fully mature dendritic cells: which signals induce tolerance or immunity? Trends Immunol 23:445–449

Maldonado-Lopez R et al (1999) CD8alpha+ and CD8alpha- subclasses of dendritic cells direct the development of distinct T helper cells in vivo. J Exp Med 189:587–592
Mapara MY et al (2002) Donor lymphocyte infusions mediate superior graft-versus-leukemia effects in mixed compared to fully allogeneic chimeras: a critical role for host antigen-presenting cells. Blood 100:1903–1909
Matte CC et al (2004) Donor APCs are required for maximal GVHD but not for GVL. Nat Med 10:987–992
McCarthy PL et al (2012) Lenalidomide after stem-cell transplantation for multiple myeloma. N Engl J Med 366:1770–1781
Merad M et al (2002) Langerhans cells renew in the skin throughout life under steady-state conditions. Nat Immunol 3:1135–1141
Merad M et al (2004) Depletion of host Langerhans cells before transplantation of donor alloreactive T cells prevents skin graft-versus-host disease. Nat Med 10:510–517
Munn DH et al (2002) Potential regulatory function of human dendritic cells expressing indoleamine 2,3-dioxygenase. Science 297:1867–1870
Munz C et al (2005) Mature myeloid dendritic cell subsets have distinct roles for activation and viability of circulating human natural killer cells. Blood 105:266–273
Nestle FO, Zheng XG, Thompson CB, Turka LA, Nickoloff BJ (1993) Characterization of dermal dendritic cells obtained from normal human skin reveals phenotypic and functionally distinctive subsets. J Immunol 151:6535–6545
Noonan K et al (2012) Lenalidomide-induced immunomodulation in multiple myeloma: impact on vaccines and antitumor responses. Clin Cancer Res 18:1426–1434
Palucka AK et al (2006) Dendritic cells loaded with killed allogeneic melanoma cells can induce objective clinical responses and MART-1 specific CD8+ T-cell immunity. J Immunother 29:545–557
Palucka K, Banchereau J (2002) How dendritic cells and microbes interact to elicit or subvert protective immune responses. Curr Opin Immunol 14:420–431
Palucka K, Banchereau J (2012) Cancer immunotherapy via dendritic cells. Nat Rev Cancer 12:265–277
Palumbo A et al (2014) Autologous transplantation and maintenance therapy in multiple myeloma. N Engl J Med 371:895–905
Pulendran B, Palucka K, Banchereau J (2001) Sensing pathogens and tuning immune responses. Science 293:253–256
Pulendran B et al (1999) Distinct dendritic cell subsets differentially regulate the class of immune response in vivo. Proc Natl Acad Sci U S A 96:1036–1041
Qi H, Egen JG, Huang AY, Germain RN (2006) Extrafollicular activation of lymph node B cells by antigen-bearing dendritic cells. Science 312:1672–1676
Ratzinger G, Reagan JL, Heller G, Busam KJ, Young JW (2003) Differential CD52 expression by distinct myeloid dendritic cell subsets: implications for alemtuzumab activity at the level of antigen presentation in allogeneic graft-host interactions in transplantation. Blood 101:1422–1429
Ratzinger G et al (2004) Mature human Langerhans cells derived from CD34+ hematopoietic progenitors stimulate greater cytolytic T lymphocyte activity in the absence of bioactive IL-12p70, by either single peptide presentation or cross-priming, than do dermal-interstitial or monocyte-derived dendritic cells. J Immunol 173:2780–2791
Reddy V et al (2004) Low dendritic cell count after allogeneic hematopoietic stem cell transplantation predicts relapse, death, and acute graft-versus-host disease. Blood 103:4330–4335
Reichardt VL et al (1999) Idiotype vaccination using dendritic cells after autologous peripheral blood stem cell transplantation for multiple myeloma--a feasibility study. Blood 93:2411–2419
Reis e Sousa C (2006) Dendritic cells in a mature age. Nat Rev Immunol 6:476–483
Reizis B, Bunin A, Ghosh HS, Lewis KL, Sisirak V (2011) Plasmacytoid dendritic cells: recent progress and open questions. Annu Rev Immunol 29:163–183
Romano E et al (2011) Peptide-Loaded Langerhans cells, despite increased IL15 secretion and T-cell activation in vitro. Elicit antitumor T-cell responses comparable to peptide-loaded monocyte-derived dendritic cells in vivo. Clin Cancer Res 17:1984–1997

Romano E et al (2012) Human Langerhans cells use an IL-15R-alpha/IL-15/pSTAT5-dependent mechanism to break T-cell tolerance against the self-differentiation tumor antigen WT1. Blood 119:5182–5190
Rosenblatt J et al (2013) Vaccination with dendritic cell/tumor fusions following autologous stem cell transplant induces immunologic and clinical responses in multiple myeloma patients. Clin Cancer Res 19:3640–3648
Shaw J, Wang YH, Ito T, Arima K, Liu YJ (2010) Plasmacytoid dendritic cells regulate B-cell growth and differentiation via CD70. Blood 115:3051–3057
Sherman LA, Chattopadhyay S (1993) The molecular basis of allorecognition. Annu Rev Immunol 11:385–402
Shlomchik WD et al (1999) Prevention of graft versus host disease by inactivation of host antigen-presenting cells. Science 285:412–415
Siegal FP et al (1999) The nature of the principal type 1 interferon-producing cells in human blood. Science 284:1835–1837
Steinman RM (2012) Decisions about dendritic cells: past, present, and future. Annu Rev Immunol 30:1–22
Steinman RM, Banchereau J (2007) Taking dendritic cells into medicine. Nature 449:419–426
Steinman RM, Hawiger D, Nussenzweig MC (2003) Tolerogenic dendritic cells. Annu Rev Immunol 21:685–711
Takeda K, Kaisho T, Akira S (2003) Toll-like receptors. Annu Rev Immunol 21:335–376
Takeuchi O, Akira S (2010) Pattern recognition receptors and inflammation. Cell 140:805–820
Tatsugami K et al (2004) Dendritic-cell therapy after non-myeloablative stem-cell transplantation for renal-cell carcinoma. Lancet Oncol 5:750–752
Timmerman JM et al (2002) Idiotype-pulsed dendritic cell vaccination for B-cell lymphoma: clinical and immune responses in 35 patients. Blood 99:1517–1526
Toubai T et al (2013) Host-derived CD8+ dendritic cells are required for induction of optimal graft-versus-tumor responses after experimental allogeneic bone marrow transplantation. Blood 121:4231–4241
Trombetta ES, Mellman I (2005) Cell biology of antigen processing in vitro and in vivo. Annu Rev Immunol 23:975–1028
Ueno H et al (2007) Dendritic cell subsets in health and disease. Immunol Rev 219:118–142
Ueno H et al (2010) Harnessing human dendritic cell subsets for medicine. Immunol Rev 234:199–212
Valladeau J, Saeland S (2005) Cutaneous dendritic cells. Semin Immunol 17:273–283
Valladeau J et al (2000) Langerin, a novel C-type lectin specific to Langerhans cells, is an endocytic receptor that induces the formation of Birbeck granules. Immunity 12:71–81
Walter S et al (2012) Multipeptide immune response to cancer vaccine IMA901 after single-dose cyclophosphamide associates with longer patient survival. Nat Med 18(8):1254–1261
Yuan J et al (2006) Langerhans-type dendritic cells genetically modified to express full-length antigen optimally stimulate CTLs in a CD4-dependent manner. J Immunol 176:2357–2365
Zhang H et al (2005) Lymphopenia and interleukin-2 therapy alter homeostasis of CD4+CD25+ regulatory T cells. Nat Med 11:1238–1243
Zhang Y et al (2002) APCs in the liver and spleen recruit activated allogeneic CD8+ T cells to elicit hepatic graft-versus-host disease. J Immunol 169:7111–7118
Zhang Z et al (2011) The helicase DDX41 senses intracellular DNA mediated by the adaptor STING in dendritic cells. Nat Immunol 12:959–965
Zhou LJ, Tedder TF (1995) Human blood dendritic cells selectively express CD83, a member of the immunoglobulin superfamily. J Immunol 154:3821–3835
Ziegler-Heitbrock L et al (2010) Nomenclature of monocytes and dendritic cells in blood. Blood 116:e74–e80

Mesenchymal Stem Cells: From Bench to Bedside and Back

12

John Barrett and Jacques Galipeau

12.1 Mesenchymal Stromal Cells (MSCs): The First Therapeutic Applications

Since the time when bone marrow cells were first cultured in vitro, investigators were aware that, in addition to cells responsible for blood formation, a population of adherent spindle cell colonies would grow on the flat surface of the culture vessel. These so-called bone marrow fibroblasts were first studied in detail by Friedenstein in St. Petersburg (then Leningrad). He found that these cells could differentiate under certain conditions into chondrocytes, fat cells, and osteoblasts (Friedenstein et al. 1974). Later investigators found that similar cells could be isolated from umbilical cord and dental pulp and can be differentiated from adipocytes (Chen et al. 2011). An important property for their application in hematopoietic cell transplantation (HCT) is that bone marrow-derived MSCs have immunosuppressive properties and inhibit T-lymphocyte proliferation. They also contribute to tissue repair and are of intense interest in the field of regenerative medicine (Le Blanc 2006). By accepted convention, cells from any tissue of origin, which share spindle cell morphology, plastic adherence, trilineage mesenchymal differentiation, and immunomodulatory properties, express CD109 and CD73, and lack CD45 and CD34, are called mesenchymal *stromal* cells (MSCs) (reviewed in Battiwalla and Barrett 2014).

J. Barrett (✉)
Stem Cell Allogenic Transplantation Section, National Heart, Lung and Blood Institute, National Institutes of Health, Bethesda, MD, USA
e-mail: barrettj@nhlbi.nih.gov

J. Galipeau
University of Wisconsin-Madison, Madison, WI, USA
e-mail: jgalipeau@wisc.edu

M.-A. Perales et al. (eds.), *Cell and Gene Therapies*, Advances and Controversies in Hematopoietic Transplantation and Cell Therapy,
https://doi.org/10.1007/978-3-319-54368-0_12

MSC as a form of cellular therapy were first explored in HCT recipients as the treatment of graft-versus-host disease (GvHD) and marrow failure. Faced with a young boy suffering from life-threatening refractory acute GvHD after an allogeneic stem cell transplantation (HCT) and prompted by the known immunosuppressive potential of MSC, Katarina Le Blanc in Stockholm generated MSC from the boy's mother and administered 2×10^6 MSC/kg intravenously. There was a remarkable and rapid clinical improvement in the liver and gut GvHD after the infusion, but 6 weeks later the GvHD had relapsed. A second infusion produced another prompt response and a prolonged GvHD-free survival (Le Blanc et al. 2004). About the same time, based on murine marrow repopulation experiments which suggested that MSC could enhance marrow engraftment, Lazarus and others first explored the potential of MSC to improve hematopoietic recovery after autologous HCT and confirmed the safety of infusion and possible benefit for hematopoietic recovery (Lazarus et al. 2005). These initial studies confirmed the infusional safety of MSC given to HCT recipients and have paved the way for subsequent clinical research. Today, more than a decade later, the potential of MSC to improve outcomes after allogeneic and autologous HCT represents an ongoing area of active research, reviewed in this chapter.

12.2 MSC and GvHD

12.2.1 Immunomodulatory Effects of MSC and Their Therapeutic Potential in GvHD

MSC interact with adaptive and innate immune cells in multiple ways. Of particular relevance to their application for GvHD is their powerful immunosuppressive interaction with T lymphocytes. MSC suppress the activation and proliferation of T cells responding to their cognate antigen and block alloresponses (Götherström et al. 2003; Rasmusson et al. 2003; Le Blanc and Mougiakakos 2012; Le Blanc et al. 2003). However they do not block already established cytotoxic T cells recognizing viruses, and antiviral T cell responses are retained after MSC infusion (Karlsson et al. 2008). They inhibit the generation of T cells with the cytotoxic Th17 phenotype and promote the generation of regulatory T cells (Tasso et al. 2012; Bessout et al. 2015). Several mechanisms of T cell suppression have been described (reviewed in Stagg and Galipeau 2012): MSCs produce IDO and PGE2 and through surface-bound CD73 break down AMP into adenosine and phosphate which are toxic to activated T cells (Melief et al. 2013). MSCs also suppress cytotoxic T cell development indirectly by stimulating monocytes to generate IL-10 and other anti-inflammatory cytokines (Tolar et al. 2011). The immunosuppressive action of MSC has been demonstrated in numerous animal models, but animal experiments focusing on the ability of MSC to prevent or treat GvHD have largely been carried out after the initial clinical studies. Not all investigators report efficacy in their specific models. Differences in findings relate to the tissue source of MSC and mode of preparation and administration (Gregoire-Gauthier et al. 2012). Most relevant to GvHD treatment in man are experiments in immune-deficient NGS mice developing xenograft GvHD from human lymphocytes (Melief et al. 2013; Le Blanc et al. 2008). MSC have been shown to both prevent GvHD and suppress established GvHD in these models. While a large body of data confirms that MSC have potent immunomodulatory and immunosuppressive properties, it still remains unclear which properties are most important for the therapeutic benefit in GvHD and how they may be selected and amplified. Furthermore the distribution and fate of infused MSC in man is not well established. Animal data show that MSCs first accumulate in the pulmonary circulation but can home to sites of tissue injury and inflammation, but their fate in human recipients is not well described. Recently we showed that in a murine xeno-GvHD model, MSC remained sequestered in the lungs but shed circulating exosomes which may have conferred the therapeutic effect on GvHD (Amarnath et al. 2015). Circulating exosomes were also identified in human recipients of MSC for GvHD treatment (Melief et al. 2013). The strength of preclinical data and anecdotal clinical cases serve as a backdrop to numerous investigators using MSC in clinical trials to treat or prevent acute or chronic GvHD as described below.

12.2.2 Clinical Trials of Bone Marrow MSC in GvHD

Initially used as salvage treatment in desperate cases of uncontrolled and life-threatening acute GvHD, investigators have also explored their application in early GvHD management. The use of MSC has also extended to treatment of chronic GvHD and attempts to prevent acute and chronic GvHD by co-administration of MSC with the allogeneic stem cell transplant. Since 2008, there have been 19 clinical trials using noncommercial MSC manufactured in GMP facilities to treat acute GvHD in 370 patients (Sánchez-Guijo et al. 2014; Muroi et al. 2013; von Bonin et al. 2009; Introna et al. 2014; Ringdén et al. 2006; Pérez-Simon et al. 2011; Zhao et al. 2013; Herrmann et al. 2012; Yin et al. 2014; Zhao et al. 2015; Te Boome et al. 2015; Ball et al. 2013; Resnick et al. 2013; von Bahr et al. 2012) (Table 12.1). Four further studies have been reported using a commercially manufactured industrial-scale expanded MSC product "Prochymal."

12.2.3 Early-Passage Small-Scale Expanded MSC to Treat Acute GvHD (Table 12.1)

Most investigators have used MSC as salvage treatment of steroid refractory acute GvHD. These studies in both children and adults included many patients who had not only failed at least a week of high-dose intravenous prednisone but had also failed second line, third line, or sometimes up to seven previous treatment approaches. Treatment with MSC often occurred many weeks or months following GvHD onset. With the exception of the first reported multicenter study in 55 patients in refractory GvHD (Sánchez-Guijo et al. 2014), the number of subjects treated in each series has been small, ranging between 7 and 48 with varying intervals between

Table 12.1 Noncommercial BM MSC trials for acute GvHD

Author	*N*=	Pediatric/ adult	GvHD status	Med dose × 10^6/kg	Doses	OR%	CR/ PR	TRM	Survival	Comment
Le Blanc et al. (2008)	55	19/34	SR	1.4[a]	1–5	53	30/9	37% (CR) 72% (PR/NR)	53% (CR) 16% (PR/NR)	Multicenter European study
Sánchez-Guijo et al. (2014)	25	–/25	SR	1.1	2–4	71	11/6	52% (CR/PR) 71%(NR)	80% (CR) 21% (PR/NR)	Multicenter, two MSC production centers
Muroi et al. (2013)	14	1/13	SR II–III	2.0	8	93	8/5	6 at 96 weeks	57%	Early admin. No grade IV
von Bonin et al. (2009)	13	–/13	SR III–IV	0.9	1–5	45	1/1	9 at 185 days	31%	Response includes concomitant therapy
Introna et al. (2014)	40	15/25	SR II–III	1.5	3	67.5	11/16	61.4% at 2 years	66% P 40% A	Multicenter, III/IV worse outcome
Ringdén et al. (2006)	8	–/8	SR III–IV	1.0	1–3	75	6/2	3	56% at 2–36 months	Includes 1 C-GvHD
Pérez-Simon et al. (2011)	10	–/10	SR II–IV	1.2	1–2	10	1/6	90%	1 survivor >11 months	Low infusional doses
Zhao et al. (2013)	22	NA	SR	4.8	2.5	72	12/4	50% at 8 months	55% at 8 months	Abstract
Herrmann et al. (2012)	12	–/12	SR II–IV	1.7–2.3[b]	1–4	58	7/4	6	6 (3–36 months)	Early after GvHD onset
Yin et al. (2014)	8	–/8	SR II–IV	2.0	3	78	5/1	2	5	Responses correlate with biomarkers

Zhao et al. (2015)	28 19 Ctrl	Median 26 y Median 29 y	SR II–IV	1	2–8	75 42	11/– 8	46% 74%	46.4% 26.3%	Controlled study! No sigificant differences, less C-GvHD
Te Boome et al. (2015)	48	7/41	SR II–IV	1–2	2–4	50	12/24	25%/50% (d28)	41% at 1 year	Biomarker study
Ball et al. (2013)	37	19/10	II–IV	1–2	1–13	50	12/24	17–53% (early vs late)	37% at 5 years	Retrospective multicenter study
Resnick et al. (2013)	50	25/25	SR II–IV	0.3–3.1	1–4	66	17/16		56% at >3 years	Some received intra-arterial MSC

SR steroid resistant (GvHD grades I–IV shown), *C-GvHD* chronic GvHD, *NA* not available, *Ctrl* controls, *OR* overall response, *CR* complete response, *PR* partial response, *NR* no response, *P* pediatric, *A* adult, *TRM* transplant related mortality

[a]Includes 8 autologous, 5 HLA donors

[b]Includes 1 HLA-identical donor

onset of steroid-requiring GvHD and the application of MSC. Only one study by Zhao and colleagues (Zhao et al. 2015) included a no-treatment control arm. Doses, schedules, source, and manufacture of MSC are varied: In general doses around 2×10^6 MSC/kg have been used given in one to eight infusions. In some trials efforts were made to select HLA-matched MSC donor, but mostly mismatched third-party MSC banks have been used. All 17 studies where MSCs are given in steroid refractory (SR)-GvHD report complete and partial responses with overall response rates typically around 70% but with reports as low as 10% (Perez-Simon et al. 2011. 2013) and as high as 93% (Muroi et al. 2013). Where reported, post-infusional survival is higher in responders, and in the single controlled study, both response and survival were significantly greater (75 vs 42% and 46.4 vs 26.3%, respectively) (Zhao et al. 2015). Despite the diversity and uncontrolled nature of most of this data, we can draw some tentative conclusions. Firstly, MSC infusion is safe, and (despite concerns) there is no convincing evidence that the immunomodulation that MSC may induce results in greater leukemic relapse or increased infections (Prasad et al. 2011; Kurtzberg et al. 2014). Secondly MSCs benefit patients with steroid refractory GvHD as confirmed in the controlled study. Responses are seen in patients with all grades of severity and in all affected organ systems. However the most reliably documented responses occur in gastrointestinal and liver GvHD with little evidence for response in skin GvHD. Favorable factors for response are younger age, earlier administration, lesser grades of GvHD, and use of fresh (non-cryopreserved) MSC products. Responses can occur with as little as a single dose of around a million MSC/kg; however relapse of GvHD is not uncommon, suggesting more prolonged treatment might be beneficial. One key outcome of SR-GvHD is a subsequent increase in mortality. Many studies contrast the dismal outcome for recipients failing to respond to MSC versus the MSC responders whose survival exceeds the anticipated historical mortality of over 50% in such cases.

12.2.4 Industrial-Scale Manufactured MSC

Four studies have used Prochymal originally manufactured by Osiris and subsequently by Mesoblast (Kebriaei et al. 2009; Martin et al. 2010; Maitra et al. 2004; Baron et al. 2010) (Table 12.2). Again there were no infusional toxicities or late sequelae. Responses occurred in 53–94% this latter in a study by Kebriaei administered MSC within 2 weeks of developing aGvHD (Maitra et al. 2004). The only phase III study randomizing patients to receive Prochymal or placebo at onset of GvHD was presented at the American Society of Hematology Meeting in 2010 (Baron et al. 2010). This multicenter study failed to demonstrate that MSC significantly improved overall response over the placebo. As such the primary goal of the trial was not met. However in subset analysis MSCs were found to result in significantly greater responses in liver and gut GvHD (76% vs 47% and 82% vs 68%, respectively). Overall the results with Prochymal appear very similar to the noncommercial products manufactured in diverse academic institutes worldwide, suggesting that the therapeutic effect of MSC is not closely dependent on the method of production.

Table 12.2 Prochymal MSC trials for acute GvHD

Author	*N*=	Age group (Median years)	GvHD status	Doses	Response	Survival	Comment
Prasad et al. (2011)	12	P	SR III–IV	8	53% OR	42% at 2 years	Best response in pediatric patients with GI GvHD
Kurtzberg et al. (2014)	59	P (8)	SR II–IV	2–8	64% OR	76% (Ctrl 9%) at d100	No difference between high vs low MSC dose
Kebriaei et al. (2009)	32	A (52)	II–IV	2–8	94% OR (77% CR, 16% PR)	68% at d90	De novo GvHD <2 weeks from onset
Martin et al. (2010)	163 81	A (44) Ctrl (40)	SR II–IV	2–8 +4 if PR	35% CR (30% placebo) NS Liver 76% CR (47% placebo) *p* 0.05 GI 82% CR (68% placebo) *p* 0.05	NA	Double-blind placebo. Randomized 2:1. No significant durable CR d28 compared with placebo control. But significant benefit for subsets with liver and/or GI GvHD

P pediatric, *A* adult, *Ctrl* placebo controls randomized 1:2 with MSC recipients, *SR* steroid refractory, *OR* overall response, *CR* complete response by d28, *PR* partial response, *GI* gastrointestinal GvHD, *NA* not available, *NS* not significant

12.2.5 MSC as Initial Treatment of Severe Acute GvHD

Studies with MSC in refractory GvHD suggested that patients might benefit if MSC was infused earlier in the course of GvHD evolution. Two trials appear to confirm this assumption. Kebriaei reports 93% responses in 32 recipients of MSC (Maitra et al. 2004), and Ball reported a 65% response with a lower TRM in those receiving earliest treatment (46% vs 74%) (Resnick et al. 2013). This may reflect less tissue damage in the promptly treated patients and may indicate the importance of modulating the immune response earlier in the course of the disease. More studies with MSC used as an adjunct to parenteral high-dose steroid treatment are clearly indicated.

12.2.6 MSC to Prevent GvHD

Maitra and colleagues exploring the role of coinfusion of MSC to boost marrow function observed that MSC suppressed T cell activation and might therefore play a role in mitigation of GvHD (Baron et al. 2010). Several investigators have coinfused MSC from various sources at the time of the bone marrow or umbilical cord stem cell transplant in matched and mismatched HCT with the specific aim of monitoring its impact on GvHD (Table 12.3). While GvHD might have been reduced in severity and refractoriness and some chronic GvHD was prevented, no conclusions (other than to the safety of the approach) can be drawn in the absence of a contemporaneous control group not receiving MSC (Maziarz et al. 2015; Wu et al. 2014a; Shipounova et al. 2014; Zhang et al. 2009; Weng et al. 2012).

12.2.7 Chronic GvHD

A few investigators have explored the potential of BM MSC largely derived from third-party donors to modify the course and severity of cGvHD (Zhao et al. 2013; Zhou et al. 2010; Peng et al. 2014; Herrmann et al. 2012; François et al. 2012; Nicolay et al. 2015). Six reports totaling 88 cGvHD recipients explore multiple infusions of MSC in patients with chronic GvHD refractory to at least first-line therapy. Patients mainly had extensive cGvHD, and one report specifies sclerodermatous GvHD. All investigators described around 20% complete remissions with about 70% partial responses and improvements in performance scores. However there appears to be a tendency for relapse of the cGvHD within months of initial treatment (Table 12.4). Evaluating this data is complicated by diversity of organ involvement, duration of the GvHD, its severity, and prior or current immunosuppressive treatment.

12.3 MSC in Tissue and Organ Repair Posttransplant

12.3.1 Experimental Basis

Many experimental studies (mainly in small mammals) have explored the repair properties of MSC in degenerative diseases and after damage from radiation, chemotherapy, or mechanical injury. MSC can accelerate repair both by differentiating into functional cell types and by creating a milieu promoting repair and reducing fibrosis. Relevant to HCT and the tissue targets of GvHD are studies on the role of MSC limiting radiation injury and promoting repair (Ringdén et al. 2007) and studies demonstrating reparative ability of MSC in chemotherapy-induced lung and liver injury (reviewed in Nicolay et al. 2015).

Clinical reports of attempts to treat posttransplant tissue injury are limited, but the results are provocative. Ringden and colleagues explored MSC infusion in seven patients with hemorrhagic cystitis, two with pneumomediastinum and one with inoperable peritonitis. Transfusion requirements were reduced in all seven patients with HC, and five had complete cessation of hematuria in a median of 3 days (Noort et al. 2002). In the other patients, pneumomediastinum and peritonitis resolved. However the role of MSC in their recovery and the mechanism of action of MSC are unclear.

Table 12.3 Prevention of GvHD (adult patients)

Author	*N*=	SCT	SCT	MSC	Schedule	A-GvHD	C-GvHD	NRM	REL	OS	Comment
Baron et al. (2010)	20 16 Ctrl	NMA	PBSCT	BM- 3P	1 coinf	II-IV 35%	65%	10% 1 y (37% P 0.02)	30% (25%)	80% (44%)	Significantly better outcomes than controls
Gonzalo-Daganzo et al. (2009)	9 46 Ctrl	MA	Haplo/Cord	BM- 3P	1 coinf	II 44%, III_IV 0% II 11% III_IV 13%24%	24%	11% 37%	1 6	89% 56%	Inconclusive benefit. Two GvHD responses to further MSC
Maziarz et al. (2015)	36	MA	HLA = (35)	Multistem	Day 2 × 1 (*n* = 18)	II-IV 37%	–	11% d100	8% d100	81% d00	Recipients of >100 × 10⁶/kg MSC had less GvHD (1/9 grade II)
Wu et al. (2014a)	36	MA	Haplo	UC	Weekly × 5 (*n* = 18)	III-IV 14%	37.5%	–	8.3%	77%	May have reduced relapse
Shipounova et al. (2014)	39 36 Ctrl	NA	HLA = BMT	BM - D	1 infusion at heme recovery	II–IV 4/39 (10.2%) 8/38 (20.5%)		23% 42%	23% 29%	– –	Half the incidence of A-GvHD in MSC recipients compared with controls

A adult, *NMA* non-myeloablative transplant, *MA* myeloablative transplant, *PBSCT* peripheral blood stem cell transplant, *Ctrl* historical controls, *coinf* coinfusion of MSC with stem cell transplant, *OS* overall survival, *A-GvHD* acute graft-versus-host disease, *C-GvHD* chronic graft-versus-host disease, *REL* relapse of leukemia, *NRM* non-relapse mortality, *UC* umbilical cord donor, *BM* bone marrow, *3P* third party donor, *D* matched donor, *NA* not available, *HLA* = HLA matched donor

Table 12.4 MSC for chronic GvHD

Author	N=	C-GvHD	BM-MSC donor	Med dose × 10^6/kg	Frequency	Response CR	PR	NR	Survival	Comment
Zhang et al. (2009)	12	Refractory	14 HLA= 10 HLA≠	1.2 (0.27–2.5)	1–3	3	6	3	75%	Raised CD4/CD8 ratio and T_{regs}
Weng et al. (2012)	19	Refractory/ progressive	3P	0.6	1–5 (med 2)	4	10	5	77.7% at 2 year	I/S tapered in <50%. Increased CD5+ B cells and CD28- CD8 cells
Zhou et al. (2010)	4	Sclerodermatous	3P	Total dose 1–2 × 10^7	4–8	>70% improved RS score[a]			100% at 4–23 months	Symptomatic improvement Increased Th1/Th2 ratio
Peng et al. (2014)	38	Extensive/ refractory	3P	1.0	≥2	5	23	10	≥12 months follow up	Max response reported, relapses occurred between 2 and 10 months
Pérez-Simon et al. (2011)	8	3–5 previous lines of Rx	D/Haplo/3P	0.2–1.2	1–4	1	2	5	62.5% 1 y med	CR patient: thrombocytopenia resolved
Herrmann et al. (2012)	7	Extensive, refractory	3P/HLA=	1.7–2.3	2–11	1	2	3	28% (inc 1 relapse)	Same paper reports 12 A-GvHD patients

Rx treatment, *D* transplant donor, *3P* third party donor, *Haplo* haploidentical family donor, T_{regs} regulatory T cells, *HLA=/HLA≠* HLA-matched/HLA-mismatched donor, *CR* complete response, *PR* partial response, *NR* no response, *A-GvHD* acute GvHD

[a]RS score: Rodnan skin score for severity of scleroderma

A beneficial role for MSC in severe late-onset HC involving BK virus is supported by a further study by Wang et al. (2015). Five of seven patients given one or more umbilical cord-derived MSC infusions promptly responded with cessation of hematuria between 2 and 12 days after first infusion. The time course of HC resolution in these patients was much more rapid than in 26 historical controls not given MSC. Further exploration in HC and other posttransplant tissue damage would benefit from the use of controls and extensive profiling of biomarkers of tissue damage and repair.

12.4 MSC to Boost Marrow Function

12.4.1 Experimental Basis

The niche function of MSC identified in murine studies was the basis for studies where human MSC was used to promote engraftment and possibly reduce GvHD in immune-deficient mice (Kim et al. 2006). In 2002 Noort and colleagues found that MSC derived from the human lung could enhance engraftment of umbilical cord CD34 cells (Lee et al. 2008). Subsequently Maitra and colleagues found that human (but not mouse) MSC promoted engraftment when coinfused with limiting numbers of human hematopoietic progenitors in NOD/SCID mice (Gonzalo-Daganzo et al. 2009). This property was restricted to MSC (not fibroblasts). The coincident suppression of human T cells also suggested a possible benefit of MSC coinfusion limiting GvHD. Further studies have confirmed a beneficial effect of human MSC when cotransplanted with human $CD34^+$ cells in NOD/SCID mice (Le Blanc et al. 2007; Ball et al. 2007).

12.4.2 Clinical Trials

A year later Lazarus and colleagues reported the first attempts in human HCT to boost engraftment and modulate GvHD (Lazarus et al. 2005). MSCs were expanded from the HLA-identical sibling stem cell transplant donors after myeloablative therapy. MSCs at a dose of $1.0–5.0 \times 10^6$ cells/kg of recipient weight were infused immediately prior to bone marrow or peripheral blood stem cells and standard GvHD prophylaxis. Forty-six adult patients were enrolled in the study. Hematological engraftment was prompt (median times to neutrophil counts $>0.5 \times 10^9$/L and platelets $>20 \times 10^9$/L were 14.0 and 20 days, respectively). There was a 28% incidence of grades II to IV acute GvHD and a 61% incidence of chronic GvHD and a progression-free survival at 2 years of 53%. While this study confirmed the safety of MSC infusion at transplant, the hematopoietic recovery, GvHD rates, and disease-free survival were not outside the expected outcomes for such a patient group and did not clearly identify a therapeutic benefit for MSC. Subsequently 10 further studies in a total of 141 patients have explored the potential benefit of infusing either BM- or UC-derived MSC at the time of transplant (Macmillan et al. 2009; Zhang et al. 2010; Liu et al. 2011; Wu et al. 2013a; Wu et al. 2013b; Meuleman et al. 2009; Liu et al. 2014; Lee et al. 2013; Wang et al. 2013; Wu et al. 2014b; Xu et al. 2014) (Table 12.5).

Table 12.5 MSC to improve stem cell engraftment

Author	*N*=	Donor	Strategy	Conditioning	MSC source	Engraftment/ recovery	GvHD A/C	Death/ Relapse	Survival	Comment
Lazarus et al. (2005)	46	HLA = sib	Coinf	MA	BM	All engrafted N 14 P20	A:II–IV 13 (28%) C: 22 (16%)	11 (24%) Rel	2 y DFS 53%	First report
Le Blanc et al. (2007)	7	HLA=	4 coinf 3 PGF	MA/RIC	BM	All engrafted N 12 P12	A: 0–I:5/C:1	1 NRM	6 survive	Promising strategy for GF
Ball et al. (2007)	14 47 Ctrl	Haplo	Coinf	MA	BM	All engrafted 7/47 engrafted	A: II 2/C:1 A:II–IV8/C:6	2 NRM 2 Rel 2 NRM 7 Rel	72% 63%	Pediatric haplo-T cell-depleted SCT MSC may improve outcome
Macmillan et al. (2009)	11 23 Ctrl	UCB	Coinf + d21	MA	BM	N 19 P75% 6 months N 15 P74% 6 months	A II–IV 38% C 72% A: II–IV 22% C 72%	5 NRM 1 Rel	75% at 1 y	No significant difference from controls
Zhang et al. (2010)	12	HLA = sib	Coinf	MA	BM	N 11 P13.5	A: II–IV 2 / C: 2	2 NRM 4 Rel	7 alive >2 y	Commercial MSC
Liu et al. (2011)	27 28 Ctrl	Haplo	Coinf	MA	BM	{	A: II–III 9/C:20 A: II–III 16/ C:2	6 NRM 2 Rel 8 NRM 1 Rel	69.7% 64.3%	Possible benefit for MSC
Wu et al. (2013a)	50	Haplo	Coinf	MA	UCB	All engrafted N 12 P15	A: II–IV 12 / C:17	1 Rel	2 year DFS 66%	Failure to show benefit
Wu et al. (2013b)	8 12 Ctrl	UCB	Coinf	MA	UCB	N 12 P30 N 21 P73	A: I–II 4 NA	2 Rel 2 NRM 2 Rel	6 at >1 year 8 at >1 year	Superior outcome for MSC

Kharbanda et al. (2014)	6	UCB 4 MUD 2	Coinf	RIC	BM	3/6 engrafted 2 autorec, 1 GF	A: II–III 2	4 NRM	2 at >1 year	Hemoglobinopathy RIC SCT
Meuleman et al. (2009)	6	3HLA = 3Haplo	PGF	MA	BM	2/6 engrafted 15 N 1.5 P 50	NA	5 NRM 1Rel	0%	High risk patients, no benefit in poor graft function
Liu et al. (2014)	20	4 HLA = 16≠	7 1° GF 13 2° GF	MA	BM	5 PR/NR	A: 4/C: 2	11 (inc 5 PR/NR)	9 at >500 days	Mixed patient group
Lee et al. (2013)	7 9 Ctrl	UCB	Coinf	MA	UCB	N 19 P 47 N 24 P57	A: I–IV 71%/C:1 A: 1–IV 62.5%/C:3	0 2 NRM	85.7% 55.6%	Benefit over hist. controls No difference in GvHD

Ped pediatric, *Coinf* coinfusion with stem cells, *Ctrl* controls, *PGF* poor graft function, *1°/2° GF* primary/secondary graft failure, *PR/NR* partial/no hematopoietic recovery, *MA* myeloablative, *RIC* reduced intensity conditioning, *SCT* stem cell transplant, *BM* bone marrow MSC, *UCB* umbilical cord blood MSC, *HLA=/HLA≠* HLA-matched/HLA-mismatched donor, *Haplo* haploidentical family donor, *MUD* matched unrelated donor MSC, *N* day neutrophils $>0.5 \times 10^9$/l, *Pt* day platelets $>20 \times 10^9$/l, *autorec* autologous hematopoietic recovery, *GF* graft failure, *DFS* disease free survival, *Rel* relapsed malignancy, *NA* not reported

Some investigators used MSC during a second transplant attempt after the first graft was rejected. Engraftment was achieved in most patients; failure mainly occurred in some recipients grafted a second time and in a series of patients with hemoglobinopathies receiving a reduced intensity conditioning. Several studies report rapid engraftment, but the true potential of MSC to accelerate engraftment can only be assessed in the single study where MSC coinfusion at transplant was compared in 8 patients versus 12 controls receiving UCB alone. In this study MSC infusion was associated with more rapid neutrophil and platelet recovery.

Overall the results indicate at best a modest benefit on engraftment and hematological recovery. It is possible that the benefit might be more apparent (and of greater clinical benefit) after UCB transplantation where recovery of marrow function is typically slower. However, only a large prospective randomized study could establish a clear role for MSC in this context.

12.5 Improving Engraftment After HLA-Haploidentical HCT for Aplastic Anemia

Hematopoietic cell transplantation for SAA is complicated by an increased risk of graft rejection consequent upon sensitization to multiple transfusions in conjunction with the irradiation-free conditioning regimens usually employed. Engraftment is further compromised when HCT are attempted from haploidentical family donors. Confronted with the relative frequency of SAA and the problem of finding HLA-matched family donors, investigators from several centers in China have explored the use of MSC to enhance engraftment in SAA recipients of haploidentical stem cells. Five reports in a total of 105 patients describe this unique experience from China (Li et al. 2014; Si et al. 2014; de Lima et al. 2012; Robinson et al. 2011; Fan et al. 2013) (Table 12.6).

Both adult and pediatric patients received HCT from either BM or PB. Conditioning typically used fludarabine and cytoxan with or without ATG, and GvHD prophylaxis was very similar across institutes involving CSA, MTX, and MMF, with or without other agents such as anti-CD25. Notably, engraftment occurred in all patients with prompt neutrophil and platelet recovery. There is some suggestion that GvHD may be mitigated with reported rates of GvHDs II–IV varying from 12.5 to 46%. Overall outcome in the context of haploidentical HCT for SAA was favorable (in the region of 75%), but without contemporaneous controls receiving stem cells alone, the definite benefit of MSC infusion on engraftment and survival awaits a prospective randomized study.

12.6 MSC to Expand UCB Ex Vivo

The slow engraftment achieved with umbilical cord blood HCT has been a limitation to the widespread acceptance of this stem cell source. Investigators have attempted to overcome the problem with double cord infusions and in vitro

Table 12.6 Coinfusion of umbilical cord MSC with haploidentical SCT for aplastic anemia

Author	*N*=	Donor	HSC	Conditioning	GVH PPX	Med dose × 10^6/kg	Engraftment	GvHD	Death/relapse	Survival	Comment
Wang et al. (2013)	22	8 Haplo 6 HLA= 8 URD	PB ± BM	Flu/Cy	CSA MTX MMF +/– CD25	1.2 (0.27–2.5)	All N 14 P 20	A: I–II 7 C: 0	1 TRM	21 > 15 months med	First report
Wu et al. (2014b)	21	Haplo	PB + BM	Flu or Bu/ CyATG	CSA MMF +/– CD25	0.5	All N 9–16 P 10–23	A: II–IV 9 C: 8	4 TRM	81% at 2 year	Low incidence of GvHD
Xu et al. (2014)	8	Haplo	PB + BM	Flu/Cy ATG ± Bu	CSA MTX MMF +/– ATG	1.0	All N 11 P 14	A: I–II 25% II–IV 12.5% C: 0	2 TRM	6 survive	–
Li et al. (2014)	17	Haplo	PB + BM	Flu/CyATG	CSA MMF CD25	2.8–10	1 graft failure N 12 P 14	A: III–IV 24% C: 14.2%	5 TRM	76% at 6 months Med surv 56mo	Age 4–29 RIC
Si et al. (2014)	37	10 HLA = 27 Haplo	PB ± BM	Flu/Cy ATG	CSA MTX MMF ATG	2.8 (0.8–3.4)	All N 14 P 19	A: II–IV 46% (17/37) C: 18.9 (7/37)	7 GvHD 1 fungal infection 1 renal failure	74.2% at 3 year	Favorable outcome in high risk

Ped pediatric, *HLA* HLA-matched donor, *Haplo* haploidentical matched family donor, *URD* unrelated donor, *PB* peripheral blood stem cell transplant, *BM* bone marrow transplant, *Flu* fludarabine, *Cy* cyclophosphamide, *ATG* antithymocyte globulin, *CSA* cyclosporine, *MMF* mycophenolate mofetil, *MTX* methotrexate, *CD25* anti-CD25 antibody, *A* acute, *C* chronic GvHD, *RIC* reduced intensity conditioning, *N* day neutrophils >0.5 × 10^9/l, *Pt* day platelets >20 × 10^9/l, *GF* graft failure, *DFS* disease-free survival, *Rel* relapsed malignancy, *Hbopathy* hemoglobinopathy

strategies to expand cord blood CD34 cells without losing their "stemness." Co-culture of cord blood with MSC to exploit the stem cell supportive properties of MSC has successfully been developed by Shpall's group (de Lima et al. 2012) and reviewed in (Robinson et al. 2011). In a clinical trial where MSC-cultured CD34 cells were coinfused with unmanipulated cells, platelet and neutrophil recovery was significantly faster than that documented in the large CIBMTR database of comparable cord blood transplants. Furthermore Fan et al. report that MSC co-culture enhances T_{regs} and suppresses GvHD in NOD/SCID mice (Xie et al. 2016). These data suggest that MSC may have greater efficacy in boosting engraftment and mitigating GvHD when cultured ex vivo with the stem cell transplant.

12.7 Where Does the Field Go from Here?

Since 2004, early-phase clinical trials of MSC used in conjunction with HCT have explored acute and chronic GvHD, engraftment and graft failure, and tissue repair in over 1000 patients. All studies confirm the safety of infusion, and although there has been concern that MSC might increase the risk of infection or disease relapse because of their immunosuppressive nature, there is no clear evidence that MSCs are detrimental in this way (Prasad et al. 2011; Kurtzberg et al. 2014). It is frustrating, therefore, that while there is strong evidence that MSCs are beneficial in GvHD and in tissue repair and possibly enhance engraftment, no clinical study to date has been rigorous enough to fully confirm a therapeutic role for MSC given to HCT recipients. This is in large part due to the small size of the case series and rarity of randomized studies. The situation is further complicated by the unpublished report of the only phase III trial using a commercial MSC product (Prochymal). In this prospective multicenter controlled study involving 244 patients, recipients randomized to MSC administered at the time of onset of GvHD fared no better than the controls receiving placebo. Although there was a significant benefit in a pediatric subgroup with gastrointestinal GvHD, the study failed to meet the criteria for therapeutic benefit defined in the protocol. The disappointing results from this study have reduced enthusiasm for large trials of MSC in GvHD (Galipeau 2013). However it is premature to abandon MSC for treating GvHD without considering the limitations that have applied to all investigations to date, whether as treatment for GvHD, tissue repair, or marrow function (Wu et al. 2014c). These limitations are due to the diversity of the MSC source and mode of preparation, the variations in dose and schedule used, and the multiple ways in which MSC is applied either prophylactically, at the onset of the complication, or as a salvage treatment. Attempts to evaluate response in GvHD are also hampered by the imprecise classical grading criteria applied to GvHD which do not accurately associate the grade of GvHD with steroid responsiveness and overall survival. Moreover, a fundamental constraint to the rational application of MSC to improve HCT outcome is that the mechanism of action of MSC is not fully understood—for example, it is not clear how much the benefit described in GvHD is attributable to immunomodulation versus tissue repair. Advances in the field of MSC therapeutics require new approaches to confront these problems addressing the variables in MSC source and manufacture, and a fuller understanding of the biology underlying the therapeutic impact of MSC.

12.7.1 MSC Source

Although MSCs have largely been derived from the bone marrow and the UC, adipose-derived MSCs are also readily manufactured, and other sources (e.g., placenta and dental pulp) are also under investigation (Jang et al. 2013; Bernardo et al. 2011). Adipose-derived MSCs have been claimed to have greater immunosuppressive potential than BM-derived MSC (Pérez-Ilzarbe et al. 2009). However, until the required properties needed for a specific application are known in detail, it is not possible to identify the relative qualities of one MSC source over another.

12.7.2 Defining the MSC Product

Unlike the CD34 marker which defines a group of hematopoietic progenitors with predictable potential, MSCs usually identified by their property of being negative for CD45 and CD34 and positive for CD105 and CD73 appear to have much greater variability in their properties. This extends from one donor to the next with older donors yielding inferior MSC (Chinnadurai et al. 2016). Another factor believed to strongly affect the nature and therapeutic potential of MSC is the number of passages used to expand the product (Galipeau et al. 2016). Since MSC can grow almost indefinitely, commercial products tend to be derived from massive expansions of a single donation over many doublings. Such MSC may lose immunosuppression, and furthermore the characteristics of such proprietary products are not known in detail (Wu et al. 2014c). To avoid incorporation of animal serum in the MSC product, many investigators substitute platelet lysate for fetal calf serum. Numerous studies attest to the comparability of these culture approaches (Salem et al. 2015). More important is the effect of thawing of the frozen MSC product on its function. Immediate infusion of MSC risks giving a product with significantly reduced biological activity while MSC rested in culture can recover overnight after thawing and may have better therapeutic efficacy when preincubated with interferon gamma (Vander Lugt et al. 2013).

Leaving aside inter-individual differences, these considerations indicate the possibility of great disparities in the therapeutic potential of MSC from different sources and methods of production and administration. A potency assay would be a prerequisite to fully define the therapeutic potential of MSC but would need to be defined according to the therapeutic outcome sought (Ponce et al. 2015). For GvHD treatment we developed a standardized T cell suppression assay that could be used to validate MSC immunosuppression, but detailed characterization of MSC function awaits a better understanding of the mechanism of action of MSC in GvHD (Jitschin et al. 2013).

12.7.3 Biomonitoring

Advances in the identification of biomarkers of disease severity are beginning to revolutionize the management of acute GvHD. Of particular relevance for future trials of MSC in GvHD is the biomarker ST2. Critically an elevated ST2 at the onset of GvHD predicts for steroid refractoriness and poorer posttransplant survival. Moreover ST2 has emerged as a more reliable predictive marker of GvHD outcome than conventional grading such that some patients with grades III–IV GvHD severity and low ST2 have favorable outcomes, while rare patients with grade I GvHD but high ST2 have the unfavorable outcome and steroid refractoriness more usually ascribed to high-grade GvHD. Because of their robustness, such biomarkers could improve the precision of risk stratification and finesse the evaluation of experimental MSC treatments (Reviewed by Paczesny 2018).

12.7.4 Clinical Trial Design

To shed clarity on a therapeutic role for MSC in transplant recipients, future studies must not fall into the trap of repeating the mistakes of the past (Wu et al. 2014c). Prospective randomized trials involving large patient numbers using a defined MSC product characterized by at least some form of potency measurement are urgently needed to advance the acceptability of MSC as a form of cell therapy to improve the outcome of allogeneic HCT. Trials evaluating MSC up front rather than as salvage treatment after diverse forms of treatment failure should be preferred. The source and manufacture of MSC should be standardized within each study, and clinical measurements of therapy should be backed up by intensive biomonitoring of the patient to include markers such as ST2 for GvHD and angiopoietin 2 for tissue damage (Paczesny 2018). Immune monitoring – especially quantifying regulatory T cells – has shown a shift toward a more tolerogenic immune milieu with increased circulating T_{regs} associated with higher IL-2 levels (known to promote T_{regs}) and higher levels of the anti-inflammatory cytokine IL-10 (Matsuoka 2018). Two studies have especially focused on biomarkers to better define immune response. Te Boom (Ball et al. 2013) used a comprehensive panel of soluble and cellular biomarkers to track clinical GvHD responses after MSC infusion. They showed that ST2 among other biomarkers was predictive for mortality after MSC infusion, while increases in immature dendritic cells were associated with decreased mortality. They emphasize the value of biomarkers in better monitoring response to MSC and their value in understanding mechanisms of action. Yin et al. noted prompt reduction in proinflammatory GvHD biomarkers and a rise or preservation of biomarkers characterizing growth factors in responders to MSC infusions (Zhao et al. 2015). Furthermore MSC-derived exosomes with T cell immunosuppressive capacity were found to circulate briefly after infusion, suggesting that sustained T cell control might be better achieved with MSC infusions spaced only 2–3 days apart (Melief et al. 2013). Such studies should serve to help us better understand mechanisms of action of these enigmatic cells and thereby both broaden and define their therapeutic scope.

References

Amarnath S, Foley JE, Farthing DE, Gress RE, Laurence A, Eckhaus MA, Métais JY, Rose JJ, Hakim FT, Felizardo TC, Cheng AV, Robey PG, Stroncek DE, Sabatino M, Battiwalla M, Ito S, Fowler DH, Barrett AJ (2015) Bone marrow-derived mesenchymal stromal cells harness purinergenic signaling to tolerize human Th1 cells in vivo. Stem Cells 33(4):1200–1212

Ball LM, Bernardo ME, Roelofs H, Lankester A, Cometa A, Egeler RM, Locatelli F, Fibbe WE (2007) Cotransplantation of ex vivo expanded mesenchymal stem cells accelerates lymphocyte recovery and may reduce the risk of graft failure in haploidentical hematopoietic stem-cell transplantation. Blood 110(7):2764–2767 Epub 2007 Jul 16.

Ball LM, Bernardo ME, Roelofs H, van Tol MJ, Contoli B, Zwaginga JJ, Avanzini MA, Conforti A, Bertaina A, Giorgiani G, Jol-van der Zijde CM, Zecca M, Le Blanc K, Frassoni F, Egeler RM, Fibbe WE, Lankester AC, Locatelli F (2013) Multiple infusions of mesenchymal stromal cells induce sustained remission in children with steroid-refractory, grade III-IV acute graft-versus-host disease. Br J Haematol 163(4):501–509

Baron F, Lechanteur C, Willems E, Bruck F, Baudoux E, Seidel L, Vanbellinghen JF, Hafraoui K, Lejeune M, Gothot A, Fillet G, Beguin Y (2010) Cotransplantation of mesenchymal stem cells might prevent death from graft-versus-host disease (GvHD) without abrogating graft-versus-tumor effects after HLA-mismatched allogeneic transplantation following nonmyeloablative conditioning. Biol Blood Marrow Transplant 16(6):838–847

Battiwalla M, Barrett AJ (2014) Bone marrow mesenchymal stromal cells to treat complications following allogeneic stem cell transplantation. Tissue Eng Part B Rev 20(3):211–217

Bernardo ME, Cometa AM, Pagliara D, Vinti L, Rossi F, Cristantielli R, Palumbo G, Locatelli F (2011) Ex vivo expansion of mesenchymal stromal cells. Best Pract Res Clin Haematol 24(1):73–81

Bessout R, Demarquay C, Moussa L, René A, Doix B, Benderitter M, Sémont A, Mathieu N (2015) TH17 predominant T-cell responses in radiation-induced bowel disease are modulated by treatment with adipose-derived mesenchymal stromal cells. J Pathol 237(4):435–446

Chen PM, Yen ML, Liu KJ, Sytwu HK, Yen BL (2011) Immunomodulatory properties of human adult and fetal multipotent mesenchymal stem cells. J Biomed Sci 18:49

Chinnadurai R, Copland IB, Garcia MA, Petersen CT, Lewis CN, Waller EK, Kirk AD, Galipeau J (2016) Cryopreserved Mesenchymal stromal cells are susceptible to T-cell mediated apoptosis which is partly rescued by IFNγ licensing. Stem Cells 34(9):2429–2442

de Lima M, McNiece I, Robinson SN, Munsell M, Eapen M, Horowitz M, Alousi A, Saliba R, McMannis JD, Kaur I, Kebriaei P, Parmar S, Popat U, Hosing C, Champlin R, Bollard C, Molldrem JJ, Jones RB, Nieto Y, Andersson BS, Shah N, Oran B, Cooper LJ, Worth L, Qazilbash MH, Korbling M, Rondon G, Ciurea S, Bosque D, Maewal I, Simmons PJ, Shpall EJ (2012) Cord-blood engraftment with ex vivo mesenchymal-cell coculture. N Engl J Med 367(24):2305–2315

Fan X, Gay FP, Ong SY, Ang JM, Chu PP, Bari S, Lim TK, Hwang WY (2013) Mesenchymal stromal cell supported umbilical cord blood ex vivo expansion enhances regulatory T cells and reduces graft versus host disease. Cytotherapy 15(5):610–619

François M, Birman E, Forner KA, Gaboury L, Galipeau J (2012) Adoptive transfer of mesenchymal stromal cells accelerates intestinal epithelium recovery of irradiated mice in an interleukin-6-dependent manner. Cytotherapy 14(10):1164–1170

Friedenstein AJ, Deriglasova UF, Kulagina NN, Panasuk AF, Rudakowa SF, Luriá EA, Ruadkow IA (1974) Precursors for fibroblasts in different populations of hematopoietic cells as detected by the in vitro colony assay method. Exp Hematol 2(2):83–92

Galipeau J (2013) The mesenchymal stromal cells dilemma--does a negative phase III trial of random donor mesenchymal stromal cells in steroid-resistant graft-versus-host disease represent a death knell or a bump in the road? Cytotherapy 15(1):2–8

Galipeau J, Krampera M, Barrett J, Dazzi F, Deans RJ, DeBruijn J, Dominici M, Fibbe WE, Gee AP, Gimble JM, Hematti P, Koh MB, LeBlanc K, Martin I, McNiece IK, Mendicino M, Oh S, Ortiz L, Phinney DG, Planat V, Shi Y, Stroncek DF, Viswanathan S, Weiss DJ, Sensebe L

(2016) International Society for Cellular Therapy perspective on immune functional assays for mesenchymal stromal cells as potency release criterion for advanced phase clinical trials. Cytotherapy 18(2):151–159

Gonzalo-Daganzo R, Regidor C, Martín-Donaire T, Rico MA, Bautista G, Krsnik I, Forés R, Ojeda E, Sanjuán I, García-Marco JA, Navarro B, Gil S, Sánchez R, Panadero N, Gutiérrez Y, García-Berciano M, Pérez N, Millán I, Cabrera R, Fernández MN (2009) Results of a pilot study on the use of third-party donor mesenchymal stromal cells in cord blood transplantation in adults. Cytotherapy 11(3):278–288

Götherström C, Ringdén O, Westgren M, Tammik C, Le Blanc K (2003) Immunomodulatory effects of human foetal liver-derived mesenchymal stem cells. Bone Marrow Transplant 32(3):265–272

Gregoire-Gauthier J, Selleri S, Fontaine F, Dieng MM, Patey N, Despars G, Beauséjour CM, Haddad E (2012) Therapeutic efficacy of cord blood-derived mesenchymal stromal cells for the prevention of acute graft-versus-host disease in a xenogenic mouse model. Stem Cells Dev 21(10):1616–1626

Herrmann R, Sturm M, Shaw K, Purtill D, Cooney J, Wright M, Phillips M, Cannell P (2012) Mesenchymal stromal cell therapy for steroid-refractory acute and chronic graft versus host disease: a phase 1 study. Int J Hematol 95(2):182–188

Introna M, Lucchini G, Dander E, Galimberti S, Rovelli A, Balduzzi A, Longoni D, Pavan F, Masciocchi F, Algarotti A, Micò C, Grassi A, Deola S, Cavattoni I, Gaipa G, Belotti D, Perseghin P, Parma M, Pogliani E, Golay J, Pedrini O, Capelli C, Cortelazzo S, D'Amico G, Biondi A, Rambaldi A, Biagi E (2014) Treatment of graft versus host disease with mesenchymal stromal cells: a phase I study on 40 adult and pediatric patients. Biol Blood Marrow Transplant 20(3):375–381

Jang MJ, Kim HS, Lee HG, Kim GJ, Jeon HG, Shin HS, Chang SK, Hur GH, Chong SY, Oh D, Chung HM (2013) Placenta-derived mesenchymal stem cells have an immunomodulatory effect that can control acute graft-versus-host disease in mice. Acta Haematol 129(4):197–206

Jitschin R, Mougiakakos D, Von Bahr L, Völkl S, Moll G, Ringden O, Kiessling R, Linder S, Le Blanc K (2013) Alterations in the cellular immune compartment of patients treated with third-party mesenchymal stromal cells following allogeneic hematopoietic stem cell transplantation. Stem Cells 31(8):1715–1725

Karlsson H, Samarasinghe S, Ball LM, Sundberg B, Lankester AC, Dazzi F, Uzunel M, Rao K, Veys P, Le Blanc K, Ringdén O, Amrolia PJ (2008) Mesenchymal stem cells exert differential effects on alloantigen and virus-specific T-cell responses. Blood 112(3):532–541

Kebriaei P, Isola L, Bahceci E, Holland K, Rowley S, McGuirk J, Devetten M, Jansen J, Herzig R, Schuster M, Monroy R, Uberti J (2009) Adult human mesenchymal stem cells added to corticosteroid therapy for the treatment of acute graft-versus-host disease. Biol Blood Marrow Transplant 15(7):804–811

Kharbanda S, Smith AR, Hutchinson SK, McKenna DH, Ball JB, Lamb LS Jr, Agarwal R, Weinberg KI, Wagner JE Jr (2014) Unrelated donor allogeneic hematopoietic stem cell transplantation for patients with hemoglobinopathies using a reduced-intensity conditioning regimen and third-party mesenchymal stromal cells. Biol Blood Marrow Transplant 20(4):581–586

Kim DH, Yoo KH, Yim YS, Choi J, Lee SH, Jung HL, Sung KW, Yang SE, Oh WI, Yang YS, Kim SH, Choi SY, Koo HH (2006) Cotransplanted bone marrow derived mesenchymal stem cells (MSC) enhanced engraftment of hematopoietic stem cells in a MSC-dose dependent manner in NOD/SCID mice. J Korean Med Sci 21(6):1000–1004

Kurtzberg J, Prockop S, Teira P, Bittencourt H, Lewis V, Chan KW, Horn B, Yu L, Talano JA, Nemecek E, Mills CR, Chaudhury S (2014) Allogeneic human Mesenchymal stem cell therapy (Remestemcel-L, Prochymal) as a rescue agent for severe refractory acute graft-versus-host disease in pediatric patients. Biol Blood Marrow Transplant 20:229–235

Lazarus HM, Koc ON, Devine SM, Curtin P, Maziarz RT, Holland HK, Shpall EJ, McCarthy P, Atkinson K, Cooper BW, Gerson SL, Laughlin MJ, Loberiza FR Jr, Moseley AB, Bacigalupo A (2005) Cotransplantation of HLA-identical sibling culture-expanded mesenchymal stem

cells and hematopoietic stem cells in hematologic malignancy patients. Biol Blood Marrow Transplant 11(5):389–398
Le Blanc K (2006) Mesenchymal stromal cells: tissue repair and immune modulation. Cytotherapy 8(6):559–561
Le Blanc K, Mougiakakos D (2012) Multipotent mesenchymal stromal cells and the innate immune system. Nat Rev Immunol 12(5):383–396
Le Blanc K, Tammik L, Sundberg B, Haynesworth SE, Ringdén O (2003) Mesenchymal stem cells inhibit and stimulate mixed lymphocyte cultures and mitogenic responses independently of the major histocompatibility complex. Scand J Immunol 57(1):11–20
Le Blanc K, Rasmusson I, Sundberg B, Götherström C, Hassan M, Uzunel M, Ringdén O (2004) Treatment of severe acute graft-versus-host disease with third party haploidentical mesenchymal stem cells. Lancet 363(9419):1439–1441
Le Blanc K, Samuelsson H, Gustafsson B, Remberger M, Sundberg B, Arvidson J, Ljungman P, Lönnies H, Nava S, Ringdén O (2007) Transplantation of mesenchymal stem cells to enhance engraftment of hematopoietic stem cells. Leukemia 21(8):1733–1738
Le Blanc K, Frassoni F, Ball L, Locatelli F, Roelofs H, Lewis I, Lanino E, Sundberg B, Bernardo ME, Remberger M, Dini G, Egeler RM, Bacigalupo A, Fibbe W, Ringdén O, Developmental Committee of the European Group for Blood and Marrow Transplantation (2008) Mesenchymal stem cells for treatment of steroid-resistant, severe, acute graft-versus-host disease: a phase II study. Lancet 371(9624):1579–1586
Lee ST, Maeng H, Chwae YJ, Oh DJ, Kim YM, Yang WI (2008) Effect of mesenchymal stem cell transplantation on the engraftment of human hematopoietic stem cells and leukemic cells in mice model. Int J Hematol 87(3):327–337
Lee SH, Lee MW, Yoo KH, Kim DS, Son MH, Sung KW, Cheuh H, Choi SJ, Oh W, Yang YS, Koo HH (2013) Co-transplantation of third-party umbilical cord blood-derived MSCs promotes engraftment in children undergoing unrelated umbilical cord blood transplantation. Bone Marrow Transplant 48(8):1040–1045
Li XH, Gao CJ, Da WM, Cao YB, Wang ZH, Xu LX, Wu YM, Liu B, Liu ZY, Yan B, Li SW, Yang XL, Wu XX, Han ZC (2014) Reduced intensity conditioning, combined transplantation of haploidentical hematopoietic stem cells and mesenchymal stem cells in patients with severe aplastic anemia. PLoS One 9(3):e89666
Liu K, Chen Y, Zeng Y, Xu L, Liu D, Chen H, Zhang X, Han W, Wang Y, Zhao T, Wang J, Wang J, Han Q, Zhao C, Huang X (2011) Coinfusion of mesenchymal stromal cells facilitates platelet recovery without increasing leukemia recurrence in haploidentical hematopoietic stem cell transplantation: a randomized, controlled clinical study. Stem Cells Dev 20(10):1679–1685
Liu X, Wu M, Peng Y, Chen X, Sun J, Huang F, Fan Z, Zhou H, Wu X, Yu G, Zhang X, Li Y, Xiao Y, Song C, Xiang AP, Liu Q (2014) Improvement in poor graft function after allogeneic hematopoietic stem cell transplantation upon administration of mesenchymal stem cells from third-party donors: a pilot prospective study. Cell Transplant 23(9):1087–1098
Macmillan ML, Blazar BR, DeFor TE, Wagner JE (2009) Transplantation of ex-vivo culture-expanded parental haploidentical mesenchymal stem cells to promote engraftment in pediatric recipients of unrelated donor umbilical cord blood: results of a phase I-II clinical trial. Bone Marrow Transplant 43(6):447–454
Maitra B, Szekely E, Gjini K, Laughlin MJ, Dennis J, Haynesworth SE, Koç ON (2004) Human mesenchymal stem cells support unrelated donor hematopoietic stem cells and suppress T-cell activation. Bone Marrow Transplant 33(6):597–604
Martin PJ, Uberti JP, Soiffer RJ et al (2010) Prochymal improves response rates in patients with steroid-refractory acute graft versus host disease (SR-GvHD) involving the liver and gut: results of a randomized, placebo-controlled, multicenter phase III trial in GvHD. Biol Blood Marrow Transplant 16:S169–S170
Matsuoka KI (2018) Low dose interleukin-2 as a modulator of Treg homeostasis after HSCT: current understanding and future perspectives. Int J Hematol 107(2):130–137
Maziarz RT, Devos T, Bachier CR, Goldstein SC, Leis JF, Devine SM, Meyers G, Gajewski JL, Maertens J, Deans RJ, Van't Hof W, Lazarus HM (2015) Single and multiple dose MultiStem

(multipotent adult progenitor cell) therapy prophylaxis of acute graft-versus-host disease in myeloablative allogeneic hematopoietic cell transplantation: a phase 1 trial. Biol Blood Marrow Transplant 21(4):720–728

Melief SM, Schrama E, Brugman MH, Tiemessen MM, Hoogduijn MJ, Fibbe WE, Roelofs H (2013) Multipotent stromal cells induce human regulatory T cells through a novel pathway involving skewing of monocytes toward anti-inflammatory macrophages. Stem Cells 31(9):1980–1991

Meuleman N, Tondreau T, Ahmad I, Kwan J, Crokaert F, Delforge A, Dorval C, Martiat P, Lewalle P, Lagneaux L, Bron D (2009) Infusion of mesenchymal stromal cells can aid hematopoietic recovery following allogeneic hematopoietic stem cell myeloablative transplant: a pilot study. Stem Cells Dev 18(9):1247–1252

Muroi K, Miyamura K, Ohashi K, Murata M, Eto T, Kobayashi N, Taniguchi S, Imamura M, Ando K, Kato S, Mori T, Teshima T, Mori M, Ozawa K (2013) Unrelated allogeneic bone marrow-derived mesenchymal stem cells for steroid-refractory acute graft-versus-host disease: a phase I/II study. Int J Hematol 98(2):206–213

Nicolay NH, Lopez Perez R, Debus J, Huber PE (2015) Mesenchymal stem cells – a new hope for radiotherapy-induced tissue damage? Cancer Lett 366(2):133–140

Noort WA, Kruisselbrink AB, in't Anker PS, Kruger M, van Bezooijen RL, de Paus RA, Heemskerk MH, Löwik CW, Falkenburg JH, Willemze R, Fibbe WE (2002) Mesenchymal stem cells promote engraftment of human umbilical cord blood-derived CD34(+) cells in NOD/SCID mice. Exp Hematol 30(8):870–878

Paczesny S (2018) Biomarkers for posttransplantation outcomes. Blood 131(20):2193–2204

Peng Y, Chen X, Liu Q, Xu D, Zheng H, Liu L, Liu Q, Liu M, Fan Z, Sun J, Li X, Zou R, Xiang AP (2014) Alteration of naïve and memory B-cell subset in chronic graft-versus-host disease patients after treatment with mesenchymal stromal cells. Stem Cells Transl Med 3(9):1023–1031

Pérez-Ilzarbe M, Díez-Campelo M, Aranda P, Tabera S, Lopez T, del Cañizo C, Merino J, Moreno C, Andreu EJ, Prósper F, Pérez-Simón JA (2009) Comparison of ex vivo expansion culture conditions of mesenchymal stem cells for human cell therapy. Transfusion 49(9):1901–1910

Pérez-Simon JA, López-Villar O, Andreu EJ, Rifón J, Muntion S, Diez Campelo M, Sánchez-Guijo FM, Martinez C, Valcarcel D, Cañizo CD (2011) Mesenchymal stem cells expanded in vitro with human serum for the treatment of acute and chronic graft-versus-host disease: results of a phase I/II clinical trial. Haematologica 96(7):1072–1076

Ponce DM, Hilden P, Mumaw C, Devlin SM, Lubin M, Giralt S, Goldberg JD, Hanash A, Hsu K, Jenq R, Perales MA, Sauter C, van den Brink MR, Young JW, Brentjens R, Kernan NA, Prockop SE, O'Reilly RJ, Scaradavou A, Paczesny S, Barker JN (2015) High day 28 ST2 levels predict for acute graft-versus-host disease and transplant-related mortality after cord blood transplantation. Blood 125(1):199–205

Prasad VK, Lucas KG, Kleiner GI, Talano JA, Jacobsohn D, Broadwater G, Monroy R, Kurtzberg J (2011) Efficacy and safety of ex vivo cultured adult human mesenchymal stem cells (Prochymal™) in pediatric patients with severe refractory acute graft-versus-host disease in a compassionate use study. Biol Blood Marrow Transplant 17(4):534–541

Rasmusson I, Ringdén O, Sundberg B, Le Blanc K (2003) Mesenchymal stem cells inhibit the formation of cytotoxic T lymphocytes, but not activated cytotoxic T lymphocytes or natural killer cells. Transplantation 76(8):1208–1213

Resnick IB, Barkats C, Shapira MY, Stepensky P, Bloom AI, Shimoni A, Mankuta D, Varda-Bloom N, Rheingold L, Yeshurun M, Bielorai B, Toren A, Zuckerman T, Nagler A, Or R (2013) Treatment of severe steroid resistant acute GvHD with mesenchymal stromal cells (MSC). Am J Blood Res 3(3):225–238

Ringdén O, Uzunel M, Rasmusson I, Remberger M, Sundberg B, Lönnies H, Marschall HU, Dlugosz A, Szakos A, Hassan Z, Omazic B, Aschan J, Barkholt L, Le Blanc K (2006) Mesenchymal stem cells for treatment of therapy-resistant graft-versus-host disease. Transplantation 81(10):1390–1397

Ringdén O, Uzunel M, Sundberg B, Lönnies L, Nava S, Gustafsson J, Henningsohn L, Le Blanc K (2007) Tissue repair using allogeneic mesenchymal stem cells for hemorrhagic cystitis, pneumomediastinum and perforated colon. Leukemia 21(11):2271–2276

Robinson SN, Simmons PJ, Yang H, Alousi AM, Marcos de Lima J, Shpall EJ (2011) Mesenchymal stem cells in ex vivo cord blood expansion. Best Pract Res Clin Haematol 24(1):83–92

Salem B, Miner S, Hensel NF, Battiwalla M, Keyvanfar K, Stroncek DF, Gee AP, Hanley PJ, Bollard CM, Ito S, Barrett AJ (2015) Quantitative activation suppression assay to evaluate human bone marrow-derived mesenchymal stromal cell potency. Cytotherapy 17(12):1675–1686

Sánchez-Guijo F, Caballero-Velázquez T, López-Villar O, Redondo A, Parody R, Martínez C, Olavarría E, Andreu E, Prósper F, Díez-Campelo M, Regidor C, Villaron E, López-Corral L, Caballero D, Cañizo MC, Pérez-Simon JA (2014) Sequential third-party mesenchymal stromal cell therapy for refractory acute graft-versus-host disease. Biol Blood Marrow Transplant 20(10):1580–1585

Shipounova IN, Petinati NA, Bigildeev AE, Zezina EA, Drize NI, Kuzmina LA, Parovichnikova EN, Savchenko VG (2014) Analysis of results of acute graft-versus-host disease prophylaxis with donor multipotent mesenchymal stromal cells in patients with hemoblastoses after allogeneic bone marrow transplantation. Biochemistry (Mosc) 79(12):1363–1370

Si Y, Yang K, Qin M, Zhang C, Du Z, Zhang X, Liu Y, Yue Y, Feng Z (2014) Efficacy and safety of human umbilical cord derived mesenchymal stem cell therapy in children with severe aplastic anemia following allogeneic hematopoietic stem cell transplantation: a retrospective case series of 37 patients. Pediatr Hematol Oncol 31(1):39–49

Stagg J, Galipeau J (2012) Mechanisms of immune modulation by mesenchymal stromal cells and clinical translation. Biol Blood Marrow Transplant 18(4):557–564

Tasso R, Ilengo C, Quarto R, Cancedda R, Caspi RR, Pennesi G (2012) Mesenchymal stem cells induce functionally active T-regulatory lymphocytes in a paracrine fashion and ameliorate experimental autoimmune uveitis. Invest Ophthalmol Vis Sci 53(2):786–793

Te Boome LC, Mansilla C, van der Wagen LE, Lindemans CA, Petersen EJ, Spierings E, Thus KA, Westinga K, Plantinga M, Bierings M, Broers AE, Cuijpers ML, van Imhoff GW, Janssen JJ, Huisman C, Zeerleder S, Huls G, Boelens JJ, Wulffraat NM, Slaper-Cortenbach IC, Kuball J (2015) Biomarker profiling of steroid-resistant acute GvHD in patients after infusion of mesenchymal stromal cells. Leukemia 29(9):1839–1846

Tolar J, Villeneuve P, Keating A (2011) Mesenchymal stromal cells for graft-versus-host disease. Hum Gene Ther 22(3):257–262

Vander Lugt MT, Braun TM, Hanash S, Ritz J, Ho VT, Antin JH, Zhang Q, Wong CH, Wang H, Chin A, Gomez A, Harris AC, Levine JE, Choi SW, Couriel D, Reddy P, Ferrara JL, Paczesny S (2013) ST2 as a marker for risk of therapy-resistant graft-versus-host disease and death. N Engl J Med 369(6):529–539

von Bahr L, Sundberg B, Lönnies L, Sander B, Karbach H, Hägglund H, Ljungman P, Gustafsson B, Karlsson H, Le Blanc K, Ringdén O (2012) Long-term complications, immunologic effects, and role of passage for outcome in mesenchymal stromal cell therapy. Biol Blood Marrow Transplant 18(4):557–564

von Bonin M, Stölzel F, Goedecke A, Richter K, Wuschek N, Hölig K, Platzbecker U, Illmer T, Schaich M, Schetelig J, Kiani A, Ordemann R, Ehninger G, Schmitz M, Bornhäuser M (2009) Treatment of refractory acute GvHD with third-party MSC expanded in platelet lysate-containing medium. Bone Marrow Transplant 43(3):245–251

Wang H, Wang Z, Zheng X, Ding L, Zhu L, Yan H, Guo Z (2013) Hematopoietic stem cell transplantation with umbilical cord multipotent stromal cell infusion for the treatment of aplastic anemia—a single-center experience. Cytotherapy 15(9):1118–1125

Wang Y, Chen F, Gu B, Chen G, Chang H, Wu D (2015) Mesenchymal stromal cells as an adjuvant treatment for severe late-onset hemorrhagic cystitis after allogeneic hematopoietic stem cell transplantation. Acta Haematol 133(1):72–77

Weng J, He C, Lai P, Luo C, Guo R, Wu S, Geng S, Xiangpeng A, Liu X, Du X (2012) Mesenchymal stromal cells treatment attenuates dry eye in patients with chronic graft-versus-host disease. Mol Ther 20(12):2347–2354

Wu Y, Wang Z, Cao Y, Xu L, Li X, Liu P, Yan P, Liu Z, Zhao D, Wang J, Wu X, Gao C, Da W, Han Z (2013a) Cotransplantation of haploidentical hematopoietic and umbilical cord mesenchymal stem cells with a myeloablative regimen for refractory/relapsed hematologic malignancy. Ann Hematol 92(12):1675–1684

Wu KH, Tsai C, Wu HP, Sieber M, Peng CT, Chao YH (2013b) Human application of ex vivo expanded umbilical cord-derived mesenchymal stem cells: enhance hematopoiesis after cord blood transplantation. Cell Transplant 22(11):2041–2051

Wu YM, Cao YB, Li XH, Xu LX, Liu ZY, Liu B, Yan B, Yang XL, Li SW, Da WM, Gao CJ, Wu XX (2014a) Transplantation of umbilical cord mesenchymal stem cells combined with haploidentical hematopoietic stem cells for 36 patients with refractory/relapsed myeloid leukemia. Zhongguo Shi Yan Xue Ye Xue Za Zhi 22(4):1053–1057

Wu Y, Cao Y, Li X, Xu L, Wang Z, Liu P, Yan P, Liu Z, Wang J, Jiang S, Wu X, Gao C, Da W, Han Z (2014b) Cotransplantation of haploidentical hematopoietic and umbilical cord mesenchymal stem cells for severe aplastic anemia: successful engraftment and mild GvHD. Stem Cell Res 12(1):132–138

Wu LW, Wang YL, Christensen JM, Khalifian S, Schneeberger S, Raimondi G, Cooney DS, Lee WP, Brandacher G (2014c) Donor age negatively affects the immunoregulatory properties of both adipose and bone marrow derived mesenchymal stem cells. Transpl Immunol 30(4):122–127

Xie M, Qin H, Luo Q, He X, He X, Lan P, Lian L (2016) Comparison of adipose-derived and bone marrow mesenchymal stromal cells in a murine model of Crohn's disease. Dig Dis Sci 62(1):115–123

Xu LX, Liu ZY, Wu YM, Cao YB, Li XH, Yan B, Yang XL, Da WM, Wu XX (2014) Clinical observation of haploidentical-hematopoietic stem cell transplantation combined with human umbilical cord-derived mesenchymal stem cells for severe aplastic anemia-II. Zhongguo Shi Yan Xue Ye Xue Za Zhi 22(3):774–778

Yin F, Battiwalla M, Ito S, Feng X, Chinian F, Melenhorst JJ, Koklanaris E, Sabatino M, Stroncek D, Samsel L, Klotz J, Hensel NF, Robey PG, Barrett AJ (2014) Bone marrow mesenchymal stromal cells to treat tissue damage in allogeneic stem cell transplant recipients: correlation of biological markers with clinical responses. Stem Cells 32(5):1278–1288

Zhang LS, Liu QF, Huang K, Zhang Y, Fan ZP, Huang SL (2009) Mesenchymal stem cells for treatment of steroid-resistant chronic graft-versus-host disease. Zhonghua Nei Ke Za Zhi 48(7):542–546

Zhang X, Li JY, Cao K, Lu H, Hong M, Qian S, Wu H, Liu P, Xu W (2010) Cotransplantation of HLA-identical mesenchymal stem cells and hematopoietic stem cells in Chinese patients with hematologic diseases. Int J Lab Hematol 32(2):256–264

Zhao K, Huang F, Peng YW, Zhou HS, Fan ZP, Zhang X, Guo XT, Xu N, Sun J, Xiang P, Liu QF (2013) Clinical observation of mesenchymal stem cell as salvage treatment for refractory acute graft-versus-host disease. Zhonghua Xue Ye Xue Za Zhi 34(2):122–126

Zhao K, Lou R, Huang F, Peng Y, Jiang Z, Huang K, Wu X, Zhang Y, Fan Z, Zhou H, Liu C, Xiao Y, Sun J, Li Y, Xiang P, Liu Q (2015) Immunomodulation effects of Mesenchymal stromal cells on acute graft-versus-host disease after hematopoietic stem cell transplantation. Biol Blood Marrow Transplant 21:97–104

Zhou H, Guo M, Bian C, Sun Z, Yang Z, Zeng Y, Ai H, Zhao RC (2010) Efficacy of bone marrow-derived mesenchymal stem cells in the treatment of sclerodermatous chronic graft-versus-host disease: clinical report. Biol Blood Marrow Transplant 16(3):403–412

Part IV

Gene Therapy

Gene Therapy for Neoplastic Hematology in Transplant Setting

13

Januario E. Castro and Thomas J. Kipps

13.1 Introduction

Traditionally, the transfer of allogeneic cells and the replacement of the immune system using allogeneic hematopoietic cell transplant (HCT) has been the only therapy that has proven to be curative for hematological malignancies. This clinical observation highlights the remarkable power that the transferred immunological graft possesses against the tumor cells, the so-called graft-versus-tumor effect (Thomas 1982).

However, allogeneic HCT is a procedure that entitles significant risk of adverse events including infection, graft-versus-host disease (GvHD), and mortality. Hence, the search for a more specific and, hopefully, less toxic therapeutic approach using immune system cells that are redirected toward the target of interest is needed and ongoing. This could be potentially accomplished by harnessing modern molecular biology, gene therapy, and cellular engineering techniques.

Gene therapy for hematologic malignancies and other diseases is rapidly becoming one of the most actively studied and awaited treatment alternatives. It involves the manipulation of genes to achieve a desired therapeutic effect. This can be accomplished by introducing a functional sequence to replace a mutated or dysfunctional gene or by deleting/replacing a gene that is no longer functional using gene editing tools. A range of therapeutic strategies have shown significant progress over the past few years; these include approaches based on immune genes, suppressor

J. E. Castro
Adoptive Cellular Therapy CART-Cell Program, Hematology-Oncology Division, Mayo Clinic Arizona, Phoenix, AZ, USA
e-mail: Castro.Januario@mayo.edu

T. J. Kipps (✉)
Moores UCSD Cancer Center, University of California, San Diego, CA, USA

CLL Research Consortium, San Diego, CA, USA
e-mail: tkipps@ucsd.edu

M.-A. Perales et al. (eds.), *Cell and Gene Therapies*, Advances and Controversies in Hematopoietic Transplantation and Cell Therapy,
https://doi.org/10.1007/978-3-319-54368-0_13

genes, or gene replacements, gene-directed enzyme-prodrug/suicide gene therapies, gene suppression, or oncolytic viral and non-viral therapies. In this chapter, we will review the historical context of gene therapy and cellular engineering development for the treatment of hematological malignancies and, particularly, in the setting of hematopoietic cell transplantation (Table 13.1).

13.2 Origin of Gene Therapy

One of the earliest recorded attempts to turn the immune system against cancer cells came from the studies performed by William Bradley Coley in the 1890s while working at the New York Cancer Hospital (now Memorial Sloan Kettering Cancer Center). He used a pool of dead bacteria to elicit an immune inflammatory reaction in cancer patients. The cancer of most patients continued to progress; however, there were some patients who experienced tumor regression, and this offered hope with the notion that the immune system could be used to fight cancer (Decker and Safdar 2009).

Billingham developed a strategy for adoptive T-cell transfer (Billingham et al. 1954) and highlighted the need to overcome the compromised immune system of patients with cancer, particularly after treatment with conventional chemotherapy. Around this time in the 1950s, Mitchison and collaborators described their pioneering work to target cancer cells using lymphocyte adoptive transfer in mouse models (Mitchison 1955).

Subsequently, the tremendous success of childhood immunizations proved that the immune system can provide the most specific and long-lasting defense against many infectious diseases, such as polio. Additional evidence came in the late 1960s when the first non-twin allogeneic HCT was performed, opening the clinical era of adoptive cell therapies (Buckner et al. 1970). Since that time, we have learned to recognize the "good" and "bad" properties of the immune system, which can exert unparalleled cytotoxic effects on the targeted cancer cells but also render sometimes fatal rejection of normal tissues in the form of GvHD. The lack of "immunological accuracy" of allo-HCT prompted the search for more targeted and redirected strategies using the transfer of genes or engineered immune cells to decrease "off-target" adverse events.

The tools and protocols used for gene therapy have improved significantly since the mid-1980s when the first experiment using stem cell gene transfer showed their potential therapeutic promise. Scientists initially found some obstacles. First, there was difficulty in delivering a modified gene into hematopoietic stem cells (HSCs) because of their lack of cell surface receptors and their quiescent state (Vollweiler et al. 2003). Second, some patients developed vector insertional mutagenesis after receiving gene therapy for severe combined immunodeficiency (Howe et al. 2008). Over three decades, these problems have been gradually resolved, and with an array of cytokine stimulation cocktails to improve HSC receptivity to engineering, and improved viral vectors, the HSC transduction rate in humans can reach from 80% to 100%. In addition, certain agents in myeloablative conditioning (MAC) regimens (e.g., busulfan, melphalan) that decrease the number of endogenous stem cells prior to infusion of the engineered HSCs have proven to be an effective method to increase

Table 13.1 Selected gene therapy trials in neoplastic hematology

References	Year	No. patients	Disease	Conditioning regimen	Gene transfer	Target	Cell dose/kg	Response rates CR (%)	Response rates PR (%)	Comments
Locke et al. (2017)	2017	7	DLBCL	FLU/CY	Retrovirus	CD19	2×10^6 anti-C19 CAR-T cells/kg	43	29	Multicenter ZUMA-1 phase 1 study in patients with refractory DLBCL
Brudno et al. (2016)	2016	20	B-cell malignancies	None	Gamma retrovirus	CD19	$1–10 \times 10^6$	30	10	Allogeneic T cells that express an anti-CD19 chimeric antigen receptor
Kalos et al. (2011) Porter et al. (2015)	2015	14	CLL	FLU/CY, PC, Benda	Lentivirus	CD19	$0.14–11 \times 10^8$	29	28	Anti-CD19 CAR-T cells persisted for 14–19 months in some patients
Lee et al. (2015)	2015	21	ALL or NHL	FLU/CY	Retrovirus	CD19	$1–3 \times 10^6$	67	NA	Anti-CD19 CAR-T cells. ALL pediatric or young adults (1–30 years)
Kochenderfer et al. (2015)	2015	14	NHL	FLU/CY	Gamma retrovirus	CD19	$0.3–5.0 \times 10^6$	36	36	Anti-CD19 CAR-T cells. Duration of ongoing CR responses (9–22 months)
Chapuis et al. (2013)	2014	11	Leukemia	Per discretion of treating physician	WT1-specific donor-derived $CD8^+$ cytotoxic T cell	WT1	$3.3 \times 10^9/m^2–3.3 \times 10^{10}/m^2$	0	0	HLA A*0201-restricted WT1-specific donor-derived $CD8^+$ cytotoxic T-cell clones were administered post-HCT
Davila et al. (2014) Brentjens et al. (2013)	2014 2013	16	ALL	CY	Retrovirus	CD19	3×10^6	88	NA	Anti-CD19 CAR-T cells. Relapsed/refractory ALL adults. One patient received less than the study dose

(continued)

Table 13.1 (continued)

References	Year	No. patients	Disease	Conditioning regimen	Gene transfer	Target	Cell dose/kg	Response rates CR (%)	PR (%)	Comments
Maude et al. (2014)	2014	25	ALL	Per discretion of treating physician	Lentivirus	CD19	0.8–21 × 10^6	99	NA	Anti-CD19 CAR-T cells. 25 pediatric patients and 5 adult patients
Grupp et al. (2013)	2013	5								
Cruz et al. (2013)	2013	4	ALL	None	Retrovirus	CD19	3.2 × 10^7–1.1 × 10^8	75	0	Retroviral FMC63 anti-CD19 scFv—CD28-CD3
		4	CLL					0	0	
Ritchie et al. (2013)	2013	4	AML	FLU/CY	Gamma retrovirus	LeY	1.4–9.2 × 10^6	25	25	Anti-LeY CAR-T cells persisted up to 10 months
Kochenderfer et al. (2012)	2012	7	CLL/NHL	FLU/CY	Gamma retrovirus	CD19	0.3–4.0 × 10^6	43	43	Anti-CD19 CAR-T cells. CAR-T cells persisted <3 months
Till et al. (2012)	2012	3	NHL	CY	Electroporation	CD20	1 × 10^8/m^2–3.3 × 10^9/m^2	0	33	Ani-CD20 CAR-T cells. CAR-T cells persisted 9–12 months
Castro et al. (2012)	2012	15	CLL	None	Adenovirus	CD154	1 × 10^{10}–33 × 10^{10}	0	20	Patients received a single IDI of 1 × 10^{10} to 33 × 10^{10} Ad-ISF35 viral particles (vp), with a defined maximum tolerated dose as 1 × 10^{11} vp

Brentjens et al. (2011)	2011	3	CLL	None	Gamma retrovirus	CD19	1.2–3.0 × 10^7	0	0	Anti-CD19 CAR-T cells. This trial included a CAR-T cell dose escalation and also compared responses in patients treated with or without conditioning chemotherapy before CAR-T cell infusion
		4		CY	Gamma retrovirus	CD19	0.4–1.0 × 10^7	0	25	Anti-CD19 CAR-T cells. The CY dose (up to 3 g/m^2) is the lowest amount of conditioning treatment among the published trials evaluating CD19-targeted CAR-T cells for NHL
Kalos et al. (2011)	2011	3	CLL	Per discretion of treating physician	Lentivirus	CD19	1.46 × 10^5–1.6 × 10^7	100	0	Patients were given a single course of chemotherapy during the week before infusion
Savoldo et al. (2011)	2011	6	NHL	None	Retrovirus	CD19	2 × 10^7/m^2–2 × 10^8/m^2	0	0	Retroviral FMC63 anti-CD19 scFv-CD3f and anti-CD19 scFv—CD28-CD3. CAR persistence for 6 weeks

(continued)

Table 13.1 (continued)

References	Year	No. patients	Disease	Conditioning regimen	Gene transfer	Target	Cell dose/kg	Response rates CR (%)	PR (%)	Comments
Wierda et al. (2010)	2010	9	CLL	None	Adenovirus	CD154	1×10^8, 3×10^8 or 1×10^9 autologous CLL cells	0	0	Before receiving the full, intended dose, patients received a test dose of 3–6 × 10^5 autologous ISF35-transduced cells IV over 1 min and then were monitored for 10–15 min; if no reaction occurred, they received the remainder of their intended dose
Kochenderfer et al. (2010)	2010	1	Lymphoma	FLU/CY	Retrovirus	CD19	1–3 × 10^8	100	0	First use of anti-CD19 CAR
Jensen et al. (2010)	2010	2	DLBCL	FLU	Retrovirus	CD19	$2 \times 10^9/m^2$	100	0	Retroviral FMC63 anti-CD19 scFv-CD3 with thymidine kinase suicide gene
		2	FL					0	0	
Till et al. (2008)	2008	7	NHL	FLU or CY	Electroporation	CD20	$1 \times 10^8/m^2$–$3.3 \times 10^9/m^2$	29	14	Anti-CD20 CAR-T cells. CAR-T cells persisted 5–9 weeks
Wierda et al. (2000)	2000	11	CLL	None	Adenovirus	CD154	3×10^6, 1×10^9, 3×10^9 autologous Ad-CD154-transduced CLL cells	0	0	Five patients received approximately 3×10^8 (pilot group and group 1), three received approximately 1×10^9 (group 2), and three received approximately 3×10^9 (group 3) autologous Ad-CD154-transduced CLL cells

engraftment rates (Aiuti et al. 2013). Moreover, newer, safer self-inactivating (SIN) viral vectors have been developed in which viral long terminal repeats (LTR) enhancers are completely removed. Using these newer vectors, there have been no new reports of therapy-related malignancy across several clinical trials, some of which have followed patients for as long as 8 years.

Glybera (alipogene tiparvovec) is the first gene therapy treatment approved in the western world. It was approved by the EMA (European Medicines Agency) on November 2012 for the treatment of patients with lipoprotein lipase deficiency (LPLD), a rare genetic disorder that causes fat to build up in the blood leading to cardiovascular disease, diabetes, and life-threatening, recurrent bouts of pancreatitis and affects one in a million people. Glybera consists of an engineered copy of the human LPL gene packaged with a tissue-specific promoter in a non-replicating AAV1 vector, which has a particular affinity for muscle cells. In order to improve activity, Glybera uses a naturally occurring variant of the LPL gene that has higher enzyme activity than the normal version of the gene that encodes the protein. Glybera is administered as a one-time series of up to 60 intramuscular injections in the legs. The patient is administered spinal anesthesia or deep sedation during the procedure. In addition, an immunosuppressive regimen is recommended from 3 days prior to and for 12 weeks following Glybera administration.

Moreover, the recent advent of genome-editing technologies has enabled a new paradigm in which the sequence of the human genome can be precisely manipulated to achieve a therapeutic effect. This includes the correction of mutations that cause disease, the addition of therapeutic genes to specific sites in the genome, and the removal of deleterious genes or genome sequences that could be implicated in pathology. Some of those strategies include nuclease-based platforms, such as zinc finger nucleases, transcription activator-like effector nucleases (TALENs), meganucleases, and the CRISPR/Cas9 system.

Overall, gene therapy is no longer a hypothetical form of treatment. It is reaching its prime time and has become a reality with recent US Food and Drug Administration (FDA) approval of anti-CD19 chimeric antigen receptor (CAR)-T-cell therapy in ALL. Several clinical trials on this field had allowed patients to obtain clinical benefit, and in some instances these responses have extended for more than a decade.

13.3 The Tools of Gene Therapy and Cellular Engineering

13.3.1 Viral Vectors

The majority of gene therapy studies thus far have employed viral vectors, because of their high efficiency of transgene delivery into the human nucleus. The most commonly used viral vectors include retroviruses, adenoviruses, and adeno-associated viruses. For a long-term effect, genome-integrating viral vectors (e.g., retroviral vector) have been employed. However, DNA integration causing critical gene mutagenesis has raised concern about long-term safety. This concern has led to the development of persisting but non-integrating viral vectors (e.g., adenoviral vector).

Virus vectors generally are genetically modified so they cannot generate progeny except in specific cell lines. One exception to this is the oncolytic vectors, which selectively replicate in and lyse human tumor cells, providing a promising means for targeted tumor destruction.

13.3.1.1 Retroviral Vectors

Retrovirus vectors are particles containing a positive-sense single-stranded RNA that typically is in the range of 7 kilobases (kb) in length. A feature of retroviral vectors is that they have the ability to stably incorporate their viral DNA into the host genome (genome-integrating viral vector), which can result in long-term expression of the transgene. Most retroviral vectors are γ-retroviral or lentiviral vectors. Lentiviral vectors are usually HIV-1 based, or may also contain elements of simian immunodeficiency virus, and have at least three advantages over γ-retroviral vectors; first, the lentiviral vector preintegration complex is able to cross the nuclear membrane in host cells even in the absence of mitosis and, therefore, is able to transduce nondividing cells, such as HSCs. Second, the lentiviral vector preintegration complex is more stable and persists longer, which improves the likelihood of integration (Cooray et al. 2012). Third, lentiviral vectors integrate to evenly distributed genomic sites, thus reducing the likelihood of driving the expression of a deleterious gene(s) or inducing mutagenesis. Contrary to that, γ-retroviral vectors prefer to integrate near gene transcription start sites, such as the CpG islands and conserved noncoding sequences and conserved transcriptional factor binding sites, and this generates a higher potential for insertional oncogenesis and gene dysregulation (Cattoglio et al. 2010).

13.3.1.2 Adenoviral Vectors

In contrast to retrovirus vectors, adenovirus vectors do not pose a risk for insertional mutagenesis because they do not integrate into the host cell's genome. More than 50 different human adenovirus serotypes exist, but current vectors primarily are derived from serotypes 2 and 5 (Douglas 2004). Adenoviral vectors are highly effective in gene therapy because of their ability to efficiently transduce both dividing and nondividing cells and to persist relatively well in long-lived targeted cells. Adenoviral vectors also have capacity to hold large segments of DNA (e.g., 7.5 kbp); they are easily manipulated with recombinant DNA techniques and have the ability to produce high titers (Kamen and Henry 2004). However, adenoviral vector infection enlists a variety of humoral and cellular immune responses (Ahi et al. 2011). Therefore, adenoviral vector therapy may result in acute toxicity, autoimmunity, and clearance of transgene-expressing cells (Puntel et al. 2013).

13.3.1.3 Adeno-Associated Viral Vectors

The adeno-associated viral vector (AAV) is a human parvovirus that initially was discovered as a contaminant in adenovirus preparations. The AAV genome is single-stranded DNA, and vector preparations are composed of a mixture of vector particles having one of the two strands of the virus. AAV requires a helper virus, such as adenovirus, to mediate a productive infection. The AAV has the ability to infect both nondividing and dividing cells and to persist without vector integration (Nathwani et al. 2011; Xiao et al. 2012). Upon entering host cells, wild-type AAV DNA becomes episomal or integrates into the genome. In contrast, current, modified AAV vectors are designed to lose their integrating ability (Daya and Berns 2008).

AAV, however, have a major limitation, and this is their small capacity for transgene insertion (<5 kb). New vector engineering had made possible to insert very large transgenes into AAV vectors. It is feasible to have split vectors in which one construct has slight sequence overlap with a second construct so that recombination after vector nuclear entry leads to the intact transgene product being expressed (Yan et al. 2000). The increased popularity of AAV vectors reflects the appreciation of the long-term transgene expression observed in animal models and the relative lack of adverse effects noted in preclinical animal models.

13.3.2 Non-viral Vectors

Non-viral vectors use different combinations of DNA or RNA. In general, these systems are easier to produce than are viral vectors (Seow and Wood 2009). Such non-viral vectors generally lack the efficiency of virus vector-mediated gene delivery systems. However, multiple strategies are being developed to improve gene delivery by non-viral vectors, including those using cationic lipids, in vivo electroporation, hydrodynamic injection of isotonic saline, cell-penetrating peptides, liposome encapsulation, neo-glycoproteins, glycosylated plasmids, or bacterial vectors. Conceivably, any one or a combination of these techniques someday may improve the efficacy of non-viral vector systems to levels approaching those of virus-based vector delivery systems.

13.3.2.1 Plasmid Vectors

Plasmid vectors are small, circular double-stranded DNA molecules (pDNA) capable of replicating in bacterial host cells. Their size ranges from 0.8 to 120 kbp, and the capacity for transgene DNA is almost unrestricted (Linnemann and Krawetz 2009).

Generally, the transgene is placed downstream of a strong promoter, such as the heterologous cytomegalovirus promoter/enhancer region, and upstream of a polyadenylation signal sequence to allow for appropriate RNA processing and transport from the nucleus. Plasmid vectors represent an important platform for gene delivery, as they are safe, stable in storage, easy to manipulate, and comparatively inexpensive to produce. However, the gene transfer efficiency of plasmid vectors is low. Naked pDNA vectors are vulnerable for degradation and permit only transient, episomal gene expression. Thus, there is great focus on the improvement of delivery and optimization of pDNA for enhanced cellular uptake and increased gene expression. For example, the replacement of polyA with synthetic or SV40 polyA sequences was shown to extend the half-life of supercoiled pDNA (Gillet et al. 2009).

13.3.2.2 Oligonucleotides

In the last decades, oligonucleotides have attracted attention as they provide an effective way to design sequence-specific ligands for nucleic acids or DNA-binding regulatory proteins for selective interference of gene expression. Oligonucleotides can be used to regulate or silence pathogenesis.

Oligonucleotides are short pieces of synthetic single-stranded DNA that can be generated with a phosphorothioate backbone that resists degradation by nucleases.

Aptamers, also called decoys or "chemical antibodies," represent an emerging class of short DNA or RNA oligonucleotides or peptides with potential therapeutical applications. They can assume stable and specific three-dimensional shapes in vivo, thereby providing specific tight binding to protein targets. The first aptamer approved for use in clinical trials was a RNA-based molecule (Macugen, pegaptanib), which is administered into the vitreous of patients with age-related macular degeneration to target vascular endothelial growth factor (Das et al. 2009). Another aptamer with apparent clinical activity is AS1411, a 26-mer unmodified guanosine-rich oligonucleotide that can inhibit cancer cell growth (Bates et al. 2009).

Another novel and potential development in oligonucleotide technology is the gene silencing potential of the siRNA. They are short, ~20–24 bp double-stranded RNA oligonucleotides mediating the degradation of complementary mRNA target after correct antisense strand has bound into RNA-induced silencing complex (RISC) (Chen et al. 2013). Chemically modified analogs, such as 2′-OMe incorporation or backbone modification, with a better stability and efficiency, have been designed.

13.3.2.3 CRISPR-Cas-Based Gene Editing

The discovery of the CRISPR-Cas microbial adaptive immune system and its application as genome editing tool represents one of the most important developments in recent years.

In 1993 Francisco Mojica was the first researcher to characterize bacterial DNA sequences that match snippets from the bacteriophage genome and postulated that they were part of an adaptive immune system response against viral infections (Mojica et al. 1993). He coined the term clustered regularly interspaced short palindromic repeats (CRISPR) and postulated that this was an adaptive immune response mechanism with gene editing capabilities (Mojica et al. 2005). The CRISPR sequences are prokaryotic DNA containing short, repetitive base sequences. Each repetition is followed by short segments of spacer DNA derived from previous exposures to foreign DNA (e.g., a virus or plasmid). This creates a cassette of "memory DNA fragments" that can match to foreign DNA, and when that occurs the cassette DNA guides the targeted cut of the invading DNA rendering inactive or mutated.

Additional experiments during the next 5–8 years led to the unveiling of the whole genome editing system including not only the CRISPR sequences but also the CRISPR-associated system (Cas) genes and the guide RNA (g-RNA). Moreover, the CRISPR/Cas9 system has been modified to edit genomes at any desired location. The key of this process is the delivery of the Cas9 nuclease complexed with a synthetic guide RNA (gRNA) into a cell; the cell's genome can be cut at a desired location, and this allows the removal or addition of new genetic fragments (Moreno and Mali 2017).

13.3.2.4 miRNA Targeting in Hematological Malignancies

microRNAs (miRNAs) are endogenous noncoding functional RNAs approximately 18–22 nucleotides in length and ubiquitously expressed in plants and animals (Bartel 2004). Their main function is to silence target messenger RNA (mRNAs) usually through imperfect complementary base pairing to the 3′-untranslated region, and they have an ability to inhibit or promote the expression of many related genes, which can in turn affect several cell-signaling pathways essential for tumor development and progression (Iorio and Croce 2012). A global dysregulation of miRNA expression has been confirmed in most tumors, and because of their involvement in critical biological pathways, they have emerged as attractive candidates for cancer therapy (Rupaimoole and Slack 2017).

Circulating miRNAs released from cancer cells can be used as novel noninvasive biomarkers and often correlate with tumor stage and prognosis (Mitchell et al. 2008). There are a number of clinical studies that are in progress evaluating the use of miRNAs as prognostic markers (www.clinicaltrials.gov). However, the only studies that had entered phase I clinical development thus far are targeting miR-122 in hepatitis C viral infection and miR-34 in primary liver cancer and solid tumors affecting the liver (Christopher et al. 2016).

13.4 Target for Gene Insertion

13.4.1 Hematopoietic Stem Cell

Hematopoietic stem cells can be modified with gene therapy protocols to treat a variety of diseases, including primary immune deficiency disease, hemoglobinopathies, metabolic diseases, and various genetic disorders (Ott et al. 2007; Tani 2016). The main advantage of modifying hematopoietic stem cells is that these cells can undergo self-renewal and/or differentiate into mature cells of different lineages.

The initial clinical trials on the application of hematopoietic stem cells used gene marking to investigate the origin of relapse of leukemia patients subjected to autologous HCT. These studies demonstrated that clinical relapse in patients with acute myelogenous leukemia (AML) and chronic myelogenous leukemia (CML) resulted from the presence of contaminating residual leukemia cells in the transplanted stem cell collection (Tey and Brenner 2007). The data from patients treated in these early studies have provided information on the long-term safety of various approaches that could be used for therapeutic gene transfer.

13.4.2 Cellular Engineering of Other Hematopoietic Cells

The initial gene therapy clinical trials for monogenic diseases were conducted successfully on patients with severe combined immunodeficiency due to ADA deficiency (ADA-SCID) (Blaese et al. 1995).

And since then more than 200 clinical protocols for monogenic diseases have been approved, and the target diseases include ADA-SCID, X-linked severe combined immunodeficiency (SCID-X1), X-linked chronic granulomatous disease (X-CGD), hemophilia, Wiskott-Aldrich syndrome (WAS), mucopolysaccharidosis, cerebral adrenoleukodystrophy, sickle cell disease, thalassemia, metachromatic leukodystrophy, familial hypercholesterolemia, Gaucher disease, Fanconi anemia, purine nucleoside phosphorylase deficiency, leukocyte adherence deficiency, gyrate atrophy, JAK3 deficiency, and epidermolysis bullosa (Tani 2016).

13.4.2.1 Suicide Gene Therapy

Today, the most effective and well-established cellular therapy approach is allogeneic HCT, which constitutes the only curative alternative for high-risk hematological malignancies including leukemias and lymphomas. However, one major limiting factor of HCT is the presence of uncontrolled GvHD. In order to modulate the antitumoral immune response and ameliorate the effect of GvHD in patients undergoing HCT, one potential strategy is to manipulate the donor cells using suicide genes that can be turned "on or off" as needed based on the presence of clinical GvHD symptoms. Herpes simplex virus thymidine kinase (HSV-TK) is the most commonly used suicide gene and confers sensitivity to the transduced cells to ganciclovir; therefore, whenever is considered necessary, the rapidly proliferating population of GvHD T cells can be controlled with ganciclovir while preserving the antitumor efficacy of allogeneic HCT that react against the tumor (graft-versus-tumor (GvT) effect). Most recently, suicide gene therapy has reemerged as an important tool that allows the control of unwanted toxic effects induced by innovative cellular therapies including CAR-T cells (Greco et al. 2015).

13.4.2.2 Gene Therapy Using Ex Vivo Manipulated Leukemia Cell Vaccines

Both autologous and allogeneic whole tumor cells were clinically developed as another form of cellular vaccine for cancer. The advantage of using the whole tumor cell approach is that the tumor antigens do not have to be prospectively identified and multiple antigens can be simultaneously targeted.

Our team at the University of California San Diego (UCSD) conducted the first studies of cellular therapy applied to chronic lymphocytic leukemia (CLL) in the late 1990s, using autologous CLL leukemia cells transduced ex vivo with an adenovirus vector expressing chimeric (mouse/human) CD154 (Ad-CD154) (Castro et al. 2003; Wierda et al. 2000; Kato et al. 1998). The goal of these studies was to generate leukemia cell that express a homolog of CD154 so that these cells would stimulate themselves and bystander leukemia cells become proficient antigen-presenting cells capable of inducing antileukemia immune responses.

Transduction of CLL B cells with Ad-CD154 induced the leukemia cells to express immune co-stimulatory molecules (Kato et al. 1998). Eleven patients received a single infusion of autologous CLL cells transduced ex vivo with Ad-CD154 (Wierda et al. 2000). Nearly all treated patients exhibited increased serum levels of IL-12 and IFN-γ, enhanced expression of immune co-stimulatory molecules on bystander leukemia cells, increased absolute numbers of blood T cells, and reduced blood leukemia cell counts and lymph node size. After additional infusions of Ad-CD154-transduced cells, patients experienced stabilization of disease and/or regression, obviating early additional treatment. Two of the treated patients did not require additional therapy 4 years after treatment (Castro et al. 2003).

On subsequent studies we tested an adenovirus vector expressing a membrane stable humanized homolog of CD154 (Ad-ISF35) (Wierda et al. 2010). Patients with CLL received dose-escalation administration of autologous leukemia cells transduced with Ad-ISF35. Similar to what was observed in patients receiving Ad-CD154, the infusions were well tolerated, and clinical benefit was observed in most patients including those with deletions in the short arm of chromosome 17 (del17p).

We also investigated whether Ad-ISF35 could be directly injected into tumor-infiltrated lymph nodes of patients with CLL. Fifteen patients with CLL received a single ultrasound-guided injection into an enlarged lymph node of 1 to 30 × 10^{10} Ad-ISF35 viral particles in four different dose cohorts. Injections were well-tolerated with some patients developing local swelling, erythema, and "flu-like" symptoms. Ad-ISF35 intranodal injection resulted in significant reductions in blood leukemia cell counts, lymphadenopathy, and splenomegaly in the majority of patients. Although there was no evidence for dissemination of Ad-ISF35 beyond the injected lymph node, direct intranodal injection of Ad-ISF35 induced CLL cells circulating in the blood to express death receptors, pro-apoptotic proteins, and immune co-stimulatory molecules, suggesting a "bystander" systemic effect (Castro et al. 2009).

These studies using transduced autologous CLL cells with homologs of CD154 showed the potential to elicit an antileukemia immune response even in patients that have been pretreated with immunosuppressive therapy. Moreover, the antileukemia effect was associated with antibody production against a leukemia-associated surface antigen, which we identified as ROR1 (Fukuda et al. 2008). ROR1 is an onco-embryonic surface antigen and survival-signaling receptor for Wnt5a. We concluded that patients treated with Ad-CD154-transduced CLL cells had significant immune stimulation leading to a break in immune tolerance to leukemia-associated antigens, such as ROR1.

Our current efforts have focused on the development of CAR-T cells that express a scFv specific for ROR1, with the goal of engineering T cells that are cytotoxic for cells bearing this antigen, which is expressed on the neoplastic cells of a variety of human cancers, but not on normal postpartum tissues (Deniger et al. 2015). Using the Sleeping Beauty transposons system, we constructed second-generation ROR1-specific CARs, signaling through CD3 and either CD28 (designated ROR1RCD28) or CD137 (designated ROR1RCD137). After transfection, we selected and expanded T cells expressing CARs through co-culture with gamma-irradiated artificial APC (aAPC), which co-expressed ROR1 and immune co-stimulatory molecules. Such T cells produced interferon-gamma and had specific cytotoxic activity against ROR1+ tumors. Moreover, such cells could eliminate ROR1+ tumor xenografts, especially T cells expressing ROR1RCD137. We anticipate that current and future clinical trials will help us investigate the ability of ROR1-CAR-T cells to specifically eliminate tumor cells, while maintaining normal B cells, in patients with CLL and other ROR1$^+$ malignancies (NCT02194374).

13.4.2.3 Immune Stimulatory Cytokines

Human leukemia cells typically express negligible levels of CD80 and low levels of CD86, causing the cells to be ineffective at stimulating T cells in response to presented antigens. Primary human leukemic cells from patients with AML can be transduced with retrovirus vectors to express CD80. In vitro, such transduced leukemia cells could stimulate proliferation of allogeneic T cells in mixed lymphocyte culture. CLL B cells transduced with HSV-based amplicon vectors encoding CD80 can stimulate allogeneic T cells in mixed lymphocyte reactions and stimulate T cells to produce IL-2 and IFN-γ (Tolba et al. 2001).

Murine B lymphoma cells transduced to express IL-2 and the lymphotactic chemokine lymphotactin are better able to induce antitumor immunity than non-transduced lymphoma cells or lymphoma cells transduced to express IL-2 alone. Two clinical trials using transduction of IL-2 in prostate cancer have been reported (Pantuck et al. 2004).

Transduction of cells with TNF-α inhibits the development or progression of leukemia in experimental animals. However, systemic administration of TNF-α induces serious toxicities that limit its clinical application. Membrane-bound TNF molecules may lack the undesirable side effects of soluble TNF-α. Co-incubation of CLL cells expressing a membrane-stabilized form of TNF-α induced bystander CLL cells to express immune accessory molecules, such as CD80 and CD54. Conceivably, such modified forms of active TNF-α that resist cleavage from the plasma membrane may be used in gene therapy of various hematologic cancers.

Preclinical models have demonstrated the efficacy of granulocyte-monocyte colony-stimulating factor (GM-CSF)-secreting cancer immunotherapies (GVAX platform) accompanied by immunotherapy-primed lymphocytes following autologous stem cell transplant (ASCT) in hematologic malignancies. A phase II study evaluated the use of autologous leukemia cells admixed with GM-CSF-secreting K562 cells (K562/GM) followed by ASCT. Fifty-four subjects were enrolled (Borrello et al. 2009), 46 (85%) achieved a complete remission, and 28 (52%) received the pretransplantation immunotherapy. For all patients who achieved a complete response, the 3-year relapse-free survival (RFS) was 47.4% and OS was 57.4%. For the 28 immunotherapy-treated patients, the RFS and OS were 61.8 and 73.4%, respectively. Posttreatment induction of delayed-type hypersensitivity reactions to autologous leukemia cells was associated with longer 3-year RFS (100% vs. 48%). Minimal residual disease was monitored by quantitative analysis of WT1, a leukemia-associated gene.

A decrease in WT1 transcripts in blood was noted in 69% of patients following the first immunotherapy dose and was also associated with longer 3-year RFS (61% vs. 0%). Collectively, this study shows that modified K562/GM cells have potential therapeutic potential in patients with AML when used in combination with primed lymphocytes and transplant (Borrello et al. 2009; Ho et al. 2009).

Similarly, in patients with chronic myeloid leukemia (CML), better molecular responses were observed in those receiving K562/GMCSF cell vaccines in combination with imatinib mesylate compared with patients that received tyrosine kinase inhibitor alone (Smith et al. 2010).

13.4.2.4 Expert Opinion

The applications of gene therapy are expanding exponentially, bringing exciting therapeutic alternatives to patients with intractable cancers. This is reflected by the fact that 64% of all gene therapy trials worldwide are aiming at the treatment of cancer (Büning 2013). Moreover, the expectation is that immunotherapy will expand beyond oncology into areas such as infectious diseases, autoimmunity, or immune deficiency.

As we see the brisk progress in the field, we also need to realize the importance to address and resolve critical questions before translating these discoveries to the clinic.

Optimization of gene transfer methods and large-scale production and expansion of engineered cells will be required to meet future demands of these new treatments. This will require the development of new equipment and specialized facilities, implementation and optimization of standard operating procedures, and the training of expert technicians in the field. Several pharmaceutical companies had established strategic partnerships with academic institutions in an effort to lead this effort (Bender 2016).

It is likely that the development of gene therapy needs to parallel the redundancy that is observed in the normal immune system, which is used to tackle complex problems such as infection and cancer (Casadevall and Pirofski 2003). Most likely, we will need to engineer cells able to provide that immunological redundancy or infuse a mixture of engineered cells with different targets/specificities. Furthermore, we might be able to give more than one type of effector cell to generate the "perfect immunological cocktail," using redirected-engineered T cells, NK cells, macrophages, dendritic cells, etc. Most likely, "One size will not fit all," and consequently, we will need to develop tailored immune reconstitution protocols based on gene therapy and cellular engineering for each specific disease.

Availability of these new treatments is going to be limited and initially accessible only to patients in large specialized centers in the USA, Europe, Australia, Japan, and China (countries that currently have open-gene-modified cell-based protocols). Broadening the coverage of gene therapy and cellular engineering will require the development of simplified protocols, the use of more effective and safer versions of gene-modified immune cells, and most likely the availability of universal OTS products that can guarantee easier logistics and shorter times for release and shipment of the cellular product.

The cost of these novel therapies is an important factor limiting wider use. As we have observed with any new therapy approved in oncology, the cost of the new therapy is always higher than the one of its predecessor (Bender 2016). The financial aspects of drug cost and coverage may limit accessibility. In the particular case of gene therapy, we will need to take into consideration not only the cost of manufacturing and administering the engineered cells but also the cost of management of adverse events and potentially prolonged hospitalizations.

13.4.2.5 Future Directions

Although some of the most dramatic results using gene-modified immunotherapy have been seen with CAR-T cells, their main problem is that their recognition is limited to cell surface structures. Contrary to that, T-cell receptors (TCRs) can recognize intracellular proteins that could correspond to mutated, misfolded, or overexpressed cancer-associated proteins (Harris and Kranz 2016). Additional studies will be required to define the role of each one of these target-binding platforms and their applicability to cancer therapy.

Another important question is regarding the preferred source of cells for engineering immunotherapy. The majority of studies published to date have used autologous T cells. This obviates HLA matching and endogenous virus testing. However, it is not certain whether autologous T cells from cancer patients are optimal for generating effective genetically modified T-cell products. Many cancer patients are elderly, and their immune system may be debilitated due to prior therapy and the inherent biology of their disease (Frumento et al. 2006). On the other hand, healthier allogeneic T cells from younger donors may be better able to proliferate and function, particularly when barriers regarding HLA matching can be minimized by selecting haploidentical or matched unrelated donor cells that are engineered using genetic editing techniques (Qasim et al. 2015). Very likely, those genetic editing tools will make it possible to provide off-the-shelf (OTS) cellular immunotherapy for immediate administration whenever they are needed. In fact, OTS cellular therapy could solve some of the major obstacles related to immediacy, logistics, and quality consistency required to expand the use of cellular immunotherapy beyond a few academic centers.

T-cell resistance can be a potential problem due to loss of the target antigen on the surface of the tumor cell (Grupp et al. 2013). The risk for selecting tumors that lack the target antigen may be mitigated using gene-modified T cells targeting only a single antigen or epitope (Roybal et al. 2016; Hegde et al. 2013).

Overall, cellular engineering using gene-modified immune cells represents a tremendous advancement toward effective treatment of hematologic malignancies. As seen with other discoveries, now we probably have more questions than answers, and methodical research will help to address those issues. Patients in desperate need for alternative treatments already have benefited from this approach. Definitely, the road ahead looks promising for cellular-based therapies (Table 13.1). Overcoming the challenges associated with the use of this new technology should optimize the use of these powerful new weapons against cancer.

References

Ahi YS, Bangari DS, Mittal SK (2011) Adenoviral vector immunity: its implications and circumvention strategies. Curr Gene Ther 11(4):307–320

Aiuti A, Biasco L, Scaramuzza S, Ferrua F, Cicalese MP, Baricordi C et al (2013) Lentiviral hematopoietic stem cell gene therapy in patients with Wiskott-Aldrich syndrome. Science 341(6148):1233151

Bartel DP (2004) MicroRNAs: genomics, biogenesis, mechanism, and function. Cell 116(2):281–297

Bates PJ, Laber DA, Miller DM, Thomas SD, Trent JO (2009) Discovery and development of the G-rich oligonucleotide AS1411 as a novel treatment for cancer. Exp Mol Pathol 86(3):151–164

Bender E (2016) Gene therapy: industrial strength. Nature 537(7619):S57–S59

Billingham RE, Brent L, Medawar PB (1954) Quantitative studies on tissue transplantation immunity. II. The origin, strength and duration of actively and adoptively acquired immunity. Proc R Soc Lond Ser B Biol Sci 143:58–80

Blaese RM, Culver KW, Miller AD, Carter CS, Fleisher T, Clerici M et al (1995) T lymphocyte-directed gene therapy for ADA- SCID: initial trial results after 4 years. Science 270(5235):475–480

Borrello IM, Levitsky HI, Stock W, Sher D, Qin L, DeAngelo DJ et al (2009) Granulocyte-macrophage colony-stimulating factor (GM-CSF)-secreting cellular immunotherapy in combination with autologous stem cell transplantation (ASCT) as postremission therapy for acute myeloid leukemia (AML). Blood 114(9):1736–1745

Brentjens RJ, Riviere I, Park JH, Davila ML, Wang X, Stefanski J et al (2011) Safety and persistence of adoptively transferred autologous CD19-targeted T cells in patients with relapsed or chemotherapy refractory B-cell leukemias. Blood 118(18):4817–4828

Brentjens RJ, Davila ML, Riviere I, Park J, Wang X, Cowell LG et al (2013) CD19-targeted T cells rapidly induce molecular remissions in adults with chemotherapy-refractory acute lymphoblastic leukemia. Sci Transl Med 5(177):177ra38

Brudno JN, Somerville RPT, Shi V, Rose JJ, Halverson DC, Fowler DH et al (2016) Allogeneic T cells that express an anti-CD19 chimeric antigen receptor induce remissions of B-cell malignancies that progress after allogeneic hematopoietic stem-cell transplantation without causing graft-versus-host disease. J Clin Oncol 34(10):1112–1121

Buckner CD, Epstein RB, Rudolph RH, Clift RA, Storb R, Thomas ED (1970) Allogeneic marrow engraftment following whole body irradiation in a patient with leukemia. Blood 35(6):741–750

Büning H (2013) Gene therapy enters the pharma market: the short story of a long journey. EMBO Mol Med 5(1):1–3

Casadevall A, Pirofski LA (2003) Exploiting the redundancy in the immune system: vaccines can mediate protection by eliciting 'unnatural' immunity. J Exp Med 197(11):1401–1404

Castro JE, Cantwell MJ, Prussak CE, Bole J, Wierda WG, Kipps TJ (2003) Long-term follow up of chronic lymphocytic leukemia patients treated with CD40-ligand (CD154) gene therapy. Blood 102(11):491a

Castro JE, Sandoval-Sus JD, Melo-Cardenas J, Darrah D, Urquiza M, Pakbaz RS et al (2009) Phase I study of intranodal direct injection of adenovirus encoding recombinant CD40-ligand (Ad-ISF35) in patients with chronic lymphocytic leukemia. J Clin Oncol 27(15s):3003

Castro JE, Melo-Cardenas J, Urquiza M, Barajas-Gamboa JS, Pakbaz RS, Kipps TJ (2012) Gene immunotherapy of chronic lymphocytic leukemia: a phase I study of intranodally injected adenovirus expressing a chimeric CD154 molecule. Cancer Res 72(12):2937–2948

Cattoglio C, Pellin D, Rizzi E, Maruggi G, Corti G, Miselli F et al (2010) High-definition mapping of retroviral integration sites identifies active regulatory elements in human multipotent hematopoietic progenitors. Blood 116(25):5507–5517

Chapuis AG, Ragnarsson GB, Nguyen HN, Chaney CN, Pufnock JS, Schmitt TM et al (2013) Transferred WT1-reactive $CD8^+$ T cells can mediate Antileukemic activity and persist in post-transplant patients. Sci Transl Med 5(174):174ra27

Chen WX, Hu Q, Qiu MT, Zhong SL, Xu JJ, Tang JH et al (2013) miR-221/222: promising biomarkers for breast cancer. Tumour Biol 34(3):1361–1370

Christopher AF, Kaur RP, Kaur G, Kaur A, Gupta V, Bansal P (2016) MicroRNA therapeutics: discovering novel targets and developing specific therapy. Perspect Clin Res 7(2):68–74

Cooray S, Howe SJ, Thrasher AJ (2012) Retrovirus and lentivirus vector design and methods of cell conditioning. Methods Enzymol 507:29–57

Cruz CR, Micklethwaite KP, Savoldo B, Ramos CA, Lam S, Ku S et al (2013) Infusion of donor-derived CD19-redirected virus-specific T cells for B-cell malignancies relapsed after allogeneic stem cell transplant: a phase 1 study. Blood 122(17):2965–2973

Das M, Mohanty C, Sahoo SK (2009) Ligand-based targeted therapy for cancer tissue. Expert Opin Drug Deliv 6(3):285–304

Davila ML, Riviere I, Wang X, Bartido S, Park J, Curran K et al (2014) Efficacy and toxicity management of 19-28z CAR T cell therapy in B cell acute lymphoblastic leukemia. Sci Transl Med 6(224):224ra25

Daya S, Berns KI (2008) Gene therapy using adeno-associated virus vectors. Clin Microbiol Rev 21(4):583–593

Decker WK, Safdar A (2009) Bioimmunoadjuvants for the treatment of neoplastic and infectious disease: Coley's legacy revisited. Cytokine Growth Factor Rev 20(4):271–281

Deniger DC, Yu J, Huls MH, Figliola MJ, Mi T, Maiti SN et al (2015) Sleeping beauty transposition of chimeric antigen receptors targeting receptor tyrosine kinase-like orphan receptor-1 (ROR1) into diverse memory T-cell populations. PLoS One 10(6):e0128151

Douglas JT (2004) Adenovirus-mediated gene delivery: an overview. Methods Mol Biol 246:3–14

Frumento G, Piazza T, Di Carlo E, Ferrini S (2006) Targeting tumor-related immunosuppression for cancer immunotherapy. Endocr Metab Immune Disord Drug Targets 6(3):233–237

Fukuda T, Chen L, Endo T, Tang L, Lu D, Castro JE et al (2008) Antisera induced by infusions of autologous Ad-CD154-leukemia B cells identify ROR1 as an oncofetal antigen and receptor for Wnt5a. Proc Natl Acad Sci U S A 105(8):3047–3052

Gillet JP, Macadangdang B, Fathke RL, Gottesman MM, Kimchi-Sarfaty C (2009) The development of gene therapy: from monogenic recessive disorders to complex diseases such as cancer. Methods Mol Biol 542:5–54

Greco R, Oliveira G, Stanghellini MT, Vago L, Bondanza A, Peccatori J et al (2015) Improving the safety of cell therapy with the TK-suicide gene. Front Pharmacol 6:95

Grupp SA, Kalos M, Barrett D, Aplenc R, Porter DL, Rheingold SR et al (2013) Chimeric antigen receptor-modified T cells for acute lymphoid leukemia. N Engl J Med 368(16):1509–1518

Harris DT, Kranz DM (2016) Adoptive T cell therapies: a comparison of T cell receptors and chimeric antigen receptors. Trends Pharmacol Sci 37(3):220–230

Hegde M, Corder A, Chow KK, Mukherjee M, Ashoori A, Kew Y et al (2013) Combinational targeting offsets antigen escape and enhances effector functions of adoptively transferred T cells in glioblastoma. Mol Ther 21(11):2087–2101

Ho VT, Vanneman M, Kim H, Sasada T, Kang YJ, Pasek M et al (2009) Biologic activity of irradiated, autologous, GM-CSF-secreting leukemia cell vaccines early after allogeneic stem cell transplantation. Proc Natl Acad Sci U S A 106(37):15825–15830

Howe SJ, Mansour MR, Schwarzwaelder K, Bartholomae C, Hubank M, Kempski H et al (2008) Insertional mutagenesis combined with acquired somatic mutations causes leukemogenesis following gene therapy of SCID-X1 patients. J Clin Investig 118(9):3143–3150

Iorio MV, Croce CM (2012) microRNA involvement in human cancer. Carcinogenesis 33(6):1126–1133

Jensen MC, Popplewell L, Cooper LJ, DiGiusto D, Kalos M, Ostberg JR et al (2010) Antitransgene rejection responses contribute to attenuated persistence of adoptively transferred CD20/CD19-specific chimeric antigen receptor redirected T cells in humans. Biol Blood Marrow Transplant 16(9):1245–1256

Kalos M, Levine BL, Porter DL, Katz S, Grupp SA, Bagg A et al (2011) T cells with chimeric antigen receptors have potent antitumor effects and can establish memory in patients with advanced leukemia. Sci Transl Med 3(95):95ra73

Kamen A, Henry O (2004) Development and optimization of an adenovirus production process. J Gene Med 6(Suppl 1):S184–S192
Kato K, Cantwell MJ, Sharma S, Kipps TJ (1998) Gene transfer of CD40-ligand induces autologous immune recognition of chronic lymphocytic leukemia B cells. J Clin Investig 101:1133–1141
Kochenderfer JN, Wilson WH, Janik JE, Dudley ME, Stetler-Stevenson M, Feldman SA et al (2010) Eradication of B-lineage cells and regression of lymphoma in a patient treated with autologous T cells genetically engineered to recognize CD19. Blood 116(20):4099–4102
Kochenderfer JN, Dudley ME, Feldman SA, Wilson WH, Spaner DE, Maric I et al (2012) B-cell depletion and remissions of malignancy along with cytokine-associated toxicity in a clinical trial of anti-CD19 chimeric-antigen-receptor-transduced T cells. Blood 119(12):2709–2720
Kochenderfer JN, Dudley ME, Kassim SH, Somerville RP, Carpenter RO, Stetler-Stevenson M et al (2015) Chemotherapy-refractory diffuse large B-cell lymphoma and indolent B-cell malignancies can be effectively treated with autologous T cells expressing an anti-CD19 chimeric antigen receptor. J Clin Oncol 33(6):540–549
Lee DW, Kochenderfer JN, Stetler-Stevenson M, Cui YK, Delbrook C, Feldman SA et al (2015) T cells expressing CD19 chimeric antigen receptors for acute lymphoblastic leukaemia in children and young adults: a phase 1 dose-escalation trial. Lancet 385(9967):517–528
Linnemann AK, Krawetz SA (2009) Silencing by nuclear matrix attachment distinguishes cell-type specificity: association with increased proliferation capacity. Nucleic Acids Res 37(9):2779–2788
Locke FL, Neelapu SS, Bartlett NL, Siddiqi T, Chavez JC, Hosing CM et al (2017) Phase 1 results of ZUMA-1: a multicenter study of KTE-C19 anti-CD19 CAR T cell therapy in refractory aggressive lymphoma. Mol Ther 25(1):285–295
Maude SL, Frey N, Shaw PA, Aplenc R, Barrett DM, Bunin NJ et al (2014) Chimeric antigen receptor T cells for sustained remissions in leukemia. N Engl J Med 371(16):1507–1517
Mitchell PS, Parkin RK, Kroh EM, Fritz BR, Wyman SK, Pogosova-Agadjanyan EL et al (2008) Circulating microRNAs as stable blood-based markers for cancer detection. Proc Natl Acad Sci U S A 105(30):10513–10518
Mitchison NA (1955) Studies on the immunological response to foreign tumor transplants in the mouse. I. The role of lymph node cells in conferring immunity by adoptive transfer. J Exp Med 102(2):157–177
Mojica FJ, Juez G, Rodríguez-Valera F (1993) Transcription at different salinities of Haloferax mediterranei sequences adjacent to partially modified PstI sites. Mol Microbiol 9(3):613–621
Mojica FJ, Díez-Villaseñor C, García-Martínez J, Soria E (2005) Intervening sequences of regularly spaced prokaryotic repeats derive from foreign genetic elements. J Mol Evol 60(2):174–182
Moreno AM, Mali P (2017) Therapeutic genome engineering via CRISPR-Cas systems. Wiley Interdiscip Rev Syst Biol Med 9(4):e1380
Nathwani AC, Tuddenham EG, Rangarajan S, Rosales C, McIntosh J, Linch DC et al (2011) Adenovirus-associated virus vector-mediated gene transfer in hemophilia B. N Engl J Med 365(25):2357–2365
Ott MG, Seger R, Stein S, Siler U, Hoelzer D, Grez M (2007) Advances in the treatment of chronic granulomatous disease by gene therapy. Curr Gene Ther 7(3):155–161
Pantuck AJ, van Ophoven A, Gitlitz BJ, Tso CL, Acres B, Squiban P et al (2004) Phase I trial of antigen-specific gene therapy using a recombinant vaccinia virus encoding MUC-1 and IL-2 in MUC-1-positive patients with advanced prostate cancer. J Immunother 27(3):240–253
Porter DL, Hwang WT, Frey NV, Lacey SF, Shaw PA, Loren AW et al (2015) Chimeric antigen receptor T cells persist and induce sustained remissions in relapsed refractory chronic lymphocytic leukemia. Sci Transl Med 7(303):303ra139
Puntel M, GM AKM, Farrokhi C, Vanderveen N, Paran C, Appelhans A et al (2013) Safety profile, efficacy, and biodistribution of a bicistronic high-capacity adenovirus vector encoding a combined immunostimulation and cytotoxic gene therapy as a prelude to a phase I clinical trial for glioblastoma. Toxicol Appl Pharmacol 268(3):318–330
Qasim W, Amrolia PJ, Samarasinghe S, Pule M (2015) First clinical application of talen engineered universal CAR19 T cells in B-ALL. Blood 126:2046

Ritchie DS, Neeson PJ, Khot A, Peinert S, Tai T, Tainton K et al (2013) Persistence and efficacy of second generation CAR T cell against the LeY antigen in acute myeloid leukemia. Mol Ther 21(11):2122–2129

Roybal KT, Rupp LJ, Morsut L, Walker WJ, McNally KA, Park JS et al (2016) Precision tumor recognition by T cells with combinatorial antigen-sensing circuits. Cell 164(4):770–779

Rupaimoole R, Slack FJ (2017) MicroRNA therapeutics: towards a new era for the management of cancer and other diseases. Nat Rev Drug Discov 16(3):203–222

Savoldo B, Ramos CA, Liu E, Mims MP, Keating MJ, Carrum G et al (2011) CD28 costimulation improves expansion and persistence of chimeric antigen receptor-modified T cells in lymphoma patients. J Clin Investig 121(5):1822–1826

Seow Y, Wood MJ (2009) Biological gene delivery vehicles: beyond viral vectors. Mol Ther 17(5):767–777

Smith BD, Kasamon YL, Kowalski J, Gocke C, Murphy K, Miller CB et al (2010) K562/GM-CSF immunotherapy reduces tumor burden in chronic myeloid leukemia patients with residual disease on imatinib mesylate. Clin Cancer Res 16(1):338–347

Tani K (2016) Current status of ex vivo gene therapy for hematological disorders: a review of clinical trials in Japan around the world. Int J Hematol 104(1):42–72

Tey SK, Brenner MK (2007) The continuing contribution of gene marking to cell and gene therapy. Mol Ther 15(4):666–676

Thomas ED (1982) Allogeneic bone marrow transplantation for blood cell disorders. Birth Defects Orig Artic Ser 18(7):361–369

Till BG, Jensen MC, Wang J, Chen EY, Wood BL, Greisman HA et al (2008) Adoptive immunotherapy for indolent non-Hodgkin lymphoma and mantle cell lymphoma using genetically modified autologous CD20-specific T cells. Blood 112(6):2261–2271

Till BG, Jensen MC, Wang J, Qian X, Gopal AK, Maloney DG et al (2012) CD20-specific adoptive immunotherapy for lymphoma using a chimeric antigen receptor with both CD28 and 4-1BB domains: pilot clinical trial results. Blood 119(17):3940–3950

Tolba KA, Bowers WJ, Hilchey SP, Halterman MW, Howard DF, Giuliano RE et al (2001) Development of herpes simplex virus-1 amplicon-based immunotherapy for chronic lymphocytic leukemia. Blood 98(2):287–295

Vollweiler JL, Zielske SP, Reese JS, Gerson SL (2003) Hematopoietic stem cell gene therapy: progress toward therapeutic targets. Bone Marrow Transplant 32(1):1–7

Wierda WG, Cantwell MJ, Woods SJ, Rassenti LZ, Prussak CE, Kipps TJ (2000) CD40-ligand (CD154) gene therapy for chronic lymphocytic leukemia. Blood 96(9):2917–2924

Wierda WG, Castro JE, Aguillon R, Sampath D, Jalayer A, McMannis J et al (2010) A phase I study of immune gene therapy for patients with CLL using a membrane-stable, humanized CD154. Leukemia 24(11):1893–1900

Xiao PJ, Lentz TB, Samulski RJ (2012) Recombinant adeno-associated virus: clinical application and development as a gene-therapy vector. Ther Deliv 3(7):835–856

Yan Z, Zhang Y, Duan D, Engelhardt JF (2000) Trans-splicing vectors expand the utility of adeno-associated virus for gene therapy. Proc Natl Acad Sci U S A 97(12):6716–6721

Gene Therapy for Nonmalignant Hematology

14

Xiuyan Wang and Isabelle Rivière

14.1 Introduction

Hematopoietic stem cells (HSCs) are long-lived, multipotent, self-renewing cells that are capable of generating all types of cells in the myeloid and lymphoid lineages (Bryder et al. 2006). Since the initial retroviral transfer of genetic materials into hematopoietic stem and progenitor cells 30 years ago, HSCs have been the prime cellular compartment for the correction of several inherited blood disorders and monogenic metabolic diseases using gene therapy (Booth et al. 2016; Cicalese and Aiuti 2015; Biffi et al. 2011). Despite the dogmatic acceptance of allogeneic transplantation as the first line of therapy with continuous improved outcomes (Buckley 2011; Pai et al. 2014), studies in several immunodeficiency diseases have clearly demonstrated that gene therapy can have long-lasting, curative effects alleviating the need to search for allogeneic donors and eliminating the risk of graft-versus-host disease (Booth et al. 2016; Cicalese and Aiuti 2015; Cavazzana et al. 2016).

Up to date, more than 150 patients affected with monogenic blood disorders and without matched donors have been treated with genetically modified $CD34^+$ HSPCs worldwide. The majority of these patients have clinically benefited from this approach. Moreover, the maturation of gene-editing technologies offers the prospect that targeted gene correction may become a viable approach for hematopoietic stem cell gene therapy in the upcoming years (Rahman et al. 2011; Mussolino and Cathomen 2012; Sander and Joung 2014).

X. Wang · I. Rivière (✉)
Michael G. Harris Cell Therapy and Cell Engineering Facility, Center for Cell Engineering, New York, NY, USA

Molecular Pharmacology Program, Memorial Sloan-Kettering Cancer Center, New York, NY, USA
e-mail: wangx1@mskcc.org; rivierei@mskcc.org

M.-A. Perales et al. (eds.), *Cell and Gene Therapies*, Advances and Controversies in Hematopoietic Transplantation and Cell Therapy,
https://doi.org/10.1007/978-3-319-54368-0_14

14.2 HSC Gene Therapy in Primary Monogenic Immunodeficiencies

PIDs are rare inherited genetic disorders that affect the development and function of the immune system, typically resulting in multiple, recurrent, and opportunistic infections with early onset. Patients may also suffer severe outcomes including not only autoimmunity, allergy, and cancer but also autoinflammation, hemophagocytosis, microangiopathies, angioedema, alveolar proteinosis, granuloma formation, and macular degeneration (Capucine Picard 2014). The gold standard therapy for patients with the most severe forms of PIDs who have a suitable donor is allogeneic hematopoietic cell transplantation (allo-HCT); the donor normal HSCs or hematopoietic progenitor cells can replace the dysfunctional hematopoietic lineages with normal cells and correct the adaptive and innate immune system (Slatter and Gennery 2013). However, allo-HCT is associated with several serious adverse events, including the toxicity of myeloablative chemotherapy and graft-versus-host disease. Delivery of a corrective gene to the patient autologous HSCs through gene delivery is an appealing therapeutic approach for a patient without an appropriate donor. Clinical studies performed in the past 20 years have validated this prediction (Booth et al. 2016; Williams and Thrasher 2014).

14.2.1 HSC Gene Therapy for SCID-X1: A Seminal Proof of Efficacy Study

SCID-X1 is an X-chromosome-linked inherited condition caused by defects in *IL2RG*, the gene encoding interleukin (IL)-2 receptor γ chain (γc). The IL-2 receptor γc is a common subunit for several hematopoietic cytokine receptors, including the IL-2, IL-4, IL-7, IL-9, IL-15, and IL-21 receptors (Sugamura et al. 1996). Defective IL-7 signaling pathway is responsible for the lack of T-cell differentiation, defective IL-15 signaling pathway is responsible for the early block in natural killer (NK) cell differentiation, and defective IL-21 signaling pathway affects the survival and proliferation of memory B cells. Patients with SCID-X1 are characterized by the absence of mature T cells and NK cells and poorly functional B cells (Leonard 1996). Spontaneous reversion of the mutation in the *IL2RG* gene led to significant correction of the immune deficiency (Stephan et al. 1996), which suggested that SCID-X1 would be an attractive and accurate model to assess the potential benefits of a gene therapy approach.

The first clinical trial of gene therapy for SCID-X1 was conducted in Paris in ten children under 1 year of age using a conventional amphotropic murine leukemia virus-based γ-retroviral vector, in which γc gene expression was driven by the LTR (Cavazzana-Calvo et al. 2000; Hacein-Bey-Abina et al. 2002). A similar trial was conducted in infants using a gibbon ape leukemia virus-pseudotyped retroviral vector in the UK (Gaspar et al. 2004). Patients enrolled in both trials did not receive any preconditioning prior to the genetically modified HSCs. Clinical outcomes for these patients are convincingly encouraging with 17 out of the 20 patients demonstrating a stable corrected phenotype after 10 years of follow-up (Hacein-Bey-Abina et al. 2010; Gaspar et al. 2011a). The majority of the patients achieved a rapid normalization of T-cell numbers and maintained a highly diverse functional T-cell repertoire. The robustness of the T lymphocyte reconstitution appeared to be directly correlated with the number of γc-corrected CD34$^+$ cells regardless of patient's disease status. The reconstitution of NK cell compartment was however less complete with only 10% of the control value—when compared to the reconstitution of the T-cell compartment 1 year after treatment. The patients' humoral responses were partially restored without detectable level of transduced B cells. However, the memory B-cell population remained defective in all patients who cannot produce high-affinity antibodies and mount poor recall responses against previously encountered antigens (Cavazzana et al. 2016; Hacein-Bey-Abina et al. 2010). Attempts to treat older patients (10–20 years old) as a rescue treatment option for HSCT failure did not achieve any significant clinical benefit, most likely due to age-related irrecoverable loss of thymic activity or a history of graft-versus-host disease (Thrasher et al. 2005; Chinen et al. 2007) (Table 14.1).

Despite these encouraging results, a total of five patients, four patients in the French study and one patient in the UK study, developed T-cell leukemia 31–68 months post-gene therapy, which resulted in the discontinuation of the trials (Hacein-Bey-Abina et al. 2008). In all cases, the severe adverse event (SAE) was due to insertional oncogenesis caused by the integration of retroviral vector within or near tumor-promoting genes, such as the *LMO2* gene. The enhancer activity of the LTR of the retroviral vector deregulated the proto-oncogenes and led to their transcriptional activation (Hacein-Bey-Abina et al. 2003; Howe et al. 2008). To improve the safety profile, a self-inactivating (SIN) γ-retroviral vector for X-SCID was developed, in which *IL2RG* cDNA was under the control of the weaker elongation factor (EF)-1α short promoter combined with the deletion of the enhancer element in the LTR (Thornhill et al. 2008; Zychlinski et al. 2008). A clinical trial using this SIN γ-retroviral vector started to recruit patient by the end of 2010. Eight out of nine patients (3.9–10.5 months old) treated with the SIN γ-retroviral vector are alive and well up to 4 years of follow-up except one who died of viral infection 4 months after infusion. In seven out of the eight remaining patients, full T-cell reconstitution and normalized T-cell proliferation were attained at the same rate as in the previous trials without insertional mutagenesis-related SAE to date (Hacein-Bey-Abina et al. 2014). A SIN lentiviral vector pseudotyped with VSVG and containing chicken β-globin chromatin insulator element was recently used for HSC gene therapy clinical trials for older SCID-X1 (7–23 years old) patients preconditioned with non-myeloablative low-dose busulfan, an alkylating agent that creates space in the bone marrow to facilitate engraftment. Patients with 2–3 years of follow-up have achieved T-cell reconstitution and sustained humoral responses without SAE (Zhou et al. 2010; De Ravin et al. 2016) (Table 14.1). These encouraging observations indicated that the newly designed SIN γ-retroviral and SIN lentiviral vectors for SCID-X1 are not only efficacious but also safer, as intended.

Table 14.1 Gene therapy clinical trials for primary immunodeficiencies

Disease (gene)	Vector (promoter)	Country	Conditioning	Nb of patients (age)	Outcome	SAEs	Ref
SCID-X1 (*IL2RG*)	γ-Retro (MLV-LTR)	France	None	10 (<1 year old)	7 patients including 3 survivors of T-ALL have stable, long-term correction of immune function in T-cell compartment	4 T-ALL	Cavazzana-Calvo et al. (2000), Hacein-Bey-Abina et al. (2010) and Hacein-Bey-Abina et al. (2008)
	γ-Retro (MLV-LTR)	UK	None	10 (<1 year old)	All patients had stable correction of immune function in T-cell compartment	1 T-ALL	Gaspar et al. (2004), Howe et al. (2008) and Gaspar et al. (2011b)
	γ-Retro (MLV-LTR)	USA	None	3 (>10 years)	No effect	None	Chinen et al. (2007)
	SIN γ-retro (EF-1α S)	France, UK, USA **NCT01410019** **NCT01129544** **NCT01175239**	None	9 + 2 (3.9–10.5 months old)	8 out of 9 patients have stable correction of immune function (T cells)	None	Booth et al. (2016) and Hacein-Bey-Abina et al. (2014)
	SIN-lenti (EF-1α S)	USA **NCT01306019**	Busulfan	5 (7–23)	Early immune recovery (T, B, and NK cells)	None	De Ravin et al. (2016)
	SIN-lenti	USA **NCT01512888**	Busulfan	0	N/A	N/A	Booth et al. (2016)

ADA-SCID (*ADA*)	γ-Retro (MLV-LTR)	Italy **NCT00599781**	Busulfan	18 (0.5–6.1 yrs)	15 out of 18 patients off ERT	None	Cicalese and Aiuti (2015) and Aiuti et al. (2009)
	γ-Retro (MLV-LTR)	UK	Melphalan or busulfan	6 (11–39 mons)	4 out 6 patients have stable recovery of immune function	None	Gaspar et al. (2011b)
	γ-Retro (MLV-LTR)	USA **NCT00018018**	Busulfan	10 (20 mons–15 yrs)	9 out of 10 patients off ERT	None	Cicalese and Aiuti (2015) and Candotti et al. (2012)
	SIN-lenti (EF-1α S)	UK, USA **NCT01380990** **NCT02022696** **NCT01852071**	Busulfan	20 (0.4–6.5 yrs)	20 out 20 patients off ERT	None	Gaspar et al. (2014), Gaspar et al. (2015), Mukherjee and Thrasher (2013) and Sadelain et al. (2015)
WAS (WASP)	γ-Retro (LTR)	Germany	Busulfan	10 (2–14)	Permanent correction of immunodeficiency achieved in majority of patients	7 leukemia, 1 AML, 4 T-ALL, and 2 primary T-ALL and secondary AML	Boztug et al. (2010) and Braun et al. (2014)
	SIN-lenti (WAS promoter)	UK, France **NCT01347242** **NCT01347346** **NCT02333760**	Busulfan and fludarabine	7 (0.8–15.5)	Six out of seven patients have stable engraftment and resolved eczema and predisposition for infection	None	Hacein-Bey Abina et al. (2015)
	SIN-lenti (WAS promoter)	Italy **NCT01515462**	CD20 mAb, busulfan, and fludarabine	8 (1.1–5.9 for the first 3 patients, no age reported for the remaining)	Stable engraftment, improved thrombocytopenia, eczema, and infectious episodes, all patients are platelet transfusion independent	None	Aiuti et al. (2013) and Scaramuzza et al. (2014)
	SIN-lenti (WAS promoter)	USA **NCT01410825**	Not reported	2 (age not reported)	Improved immune and hematologic parameters	None	Kuo and Kohn (2016)

(continued)

Table 14.1 (continued)

Disease (gene)	Vector (promoter)	Country	Conditioning	Nb of patients (age)	Outcome	SAEs	Ref
CGD (CYBB)	γ-Retro (MLV-LTR)	USA	None	5 (18–27 yrs)	No clinical benefit	None	Malech et al. (1997)
	γ-Retro (SFFV-LTR)	Germany	Busulfan	2 (25–26 years old)	Short-term rapid resolution of preexisting infections	2 MDS	Ott et al. (2006) and Stein et al. (2010)
	γ-Retro (SFFV-LTR)	Switzerland **NCT00927134**	Busulfan	1 (8.5 years old	Initial detection of gene-corrected granulocytes and neutrophils	Clonal myeloproliferation	Grez et al. (2011) and Bianchi et al. (2011)
	γ-Retro (MLV-LTR or SFFV-LTR)	UK	Melphalan	3 (5–27)	Initial and transient detection of transgene in periphery blood granulocytes	None	Grez et al. (2011)
	γ-Retro (MLV-LTR)	USA **NCT00394316**	Busulfan	3 (19–28 years old)	Initial high gene marking and sustained low-level long-term marking in 2 out of the 3 patients with fully or partially resolution of infection	None	Kang et al. (2010)
	γ-Retro (MLV-LTR)	Korea **NCT00778882**	Busulfan + fludarabine	2 (9–18)	Initial transient gene marking	None	Kang et al. (2011a)
	SIN-lenti	Europe **NCT01855685**	Myeloablative Busulfan	1	Known	Not known	Booth et al. (2016) and Kuo and Kohn (2016)
	SIN-lenti G1XCGD	USA **NCT02234934** France **NCT02757911**	Myeloablative Busulfan	1	Not known	Not known	Booth et al. (2016)
	SIN-retro	Germany **NCT01906541**	Busulfan	0	Not known	Not known	Booth et al. (2016)

CYBB gene encoding the gp91^{phox} subunit of NADPH oxidase, *SAE* serious adverse events, *retro* retrovirus, *lenti* lentivirus, *LTR* long terminal repeat, *SIN* self-inactivated, *T-ALL* T-cell acute lymphocytic leukemia, *EF1aS* elongation factor-1α short promoter, *yrs* years, *mons* months, *AML* acute myeloid leukemia, *MDS* myelodysplastic syndrome, *mAb* monoclonal antibody

14.2.2 HSC Gene Therapy for ADA-SCID: The First Approved Ex Vivo Stem Cell Therapy as a Drug by the European Medicines Agency

Adenosine deaminase (ADA) is an essential enzyme in the purine salvage pathway. ADA is ubiquitously expressed in all tissues and removes deoxyadenosine and adenosine generated during DNA and RNA degradation, respectively, under physiological circumstances. Its deficiency leads to the accumulation of toxic metabolites causing SCID phenotype due to abnormal development and function of T cells, B cells, and NK cells, as well as non-immunological abnormalities affecting the skeleton, nervous system, respiratory system, gastrointestinal tract, and liver (Dissing and Knudsen 1972). Patients with ADA-SCID typically succumb to life-threatening opportunistic infections within the first year of life due to severe immune deficiencies. Treatment options for ADA-SCID include allogeneic HSCT from matched donors, enzyme replacement therapy, and more recently gene therapy (Gaspar et al. 2009). ADA gene therapy trials conducted in the early 1990s using γ-retroviral vector delivery of corrective ADA cDNA into various cell types, including lymphocytes (Blaese et al. 1995; Onodera et al. 1998), umbilical cord blood (Kohn et al. 1995), and bone marrow (Bordignon et al. 1993; Hoogerbrugge et al. 1996), failed to produce clinical benefits, until Aiuti and colleagues reported their clinical trial in ten patients who receive a mild conditioning regimen with busulfan before the infusion of transduced HSCs (Aiuti et al. 2007, 2009) (Table 14.1). More than 40 patients with ADA-SCID have been treated with conventional γ-retroviral vector with intact LTRs since 2000, with 100% survival and approximately 75% disease-free survival without the need for enzyme replacement therapy or allo-HCT (Gaspar et al. 2011b; Candotti et al. 2012) (Table 14.1). No SAE related to insertional mutagenesis has been reported despite the similar design and integration profile of the ADA-SCID γ-retroviral vector (Aiuti et al. 2007) with the γ-retroviral vectors used in the initial SCID-X1 trials. Moreover, another γ-retroviral vector design for ADA-SCID trial was used by the UK group with LTR from the spleen focus-forming virus. No SAE due to insertional mutagenesis was found in these patients either (Gaspar et al. 2011b, 2014; Cicalese et al. 2014), although this vector design has been found to cluster at the ecotropic virus integration site 1 (EVI1) and led to myelodysplastic syndrome (MDS) (Buonamici et al. 2003). These observations suggest that the background of ADA deficiency offers a disease-specific protection against vector-related insertional mutagenesis (Williams and Thrasher 2014).

Aiming to improve the safety profile and efficacy of this promising HSC gene therapy for ADA-SCID, a SIN lentiviral vector was developed featuring the codon-optimized ADA cDNA under the control of the elongation factor 1α (EF1α) short promoter. Efficacious preclinical results were obtained (Carbonaro et al. 2012), which prompted the initiation of clinical trials using this SIN lentiviral vector (Gaspar et al. 2015). Autologous $CD34^+$ cells are harvested from the bone marrow or mobilized peripheral blood and transduced with the SIN lentiviral vector. Patients undergo bone marrow cytoreduction with 4–5 mg/kg of busulfan followed by infusion with transduced $CD34^+$ cells. The status of the first 20 patients (0.4–6.5 years of age) in these trials was reported in 2015 with follow-up ranging from 1 month to 3 years (Gaspar et al. 2015). All patients are clinically well with evident immunological and metabolic recovery. Integration site analysis revealed a polyclonal insertional pattern, and no clonal expansion of genes associated with mutagenesis was detected in any of the patients (Gaspar et al. 2015). As of May 2016, a total of 75 ADA-SCID patients have been treated using HSC gene therapy with 74 patient alive and 66 patients off enzyme replacement therapy (oral presentation by Dr. A. Fischer at ASGCT 2016). The pharmaceutical company GlaxoSmithKline (GSK) obtained approval from the European Medicines Agency to commercialize the first ex vivo HSC gene therapy to treat ADA-SCID in May 2016.

14.2.3 HSC Gene Therapy for WAS: A Work in Progress

WAS is a monogenic X-linked primary immunodeficiency caused by mutations in *WAS* gene encoding WAS protein (WASP). WASP is a crucial regulator for hematopoietic cell cytoskeletal reorganization (Bosticardo et al. 2009). The syndrome is characterized by various symptoms ranging from micro-thrombocytopenia, immune dysfunction, elevated frequency of tumor formation, and eczema depending on the types of WASP mutations (Notarangelo et al. 2008). Although allo-HCT is a curative treatment for WAS patient with suitable donor, alternative treatment options, such as HSC gene therapy, are needed for patients lacking matched donors.

The first clinical trial for WAS was conducted in Germany between 2006 and 2009. Ten patients (age 2–14 years) received autologous HSCs transduced with an LTR-driven γ-retroviral vector after reduced-intensity conditioning with busulfan. High cell dose and high transduction efficiency were achieved, which correlated with the restored WASP expression in both myeloid and lymphoid lineages, as well as in platelets (Boztug et al. 2010). Although marked clinical benefits in several of these patients were observed, seven out of ten of patients developed leukemia due to γ-retroviral vector insertional mutagenesis largely associated with dysregulation of proto-oncogenes such as LMO2, MDS1, and MN1 (Braun et al. 2014; Kuo and Kohn 2016). A SIN lentiviral vector was subsequently developed, in which WAS cDNA was put under the control of its endogenous promoter. An international multicenter phase I/II clinical trial has begun using this SIN lentiviral vector design in combination with reduced-intensity regimen. There have been seven patients treated in France and England (Hacein-Bey Abina et al. 2015), six patients treated in Italy (Aiuti et al. 2013; Scaramuzza et al. 2014), and two patients treated in the USA (Kuo and Kohn 2016) (Table 14.1). Multi-lineage engraftment of the gene-corrected cells and sustained, robust clinical improvement have been observed in these patients. Functional transduced NK cells were detectable 1 month after treatment and increased over time. Moreover, vector insertion sites are highly polyclonal without signs of clonal expansion (Hacein-Bey Abina et al. 2015; Aiuti et al. 2013; Scaramuzza et al. 2014).

14.2.4 HSC Gene Therapy for X-Linked CGD: Further Research Needed

CGD is a rare inherited immunodeficiency disorder caused by defective superoxide production in phagocytic cells. X-linked form of CGD, which accounts for about two-thirds of the CGD cases, is caused by mutations in the *CYBB* gene that encodes the $gp91^{phox}$ subunit of NADPH oxidase. The defect in formation of microbicidal oxygen species renders the phagocytes unable to fight against a wide range of organisms. Patients also experience sterile, chronic, granulomatous inflammation caused by increased production of pro-inflammation cytokines, delayed apoptosis of inflammatory cells, and deficient secretion of anti-inflammatory mediators (Kang et al. 2011b).

Allo-HCT is an effective therapy for X-CGD patient with HLA-matched donor (Gungor et al. 2014). Alternative therapies still need to be established for patients without a suitable donor. The initial clinical trials of HSC gene therapy were conducted using first-generation γ-retroviral vectors in which the $gp91^{phox}$ expression was under the control of the spleen focus-forming virus LTR. Some patients initially sustained some clinical benefit because of the corrected NADPH activity (Ott et al. 2006; Bianchi et al. 2009; Grez et al. 2011) (Table 14.1). However, the effect was only transient. This was due to either the downregulation of the transgene expression as a result of viral promoter methylation (Booth et al. 2016) or the progressive decrease in cell engraftment possibly because of $gp91^{phox}$-induced apoptosis in HSCs (Touzot et al. 2014) or immune response to the newly expressed $gp91^{phox}$ protein in CGD patients (Grez et al. 2011). Moreover, the γ-retroviral vectors were found to be inserted close to proto-oncogenes including *PRDM16*, *SETBP1*, and *MDS-EV1*. Patients with dominant MDS-EV1 clones developed myelodysplastic syndrome (Ott et al. 2006; Stein et al. 2010) (Table 14.1). Similarly, clinical trials using γ-retroviral vector with murine leukemia virus LTR to introduce $gp91^{phox}$ cDNA (Kang et al. 2010, 2011b) into $CD34^{+}$ cells also elicited a similar initial high gene marking followed by a quick decline in patients (Grez et al. 2011; Kang et al. 2010, 2011b) (Table 14.1). Safer SIN lentiviral vector with myeloid-specific promoter has been developed for X-CGD HSC gene therapy, and new clinical trials have been opened in Europe and the USA using this vector design (Kuo and Kohn 2016).

14.3 HSC Gene Therapy for Other Diseases

The encouraging results of HSC gene therapy for PIDs have promoted the expansion of HSC gene therapy repertoire to other diseases. Phase I/II clinical trials have been initiated for blood disorders, such as X-linked ALD (X-ALD), MLD, β-thalassemia, and sickle cell disease.

14.3.1 HSC Gene Therapy for ALD and MLD

X-ALD is a monogenic metabolic disease caused by inactivating mutations in the *ABCD1* gene encoding the ALD protein (ALDP). ALDP is a peroxisomal protein belonging to the ATP-binding cassette (ABC) transporter superfamily. Functional loss of ALDP is associated with abnormal peroxisomal β-oxidation and accumulation of saturated very-long-chain fatty acids (VLCFAs) in tissues and body fluids. The defect of ALDP disrupts myelin maintenances by oligodendrocytes and microglia, which results in a fatal demyelinating disease of the central nervous system (CNS) (Mosser et al. 1993; Moser et al. 2007). Allo-HCT is the only effective therapy, which can arrest the neuroinflammatory demyelinating process, provided the procedure is performed at an early stage of the disease (Aubourg et al. 1990; Shapiro et al. 2000). However, demyelination cannot be arrested if the disease has progressed past a certain stage.

The first clinical trial for ALD patients was conducted in France. The two patients without suitable HSC donor underwent a fully myeloablative conditioning regimen with busulfan and cyclophosphamide and were subsequently infused with GM-CSF-mobilized $CD34^+$ cells transduced with a SIN lentiviral vector expressing *ABCD1* cDNA under the control of a modified MND promoter (Biffi et al. 2011; Cartier et al. 2009). Clear clinical benefit from the HSC gene therapy was observed. Progression of demyelination disease was arrested 14–16-month post-gene therapy, and lesions did not further progressed up to 4 years posttreatment (Cartier et al. 2009, 2010), which is similar to those obtained in patients who had successful HSCT. No clonal skewing or dominance related to vector insertional mutagenesis was detected during the period of post-infusion follow-up (Biffi et al. 2011) (Table 14.2).

14.3.2 HSC Gene Therapy for MLD

MLD is a fatal neurodegenerative lysosomal storage disease (LSD) caused by deficiency of the lysosome enzyme arylsulfatase A (ARSA). ARSA deficiency results in a massive accumulation of its substrate, sulfatide, in oligodendrocytes, microglia, and neurons of the CNS and in Schwann cells and macrophages of the peripheral nervous system, which leads to widespread demyelination and neurodegeneration. Patients experience severe progressive motor and cognitive impairment and succumb to the disease within a few years of symptoms onset. MLD is classified into clinical variants—late infantile, early and late juveniles, and adult—based on symptoms onset; the infantile patients exhibit the worst prognosis (Gieselmann and Krageloh-Mann 2010). No effective treatments, including allo-HCT, can significantly delay the progression and the fatal outcome of this disease (Biffi et al. 2008; Musolino et al. 2014).

A phase I/II HSC gene therapy clinical trial was conducted in Italy in nine children diagnosed with early-onset disease using a SIN lentiviral vector in which the human ARSA cDNA was under the control of the human phosphoglycerate kinase (PGK)

Table 14.2 Gene therapy clinical trials for ALD and MLD

Disease (gene)	Vector (promoter)	Country	Conditioning	Nb of patients (age)	Outcome	SAEs	Ref
X-ALD (*ABCD1*)	SIN-lenti (MND promoter)	France	Busulfan and cyclophosphamide	2 (7–7.5 yrs)	Polyclonal reconstitution of both myeloid and lymphoid lineages, stable disease	None	Cartier et al. (2009) and Cartier et al. (2010)
MLD (*ARSA*)	SIN-lenti (PGK promoter)	Italy **NCT01560182**	Busulfan	9 (7–59 mons)	Stable engraftment, prevention of disease onset or progression	None	Biffi et al. (2013) and Sessa et al. (2016)
X-ALD (*ABCD1*)	Lenti-D	USA **NCT01896102 Phase 2/3**	Busulfan and cyclophosphamide	Not known	Not known	Not known	N/A
X-ALD (*ABCD1*) and MLD (*ARSA*)	Lentiviral vector	China **NCT02559830**	Not specified	Not known	Not known	Not known	N/A

ABCD1 ATP-binding cassette, subfamily D, member 1, *ALD* adrenoleukodystrophy, *MLD* metachromatic leukodystrophy, *MND* myeloproliferative sarcoma virus enhancer, negative control region deleted, dl587rev primer binding site substituted, *yrs* years old, *mons* months old, *ARSA* arylsulfatase A, *PGK* phosphoglycerate kinase

promoter (Biffi et al. 2013; Sessa et al. 2016) (Table 14.2). Autologous bone marrow-derived $CD34^+$ HSCs transduced with the SIN lentiviral vector were reinfused into patients after myeloablative conditioning with busulfan. The follow-up analysis of all nine children enrolled in this trial was reported recently with clear and convincing clinical benefits using this therapy (Sessa et al. 2016). Stable and sustained engraftment of gene-corrected HSC and a progressive reconstitution of ARSA activity in HSC and cerebrospinal fluid were documented in all patients. Eight out of the nine patients had prevention of disease onset or arrest of disease progression. Treatment resulted in protection from CNS demyelination in eight out of the nine patients and sign of remyelination in at least three patients. So far, no genotoxicity related to lentiviral vector insertion was observed in all the patients with a medium of 3-year follow-up (Sessa et al. 2016). Although long-term follow-up and larger cohort of patients are still needed, this study shed light on the first possible curative treatment for this devastating disease.

14.3.3 HSC Gene Therapy for β-Thalassemia and Sickle Cell Disease

The β-thalassemias are inherited blood disorders that result from the defective or absent production of the beta chain of hemoglobin. Beta-thalassemia major is treated with lifelong transfusions of donor red blood cells (RBCs), but transfusion therapy does not correct ineffective erythropoiesis and exacerbates systemic iron accumulation, requiring intense iron chelation therapy. The transplantation of donor HSCs in thalassemic patients is potentially curative, but this option is not available to the majority of thalassemic subjects, for whom a suitable matched related donor cannot be found (Sadelain et al. 2007). Because of the greater risks associated with HLA-matched-unrelated or mismatched transplants, most thalassemia patients undergo lifelong transfusion therapy and all of its consequences.

Sickle cell disease (SCD) is a recessive congenital blood disorder caused by an amino acid substitution at position 6 (Glu→Val) in the β-globin chain of hemoglobin (Hb) (Steinberg et al. 2001a; Pauling et al. 1949). The resulting hemoglobin, termed HbS, polymerizes causing red blood cells to sickle and eventually obstruct blood flow in small vessels. Chronic hemolysis, frequent infections, and recurring episodes of microvascular obstruction are the archetypal features of SCD. The vaso-occlusive "crises" which are responsible for damaging various organs can cause long-term disability, significantly reduced mean life span, and sometimes sudden death (Serjeant 1985; Steinberg et al. 2001b; Bunn 1997).

14.3.4 HSC Gene Therapy for β-Thalassemia: Myeloablative or Non-myeloablative Conditioning?

The report by May et al. describing the therapeutic efficiency in thalassemic mice of recombinant lentiviruses expressing the human beta-globin gene under the control of its locus control region paved the way for the treatment of hemoglobinopathies using HSC gene therapy (May et al. 2000). Trials evaluating globin gene transfer in thalassemic subjects are opened and accruing patients. The first two trials opened in Paris (LG001, (Cavazzana-Calvo et al. 2010)) and New York (NCT01639690, (Mansilla-Soto et al. 2016)), evaluating the b87/HVP569 and TNS9.3.55 vectors, respectively. Other trials subsequently opened utilizing either the BB305 vector, a variant of the β87/HPV569 vector, or the GLOBE vector (Mansilla-Soto et al. 2016; Negre et al. 2016) (Table 14.3).

Despite low engraftment of HVP569-transduced HSCs, one of the four subjects in the Paris trial showed clinical benefit, thanks to the emergence of a single myeloid progenitor clone driven by the transactivation of the HMGA2 gene at the site of vector integration (Cavazzana-Calvo et al. 2010). The erythroid progeny of this dominant clone expressed the vector-encoded b87 chain, which accounted for about one-third of the total hemoglobin starting 1 year after the infusion. Another third of the hemoglobin came from the subject himself who did have a β^+ form of the disease. Additionally, the patient had an unusually elevated and sustained expression of hemoglobin F resulting from the activation of the endogenous fetal or gamma-globin gene post-autologous transplantation. Subsequently, 13 thalassemic subjects have been infused with $CD34^+$ cells transduced with BB305 (NCT02151526, NCT01745120). Initial results have been reported at scientific meetings indicating clinical benefit in patients with β^+- or βE-thalassemia (Negre et al. 2016). The New York trial opened in 2012, enrolling adult subjects with transfusion-dependent beta- thalassemia major. The treatment is based on the administration of autologous $CD34^+$ hematopoietic cells transduced with the TNS9.3.55 vector that encodes the wild-type human β-globin gene. Importantly, this protocol calls for reduced-intensity conditioning in contrast to the fully myeloablative regimen applied in the trials described above. Indeed, in other blood disorders treated with transduced autologous $CD34^+$ cells, it was demonstrated that conditioning with busulfan at 8 mg/kg is sufficient to achieve therapeutic engraftment of modified HSCs (Ott et al. 2006). Our results to date show stable engraftment without clonal dominance in four subjects infused and one patient with significant decrease in transfusion requirements (Mansilla-Soto et al. 2016; Sadelain et al. 2015). Although there is general consensus that a non-myeloablative conditioning regimen would have many advantages, including decreased toxicity, rapid hematopoietic recovery, and shortened hospitalization, it remains to be determined whether it will be sufficient to support the efficacy of this treatment (Table 14.3).

The Milano trial utilizes another variant of TNS9 lacking the HS4 element (Miccio et al. 2008). The protocol opened recently and the first subject was infused in late 2015 (NCT02453477, (Marktel et al. 2017)). It differs from the trials described above by the cell infusion route, which is not intravenous but medullary via the iliac crest. The conditioning used by the TIGET team includes thiotepa and treosulfan.

Table 14.3 Gene therapy clinical trials for thalassemia and sickle cell disease

Disease (gene)	Vector (promoter)	Country (study #ID)	Conditioning	Nb of patients (age)	Outcome	SAEs	Ref
b-Thal (b-globin)	TNS9.3.55	USA **NCT01639690**	Non-myeloablative	4	One patient with significant decrease in transfusion requirement (unpublished data)	None	Mansilla-Soto et al. (2016)
b-Thal and SCD (b87-globin)	HPV569	France **LG001**	Myeloablative	4 Thal (P2, 18 yrs)	One bE-/b0-treated patient independent of transfusions for more than 7 years	HMGA2 activation	Cavazzana-Calvo et al. (2010)
b-Thal and SCD (b87-globin)	BB305	France, USA, Thailand, Australia **NCT02151526** **NCT01745120** **NCT02140554**	Myeloablative	4 SCD (13–19 yrs) 11 Thal (18–35 yrs)	Some benefit (unpublished data)	Not known	Mansilla-Soto et al. (2016) and Negre et al. (2016)
b-Thal (b-globin)	GLOBE	Italy **NCT02453477**	Myeloablative	1	Not known	Not known	Marktel et al. (2017)
SCD (g-globin)	sGbG	USA **NCT02186418**	Not specified	Not known	Not known	Not known	N/A
SCD (**b**AS3-globin)	Lenti/**b**AS3-FB	USA **NCT02247843**	Busulfan, dose not specified	Not known	Not known	Not known	N/A

14.3.5 HSC Gene Therapy for Sickle Cell Disease

The only available curative therapy for SCD is also allogeneic bone marrow transplantation. In the absence of a suitable donor, the genetic correction of autologous HSCs represents a highly attractive alternative. In SCD, the vector-encoded globin chain must compete against the endogenous β^s-chains for binding to α-chains. For this reason, several investigators favor the use of β-chains other than the normal β-chain for the treatment of this disease. The γ-globin chain, which has higher affinity for the α-chain than the β-chain, is therefore frequently utilized in vectors designed to treat SCD (Blouin et al. 2000). A variation on this concept is to mutagenize the human β-globin gene to introduce amino acid residues that increase α-chain affinity. Two mutant β-chains, β87 and βAS3, have increased competitive properties vis-à-vis of β^S (Pawliuk et al. 2001; Levasseur et al. 2003, 2004).

Four subjects with SCD have been treated with BB305 (β87 variant) (NCT02151526, NCT02140554) in France and in the USA in ongoing trials. Initial results have been presented at scientific meetings (Negre et al. 2016). Two additional trials have opened in the USA using either the βAS3 variant (NCT02247843) or the γ-globin cDNA (NCT02186418). Genetic approaches to treat SCD are not confined to globin gene addition and encompass a variety of other strategies. Some aim to reactivate the endogenous γ-globin gene, which is normally silenced after birth, and others to correct the sickle mutation or remove the mutated β^S-globin transcript. One important finding is that Bcl11a acts as a negative regulator of γ-globin expression, promoting the switch from fetal to adult hemoglobin production (Canver and Orkin 2016). It was demonstrated that the alteration of Bcl11a expression using a ZFN that cleaves a GATA1 motif in the Bcl11a gene results in marked increase of γ-globin transcripts associated with a corresponding decrease in Bcl11a mRNA levels (Vierstra et al. 2015). These studies have uncovered the role of Bcl11a in the complex regulation of globin gene expression and also revealed potential new genetic approaches to reverse globin switching for the treatment of hemoglobinopathies (Mansilla-Soto et al. 2016; Guda et al. 2015) (Table 14.3).

14.4 Gene Editing for HSC Gene Therapy

Tremendous headway in HSC gene therapy has been made during the past two decades owing to deeper understanding of the molecular basis of diseases in combination with safer design of vectors for viral gene delivery and improved conditioning regimen (Booth et al. 2016; Kuo and Kohn 2016). However, potential insertional mutagenesis due to incorporation of functional genes via viral vectors into diseased cells at other sites than their natural loci is still a major safety concern. The rapid development of gene-editing technologies including ZFN, TALEN, and CRISPR/Cas over the past decade presents an attracting forefront that enables targeted gene correction in situ. In theory, such targeted platforms allow the corrected target genes to be expressed under the control of their native regulatory elements and thus eliminate the risk of insertional mutagenesis.

ZFN (Urnov et al. 2010), TALEN (Joung and Sander 2013), and CRISPR/Cas (Sander and Joung 2014) are all artificial endonucleases that combine specific DNA recognition sequences, which mediate precise genomic targeting, and an endonuclease, which generates a double-stranded break (DSB) in the DNA. Following DSB, repair could be made either by the error-prone nonhomologous end-joining (NHEJ) pathway or by the high-fidelity homology-directed repair (HDR) pathway (Ott de Bruin et al. 2015). NHEJ commonly introduces insertions and deletions, which can be exploited to inactivate the dominant mutated allele. HDR pathway allows targeted editing either by integrating an expression cassette into a safe genomic harbor or correcting disease-causing mutations by inserting a functional copy of the affected gene downstream of its own promoter. ZFN is the most clinically advanced endonuclease and has been used to interrupt the CCR5 gene in T cells of HIV-positive subjects. The trial has proven to be safe and demonstrated sustained increase of engineered T cells in participating patients (Tebas et al. 2014). TALEN also entered clinical trials for engineering allogeneic CD19-targeted chimeric antigen receptor (CAR) T cells in an infant girl with refractory, relapsed B-cell acute lymphocytic leukemia (Waseem Qasim et al. 2015).

Therapeutic genome editing for β-thalassemia and SCD are also being developed for clinical evaluation. Strategies based on gene addition or gene correction, including homologous recombination for hemoglobinopathies, have been recently reviewed by Mansilla-Soto et al. (2016). Although these approaches are exciting and transferable to certain types of PIDs, the correction of diseased genes in patients HSCs is key for many inborn monogenic disorders and still remains a challenge. To this end, Genovese and colleagues have demonstrated targeted integration of corrective cDNA into the *IL2RG* locus in SCID-X1 patient $CD34^+$ cells using ZFN and long-term multi-lineage immune reconstitution in immunodeficient NSG mice after infusion of the gene-corrected $CD34^+$ cells (Genovese et al. 2014). Induced pluripotent stem cells (iPSCs) derived from CGD patients have also been used as a model to demonstrate successful genetic correction using ZFNs (Merling et al. 2015), TALENs (Dreyer et al. 2015), and CRISPR/Cas9 (Flynn et al. 2015). More recently, the therapeutic potential of CRISPR/Cas9 genome editing was further tested in vivo in a variety of murine disease models (Long et al. 2016; Nelson et al. 2016; Tabebordbar et al. 2016). Despite the exciting progress toward the clinical application of the gene-editing platforms, important technical issues (such as low transduction efficiency in HSCs), safety issues (such as off-target effects), and ethical issues (such as the use of embryo) remained to be addressed. The undesirable mutations introduced by targeted nucleases are difficult to assess, in part owing to their small size and easy escape from detection. Novel monitoring assays, however, hold the promise of advancing this field.

14.5 Concluding Remarks

HSC engineering beyond the crossroads—Over the past 20 years, more than 150 subjects with multiple disease indications have received, and most of them benefited, from HSC gene therapy. This form of therapy has made significant progress since the seminal study in patients with SCID-X1 and continues to develop at a fast pace. Up to now, HSC gene therapy has been shown to provide therapeutic benefit in primary immunodeficiencies (Booth et al. 2016; Kuo and Kohn 2016), thalassemia (Mansilla-Soto et al. 2016), and leukodystrophies (Sessa et al. 2016). The first approval of genetically modified HSCs a drug has been granted to GSK in May 2016 by the EMA in Europe for the treatment of ADA-SCID. The disease repertoire for HSC gene therapy is steadily expanding. With the continuous improvement in vector design; deeper understanding of HSC biology; more refinement in bioprocessing and manufacturing; promising new technologies, in particular the gene-editing platforms; and better conditioning regimen prior to bone marrow transplantation, HSC gene therapy is poised to become the standard of care for a spectrum of hereditary and acquired disorders. HSC engineering remains one of the most tantalizing medical research objectives for the twenty-first century.

Acknowledgments We thank Michel Sadelain, MD, PhD, for reviewing the manuscript.

References

Aiuti A, Biasco L, Scaramuzza S, Ferrua F, Cicalese MP, Baricordi C, Dionisio F, Calabria A, Giannelli S, Castiello MC, Bosticardo M, Evangelio C, Assanelli A, Casiraghi M, Di Nunzio S, Callegaro L, Benati C, Rizzardi P, Pellin D, Di Serio C, Schmidt M, Von Kalle C, Gardner J, Mehta N, Neduva V, Dow DJ, Galy A, Miniero R, Finocchi A, Metin A, Banerjee PP, Orange JS, Galimberti S, Valsecchi MG, Biffi A, Montini E, Villa A, Ciceri F, Roncarolo MG, Naldini L (2013) Lentiviral hematopoietic stem cell gene therapy in patients with Wiskott-Aldrich syndrome. Science 341:1233151

Aiuti A, Cassani B, Andolfi G, Mirolo M, Biasco L, Recchia A, Urbinati F, Valacca C, Scaramuzza S, Aker M, Slavin S, Cazzola M, Sartori D, Ambrosi A, Di Serio C, Roncarolo MG, Mavilio F, Bordignon C (2007) Multilineage hematopoietic reconstitution without clonal selection in ADA-SCID patients treated with stem cell gene therapy. J Clin Invest 117:2233–2240

Aiuti A, Cattaneo F, Galimberti S, Benninghoff U, Cassani B, Callegaro L, Scaramuzza S, Andolfi G, Mirolo M, Brigida I, Tabucchi A, Carlucci F, Eibl M, Aker M, Slavin S, Al-Mousa H, Al Ghonaium A, Ferster A, Duppenthaler A, Notarangelo L, Wintergerst U, Buckley RH, Bregni M, Marktel S, Valsecchi MG, Rossi P, Ciceri F, Miniero R, Bordignon C, Roncarolo MG (2009) Gene therapy for immunodeficiency due to adenosine deaminase deficiency. N Engl J Med 360:447–458

Aubourg P, Blanche S, Jambaque I, Rocchiccioli F, Kalifa G, Naud-Saudreau C, Rolland MO, Debre M, Chaussain JL, Griscelli C et al (1990) Reversal of early neurologic and neuroradiologic manifestations of X-linked adrenoleukodystrophy by bone marrow transplantation. N Engl J Med 322:1860–1866

Bianchi M, Hakkim A, Brinkmann V, Siler U, Seger RA, Zychlinsky A, Reichenbach J (2009) Restoration of NET formation by gene therapy in CGD controls aspergillosis. Blood 114:2619–2622

Bianchi M, Niemiec MJ, Siler U, Urban CF, Reichenbach J (2011) Restoration of anti-Aspergillus defense by neutrophil extracellular traps in human chronic granulomatous disease after gene therapy is calprotectin-dependent. J Allergy Clin Immunol 127:1243–1252 e1247

Biffi A, Aubourg P, Cartier N (2011) Gene therapy for leukodystrophies. Hum Mol Genet 20:R42–R53

Biffi A, Lucchini G, Rovelli A, Sessa M (2008) Metachromatic leukodystrophy: an overview of current and prospective treatments. Bone Marrow Transplant 42(Suppl 2):S2–S6

Biffi A, Montini E, Lorioli L, Cesani M, Fumagalli F, Plati T, Baldoli C, Martino S, Calabria A, Canale S, Benedicenti F, Vallanti G, Biasco L, Leo S, Kabbara N, Zanetti G, Rizzo WB, Mehta NA, Cicalese MP, Casiraghi M, Boelens JJ, Del Carro U, Dow DJ, Schmidt M, Assanelli A, Neduva V, Di Serio C, Stupka E, Gardner J, von Kalle C, Bordignon C, Ciceri F, Rovelli A, Roncarolo MG, Aiuti A, Sessa M, Naldini L (2013) Lentiviral hematopoietic stem cell gene therapy benefits metachromatic leukodystrophy. Science 341:1233158

Blaese RM, Culver KW, Miller AD, Carter CS, Fleisher T, Clerici M, Shearer G, Chang L, Chiang Y, Tolstoshev P, Greenblatt JJ, Rosenberg SA, Klein H, Berger M, Mullen CA, Ramsey WJ, Muul L, Morgan RA, Anderson WF (1995) T lymphocyte-directed gene therapy for ADA-SCID: initial trial results after 4 years. Science 270:475–480

Blouin MJ, Beauchemin H, Wright A, De Paepe M, Sorette M, Bleau AM, Nakamoto B, Ou CN, Stamatoyannopoulos G, Trudel M (2000) Genetic correction of sickle cell disease: insights using transgenic mouse models. Nat Med 6:177–182

Booth C, Gaspar HB, Thrasher AJ (2016) Treating Immunodeficiency through HSC Gene Therapy. Trends Mol Med 22:317–327

Bordignon C, Mavilio F, Ferrari G, Servida P, Ugazio AG, Notarangelo LD, Gilboa E, Rossini S, O'Reilly RJ, Smith CA et al (1993) Transfer of the ADA gene into bone marrow cells and peripheral blood lymphocytes for the treatment of patients affected by ADA-deficient SCID. Hum Gene Ther 4:513–520

Bosticardo M, Marangoni F, Aiuti A, Villa A, Grazia Roncarolo M (2009) Recent advances in understanding the pathophysiology of Wiskott-Aldrich syndrome. Blood 113:6288–6295

Boztug K, Schmidt M, Schwarzer A, Banerjee PP, Diez IA, Dewey RA, Bohm M, Nowrouzi A, Ball CR, Glimm H, Naundorf S, Kuhlcke K, Blasczyk R, Kondratenko I, Marodi L, Orange JS, von Kalle C, Klein C (2010) Stem-cell gene therapy for the Wiskott-Aldrich syndrome. N Engl J Med 363:1918–1927

Braun CJ, Boztug K, Paruzynski A, Witzel M, Schwarzer A, Rothe M, Modlich U, Beier R, Gohring G, Steinemann D, Fronza R, Ball CR, Haemmerle R, Naundorf S, Kuhlcke K, Rose M, Fraser C, Mathias L, Ferrari R, Abboud MR, Al-Herz W, Kondratenko I, Marodi L, Glimm H, Schlegelberger B, Schambach A, Albert MH, Schmidt M, von Kalle C, Klein C (2014) Gene therapy for Wiskott-Aldrich syndrome--long-term efficacy and genotoxicity. Sci Transl Med 6:227–233

Bryder D, Rossi DJ, Weissman IL (2006) Hematopoietic stem cells: the paradigmatic tissue-specific stem cell. Am J Pathol 169:338–346

Buckley RH (2011) Transplantation of hematopoietic stem cells in human severe combined immunodeficiency: longterm outcomes. Immunol Res 49:25–43

Bunn HF (1997) Pathogenesis and treatment of sickle cell disease. N Engl J Med 337:762–769

Buonamici S, Chakraborty S, Senyuk V, Nucifora G (2003) The role of EVI1 in normal and leukemic cells. Blood Cells Mol Dis 31:206–212

Candotti F, Shaw KL, Muul L, Carbonaro D, Sokolic R, Choi C, Schurman SH, Garabedian E, Kesserwan C, Jagadeesh GJ, Fu PY, Gschweng E, Cooper A, Tisdale JF, Weinberg KI, Crooks GM, Kapoor N, Shah A, Abdel-Azim H, Yu XJ, Smogorzewska M, Wayne AS, Rosenblatt HM, Davis CM, Hanson C, Rishi RG, Wang X, Gjertson D, Yang OO, Balamurugan A, Bauer G, Ireland JA, Engel BC, Podsakoff GM, Hershfield MS, Blaese RM, Parkman R, Kohn DB (2012) Gene therapy for adenosine deaminase-deficient severe combined immune deficiency: clinical comparison of retroviral vectors and treatment plans. Blood 120:3635–3646

Canver MC, Orkin SH (2016) Customizing the genome as therapy for the beta-hemoglobinopathies. Blood 127:2536–2545

Capucine Picard J-LC (2014) Evolution of the definition of primary immunodeficiencies. In: Etzioni A, Ochs HD (eds) Primary immunodeficiency disorders. Elsevier Inc., Oxford, pp 29–40

Carbonaro DA, Jin X, Wang X, Yu XJ, Rozengurt N, Kaufman ML, Wang X, Gjertson D, Zhou Y, Blackburn MR, Kohn DB (2012) Gene therapy/bone marrow transplantation in ADA-deficient mice: roles of enzyme-replacement therapy and cytoreduction. Blood 120:3677–3687

Cartier N, Hacein-Bey-Abina S, Bartholomae CC, Veres G, Schmidt M, Kutschera I, Vidaud M, Abel U, Dal-Cortivo L, Caccavelli L, Mahlaoui N, Kiermer V, Mittelstaedt D, Bellesme C,

Lahlou N, Lefrère F, Blanche S, Audit M, Payen E, Leboulch P, l'Homme B, Bougnères P, Von Kalle C, Fischer A, Cavazzana-Calvo M, Aubourg P (2010) Hematopoietic stem cell gene therapy with lentiviral vector in X-linked adrenoleukodystrophy. In: XVIIIth Annual Congress of the European Society of Gene and Cell Therapy. Human Gene Therapy, Milano, pp 11–12

Cartier N, Hacein-Bey-Abina S, Bartholomae CC, Veres G, Schmidt M, Kutschera I, Vidaud M, Abel U, Dal-Cortivo L, Caccavelli L, Mahlaoui N, Kiermer V, Mittelstaedt D, Bellesme C, Lahlou N, Lefrere F, Blanche S, Audit M, Payen E, Leboulch P, l'Homme B, Bougneres P, Von Kalle C, Fischer A, Cavazzana-Calvo M, Aubourg P (2009) Hematopoietic stem cell gene therapy with a lentiviral vector in X-linked adrenoleukodystrophy. Science 326:818–823

Cavazzana M, Six E, Lagresle-Peyrou C, Andre-Schmutz I, Hacein-Bey-Abina S (2016) Gene therapy for X-linked severe combined immunodeficiency: where do we stand? Hum Gene Ther 27:108–116

Cavazzana-Calvo M, Hacein-Bey S, de Saint Basile G, Gross F, Yvon E, Nusbaum P, Selz F, Hue C, Certain S, Casanova JL, Bousso P, Deist FL, Fischer A (2000) Gene therapy of human severe combined immunodeficiency (SCID)-X1 disease. Science 288:669–672

Cavazzana-Calvo M, Payen E, Negre O, Wang G, Hehir K, Fusil F, Down J, Denaro M, Brady T, Westerman K, Cavallesco R, Gillet-Legrand B, Caccavelli L, Sgarra R, Maouche-Chretien L, Bernaudin F, Girot R, Dorazio R, Mulder GJ, Polack A, Bank A, Soulier J, Larghero J, Kabbara N, Dalle B, Gourmel B, Socie G, Chretien S, Cartier N, Aubourg P, Fischer A, Cornetta K, Galacteros F, Beuzard Y, Gluckman E, Bushman F, Hacein-Bey-Abina S, Leboulch P (2010) Transfusion independence and HMGA2 activation after gene therapy of human beta-thalassaemia. Nature 467:318–322

Chinen J, Davis J, De Ravin SS, Hay BN, Hsu AP, Linton GF, Naumann N, Nomicos EY, Silvin C, Ulrick J, Whiting-Theobald NL, Malech HL, Puck JM (2007) Gene therapy improves immune function in preadolescents with X-linked severe combined immunodeficiency. Blood 110:67–73

Cicalese MP, Aiuti A (2015) Clinical applications of gene therapy for primary immunodeficiencies. Hum Gene Ther 26:210–219

Cicalese MP, Ferrua F, Pajno R, Barzaghi F, Castagnaro L, Frittoli M, Giannelli S, Dionisio F, Brigida I, Carlucci F, Tabucchi A, Hogg A, Singh K, Campanile A, Appleby J, Philipson R, Roncarolo MG, Aiuti A (2014) Long-term safety and efficacy of retroviral-mediated gene therapy for ADA-SCID. J Clin Immunol 34:S311

De Ravin SS, Wu X, Moir S, Anaya-O'Brien S, Kwatemaa N, Littel P, Theobald N, Choi U, Su L, Marquesen M, Hilligoss D, Lee J, Buckner CM, Zarember KA, O'Connor G, McVicar D, Kuhns D, Throm RE, Zhou S, Notarangelo LD, Hanson IC, Cowan MJ, Kang E, Hadigan C, Meagher M, Gray JT, Sorrentino BP, Malech HL (2016) Lentiviral hematopoietic stem cell gene therapy for X-linked severe combined immunodeficiency. Sci Transl Med 8:335–357

Dissing J, Knudsen B (1972) Adenosine-deaminase deficiency and combined immunodeficiency syndrome. Lancet 2:1316

Dreyer AK, Hoffmann D, Lachmann N, Ackermann M, Steinemann D, Timm B, Siler U, Reichenbach J, Grez M, Moritz T, Schambach A, Cathomen T (2015) TALEN-mediated functional correction of X-linked chronic granulomatous disease in patient-derived induced pluripotent stem cells. Biomaterials 69:191–200

Flynn R, Grundmann A, Renz P, Hanseler W, James WS, Cowley SA, Moore MD (2015) CRISPR-mediated genotypic and phenotypic correction of a chronic granulomatous disease mutation in human iPS cells. Exp Hematol 43:838–848 e833

Gaspar B, Buckland K, Rivat C, Booth C, Gilmour K, Carbonaro D, Cornetta K, Schmidt M, Kohn DB, Thrasher AJ (2014) Immunological and metabolic correction after lentiviral vector mediated haematopoietic stem cell gene therapy for ADA deficiency. J Clin Immunol 34:S167

Gaspar HB, Aiuti A, Porta F, Candotti F, Hershfield MS, Notarangelo LD (2009) How I treat ADA deficiency. Blood 114:3524–3532

Gaspar HB, Cooray S, Gilmour KC, Parsley KL, Adams S, Howe SJ, Al Ghonaium A, Bayford J, Brown L, Davies EG, Kinnon C, Thrasher AJ (2011a) Long-term persistence of a polyclonal T cell repertoire after gene therapy for X-linked severe combined immunodeficiency. Sci Transl Med 3:97–79

Gaspar HB, Cooray S, Gilmour KC, Parsley KL, Zhang F, Adams S, Bjorkegren E, Bayford J, Brown L, Davies EG, Veys P, Fairbanks L, Bordon V, Petropoulou T, Kinnon C, Thrasher AJ (2011b) Hematopoietic stem cell gene therapy for adenosine deaminase-deficient severe combined immunodeficiency leads to long-term immunological recovery and metabolic correction. Sci Transl Med 3:97–80

Gaspar HB, Parsley KL, Howe S, King D, Gilmour KC, Sinclair J, Brouns G, Schmidt M, Von Kalle C, Barington T, Jakobsen MA, Christensen HO, Al Ghonaium A, White HN, Smith JL, Levinsky RJ, Ali RR, Kinnon C, Thrasher AJ (2004) Gene therapy of X-linked severe combined immunodeficiency by use of a pseudotyped gammaretroviral vector. Lancet 364:2181–2187

Gaspar HB, Buckland K, Denise A, Carbonaro D, Kit Shaw PB, Davila A, Kimberly C, Gilmour CB, Terrazs D, Cornetta K, Anna MSP, Sokolic R, Candotti F, Kohn DB, Thrasher AJ (2015) Immunological and metabolic correction after lentiviral vector gene therapy for ADA deficiency. Mol Ther 23:S102–S103

Genovese P, Schiroli G, Escobar G, Di Tomaso T, Firrito C, Calabria A, Moi D, Mazzieri R, Bonini C, Holmes MC, Gregory PD, van der Burg M, Gentner B, Montini E, Lombardo A, Naldini L (2014) Targeted genome editing in human repopulating haematopoietic stem cells. Nature 510:235–240

Gieselmann V, Krageloh-Mann I (2010) Metachromatic leukodystrophy--an update. Neuropediatrics 41:1–6

Grez M, Reichenbach J, Schwable J, Seger R, Dinauer MC, Thrasher AJ (2011) Gene therapy of chronic granulomatous disease: the engraftment dilemma. Mol Ther 19:28–35

Guda S, Brendel C, Renella R, Du P, Bauer DE, Canver MC, Grenier JK, Grimson AW, Kamran SC, Thornton J, de Boer H, Root DE, Milsom MD, Orkin SH, Gregory RI, Williams DA (2015) miRNA-embedded shRNAs for lineage-specific BCL11A knockdown and hemoglobin F induction. Mol Ther 23:1465–1474

Gungor T, Teira P, Slatter M, Stussi G, Stepensky P, Moshous D, Vermont C, Ahmad I, Shaw PJ, Telles da Cunha JM, Schlegel PG, Hough R, Fasth A, Kentouche K, Gruhn B, Fernandes JF, Lachance S, Bredius R, Resnick IB, Belohradsky BH, Gennery A, Fischer A, Gaspar HB, Schanz U, Seger R, Rentsch K, Veys P, Haddad E, Albert MH, Hassan M, Inborn Errors Working Party of the European Society for blood and marrow Transplantation (2014) Reduced-intensity conditioning and HLA-matched haemopoietic stem-cell transplantation in patients with chronic granulomatous disease: a prospective multicentre study. Lancet 383:436–448

Hacein-Bey Abina S, Gaspar HB, Blondeau J, Caccavelli L, Charrier S, Buckland K, Picard C, Six E, Himoudi N, Gilmour K, McNicol AM, Hara H, Xu-Bayford J, Rivat C, Touzot F, Mavilio F, Lim A, Treluyer JM, Heritier S, Lefrere F, Magalon J, Pengue-Koyi I, Honnet G, Blanche S, Sherman EA, Male F, Berry C, Malani N, Bushman FD, Fischer A, Thrasher AJ, Galy A, Cavazzana M (2015) Outcomes following gene therapy in patients with severe Wiskott-Aldrich syndrome. JAMA 313:1550–1563

Hacein-Bey-Abina S, Garrigue A, Wang GP, Soulier J, Lim A, Morillon E, Clappier E, Caccavelli L, Delabesse E, Beldjord K, Asnafi V, MacIntyre E, Dal Cortivo L, Radford I, Brousse N, Sigaux F, Moshous D, Hauer J, Borkhardt A, Belohradsky BH, Wintergerst U, Velez MC, Leiva L, Sorensen R, Wulffraat N, Blanche S, Bushman FD, Fischer A, Cavazzana-Calvo M (2008) Insertional oncogenesis in 4 patients after retrovirus-mediated gene therapy of SCID-X1. J Clin Invest 118:3132–3142

Hacein-Bey-Abina S, Hauer J, Lim A, Picard C, Wang GP, Berry CC, Martinache C, Rieux-Laucat F, Latour S, Belohradsky BH, Leiva L, Sorensen R, Debre M, Casanova JL, Blanche S, Durandy A, Bushman FD, Fischer A, Cavazzana-Calvo M (2010) Efficacy of gene therapy for X-linked severe combined immunodeficiency. N Engl J Med 363:355–364

Hacein-Bey-Abina S, Le Deist F, Carlier F, Bouneaud C, Hue C, De Villartay JP, Thrasher AJ, Wulffraat N, Sorensen R, Dupuis-Girod S, Fischer A, Davies EG, Kuis W, Leiva L, Cavazzana-Calvo M (2002) Sustained correction of X-linked severe combined immunodeficiency by ex vivo gene therapy. N Engl J Med 346:1185–1193

Hacein-Bey-Abina S, Pai SY, Gaspar HB, Armant M, Berry CC, Blanche S, Bleesing J, Blondeau J, de Boer H, Buckland KF, Caccavelli L, Cros G, De Oliveira S, Fernandez KS, Guo D, Harris CE, Hopkins G, Lehmann LE, Lim A, London WB, van der Loo JC, Malani N, Male F, Malik P, Marinovic MA, McNicol AM, Moshous D, Neven B, Oleastro M, Picard C, Ritz J, Rivat C, Schambach A, Shaw KL, Sherman EA, Silberstein LE, Six E, Touzot F, Tsytsykova A, Xu-Bayford J, Baum C, Bushman FD, Fischer A, Kohn DB, Filipovich AH, Notarangelo LD, Cavazzana M, Williams DA, Thrasher AJ (2014) A modified gamma-retrovirus vector for X-linked severe combined immunodeficiency. N Engl J Med 371:1407–1417

Hacein-Bey-Abina S, Von Kalle C, Schmidt M, McCormack MP, Wulffraat N, Leboulch P, Lim A, Osborne CS, Pawliuk R, Morillon E, Sorensen R, Forster A, Fraser P, Cohen JI, de Saint Basile G, Alexander I, Wintergerst U, Frebourg T, Aurias A, Stoppa-Lyonnet D, Romana S, Radford-Weiss I, Gross F, Valensi F, Delabesse E, Macintyre E, Sigaux F, Soulier J, Leiva LE, Wissler M, Prinz C, Rabbitts TH, Le Deist F, Fischer A, Cavazzana-Calvo M (2003) LMO2-associated clonal T cell proliferation in two patients after gene therapy for SCID-X1. Science 302:415–419

Hoogerbrugge PM, van Beusechem VW, Fischer A, Debree M, le Deist F, Perignon JL, Morgan G, Gaspar B, Fairbanks LD, Skeoch CH, Moseley A, Harvey M, Levinsky RJ, Valerio D (1996) Bone marrow gene transfer in three patients with adenosine deaminase deficiency. Gene Ther 3:179–183

Howe SJ, Mansour MR, Schwarzwaelder K, Bartholomae C, Hubank M, Kempski H, Brugman MH, Pike-Overzet K, Chatters SJ, de Ridder D, Gilmour KC, Adams S, Thornhill SI, Parsley KL, Staal FJ, Gale RE, Linch DC, Bayford J, Brown L, Quaye M, Kinnon C, Ancliff P, Webb DK, Schmidt M, von Kalle C, Gaspar HB, Thrasher AJ (2008) Insertional mutagenesis combined with acquired somatic mutations causes leukemogenesis following gene therapy of SCID-X1 patients. J Clin Invest 118:3143–3150

Joung JK, Sander JD (2013) TALENs: a widely applicable technology for targeted genome editing. Nat Rev Mol Cell Biol 14:49–55

Kang EM, Choi U, Theobald N, Linton G, Long Priel DA, Kuhns D, Malech HL (2010) Retrovirus gene therapy for X-linked chronic granulomatous disease can achieve stable long-term correction of oxidase activity in peripheral blood neutrophils. Blood 115:783–791

Kang EM, Marciano BE, DeRavin S, Zarember KA, Holland SM, Malech HL (2011b) Chronic granulomatous disease: overview and hematopoietic stem cell transplantation. J Allergy Clin Immunol 127:1319–1326; quiz 1327-1318

Kang HJ, Bartholomae CC, Paruzynski A, Arens A, Kim S, Yu SS, Hong Y, Joo CW, Yoon NK, Rhim JW, Kim JG, Von Kalle C, Schmidt M, Kim S, Ahn HS (2011a) Retroviral gene therapy for X-linked chronic granulomatous disease: results from phase I/II trial. Mol Ther 19:2092–2101

Kohn DB, Weinberg KI, Nolta JA, Heiss LN, Lenarsky C, Crooks GM, Hanley ME, Annett G, Brooks JS, el-Khoureiy A et al (1995) Engraftment of gene-modified umbilical cord blood cells in neonates with adenosine deaminase deficiency. Nat Med 1:1017–1023

Kuo CY, Kohn DB (2016) Gene therapy for the treatment of primary immune deficiencies. Curr Allergy Asthma Rep 16:39

Leonard WJ (1996) The molecular basis of X-linked severe combined immunodeficiency: defective cytokine receptor signaling. Annu Rev Med 47:229–239

Levasseur DN, Ryan TM, Pawlik KM, Townes TM (2003) Correction of a mouse model of sickle cell disease: lentiviral/antisickling beta-globin gene transduction of unmobilized, purified hematopoietic stem cells. Blood 102:4312–4319

Levasseur DN, Ryan TM, Reilly MP, McCune SL, Asakura T, Townes TM (2004) A recombinant human hemoglobin with anti-sickling properties greater than fetal hemoglobin. J Biol Chem 279:27518–27524

Long C, Amoasii L, Mireault AA, McAnally JR, Li H, Sanchez-Ortiz E, Bhattacharyya S, Shelton JM, Bassel-Duby R, Olson EN (2016) Postnatal genome editing partially restores dystrophin expression in a mouse model of muscular dystrophy. Science 351:400–403

Malech HL, Maples PB, Whiting-Theobald N, Linton GF, Sekhsaria S, Vowells SJ, Li F, Miller JA, DeCarlo E, Holland SM, Leitman SF, Carter CS, Butz RE, Read EJ, Fleisher TA, Schneiderman RD, Van Epps DE, Spratt SK, Maack CA, Rokovich JA, Cohen LK, Gallin JI (1997) Prolonged production of NADPH oxidase-corrected granulocytes after gene therapy of chronic granulomatous disease. Proc Natl Acad Sci U S A 94:12133–12138

Mansilla-Soto J, Riviere I, Boulad F, Sadelain M (2016) Cell and gene therapy for the beta-thalassemias: advances and prospects. Hum Gene Ther 27:295–304

Marktel S, Cicalese MP, Giglio F, Scaramuzza S, Calbi V, Casiraghi M, Ciotti F, Lidonnici MR, Rossi C, Masera N, D'Angelo E, Mirra N, Origa R, Tartaglione I, Mandelli G, Milani R, Gattillo S, Coppola M, Viarengo G, Santoleri L, Calabria A, Perrotta S, Montini E, Graziadei G, Naldini L, Cappellini MD, Ciceri F, Aiuti A, Ferrari G (2017) Gene therapy for Beta Thalassemia: Preliminary Results from the PHASE I/II Tiget-Bthal Trial of autologous hematopoietic stem cells genetically modified with GLOBE lentiviral vector. Blood 130:355

May C, Rivella S, Callegari J, Heller G, Gaensler KM, Luzzatto L, Sadelain M (2000) Therapeutic haemoglobin synthesis in beta-thalassaemic mice expressing lentivirus-encoded human beta-globin. Nature 406:82–86

Merling RK, Sweeney CL, Chu J, Bodansky A, Choi U, Priel DL, Kuhns DB, Wang H, Vasilevsky S, De Ravin SS, Winkler T, Dunbar CE, Zou J, Zarember KA, Gallin JI, Holland SM, Malech HL (2015) An AAVS1-targeted minigene platform for correction of iPSCs from all five types of chronic granulomatous disease. Mol Ther 23:147–157

Miccio A, Cesari R, Lotti F, Rossi C, Sanvito F, Ponzoni M, Routledge SJ, Chow CM, Antoniou MN, Ferrari G (2008) In vivo selection of genetically modified erythroblastic progenitors leads to long-term correction of beta-thalassemia. Proc Natl Acad Sci U S A 105:10547–10552

Moser HW, Mahmood A, Raymond GV (2007) X-linked adrenoleukodystrophy. Nat Clin Pract Neurol 3:140–151

Mosser J, Douar AM, Sarde CO, Kioschis P, Feil R, Moser H, Poustka AM, Mandel JL, Aubourg P (1993) Putative X-linked adrenoleukodystrophy gene shares unexpected homology with ABC transporters. Nature 361:726–730

Mukherjee S, Thrasher AJ (2013) Gene therapy for PIDs: progress, pitfalls and prospects. Gene 525:174–181

Musolino PL, Lund TC, Pan J, Escolar ML, Paker AM, Duncan CN, Eichler FS (2014) Hematopoietic stem cell transplantation in the leukodystrophies: a systematic review of the literature. Neuropediatrics 45:169–174

Mussolino C, Cathomen T (2012) TALE nucleases: tailored genome engineering made easy. Curr Opin Biotechnol 23:644–650

Negre O, Eggimann AV, Beuzard Y, Ribeil JA, Bourget P, Borwornpinyo S, Hongeng S, Hacein-Bey S, Cavazzana M, Leboulch P, Payen E (2016) Gene therapy of the beta-hemoglobinopathies by lentiviral transfer of the beta(A(T87Q))-globin gene. Hum Gene Ther 27:148–165

Nelson CE, Hakim CH, Ousterout DG, Thakore PI, Moreb EA, Castellanos Rivera RM, Madhavan S, Pan X, Ran FA, Yan WX, Asokan A, Zhang F, Duan D, Gersbach CA (2016) In vivo genome editing improves muscle function in a mouse model of Duchenne muscular dystrophy. Science 351:403–407

Notarangelo LD, Miao CH, Ochs HD (2008) Wiskott-Aldrich syndrome. Curr Opin Hematol 15:30–36

Onodera M, Ariga T, Kawamura N, Kobayashi I, Ohtsu M, Yamada M, Tame A, Furuta H, Okano M, Matsumoto S, Kotani H, McGarrity GJ, Blaese RM, Sakiyama Y (1998) Successful peripheral T-lymphocyte-directed gene transfer for a patient with severe combined immune deficiency caused by adenosine deaminase deficiency. Blood 91:30–36

Ott de Bruin LM, Volpi S, Musunuru K (2015) Novel genome-editing tools to model and correct primary immunodeficiencies. Front Immunol 6:250

Ott MG, Schmidt M, Schwarzwaelder K, Stein S, Siler U, Koehl U, Glimm H, Kuhlcke K, Schilz A, Kunkel H, Naundorf S, Brinkmann A, Deichmann A, Fischer M, Ball C, Pilz I, Dunbar C, Du Y, Jenkins NA, Copeland NG, Luthi U, Hassan M, Thrasher AJ, Hoelzer D, von Kalle C, Seger R, Grez M (2006) Correction of X-linked chronic granulomatous disease by gene

therapy, augmented by insertional activation of MDS1-EVI1, PRDM16 or SETBP1. Nat Med 12:401–409
Pai SY, Logan BR, Griffith LM, Buckley RH, Parrott RE, Dvorak CC, Kapoor N, Hanson IC, Filipovich AH, Jyonouchi S, Sullivan KE, Small TN, Burroughs L, Skoda-Smith S, Haight AE, Grizzle A, Pulsipher MA, Chan KW, Fuleihan RL, Haddad E, Loechelt B, Aquino VM, Gillio A, Davis J, Knutsen A, Smith AR, Moore TB, Schroeder ML, Goldman FD, Connelly JA, Porteus MH, Xiang Q, Shearer WT, Fleisher TA, Kohn DB, Puck JM, Notarangelo LD, Cowan MJ, O'Reilly RJ (2014) Transplantation outcomes for severe combined immunodeficiency, 2000–2009. N Engl J Med 371:434–446
Pauling L, Itano HA, Singer SJ, Wells IC (1949) Sickle cell anemia, a molecular disease. Science 110:543–546
Pawliuk R, Westerman KA, Fabry ME, Payen E, Tighe R, Bouhassira EE, Acharya SA, Ellis J, London IM, Eaves CJ, Humphries RK, Beuzard Y, Nagel RL, Leboulch P (2001) Correction of sickle cell disease in transgenic mouse models by gene therapy. Science 294:2368–2371
Rahman SH, Maeder ML, Joung JK, Cathomen T (2011) Zinc-finger nucleases for somatic gene therapy: the next frontier. Hum Gene Ther 22:925–933
Sadelain M, Boulad F, Maggio A, Wang X, Moi P, Riviere SAI (2015) Gene therapy for beta-thalassemia major. The Memorial Sloan Kettering Experience. Cooley's Anemia Foundation Symposium, October 2015
Sadelain M, Boulad F, Galanello R, Giardina P, Locatelli F, Maggio A, Rivella S, Riviere I, Tisdale J (2007) Therapeutic options for patients with severe beta-thalassemia: the need for globin gene therapy. Hum Gene Ther 18:1–9
Sander JD, Joung JK (2014) CRISPR-Cas systems for editing, regulating and targeting genomes. Nat Biotechnol 32:347–355
Scaramuzza S, Giannelli S, Ferrua F, Castiello MC, Assanelli A, Cicalese MP, Biasco L, Ottaviano G, Casiraghi M, Rizzardi P, Bosticardo M, Finocchi A, Metin A, Albert M, Petrescu C, Banerjee PP, Orange JS, Biffi Ciceri AF, Villa A, Roncarolo MG, Naldini L, Aiuti A (2014) Persistent multilineage engraftment and WASP restored expression after lentiviral mediated CD34+ cells gene therapy for the treatment of Wiskott-Aldrich syndrome. Mol Ther 22:S88
Serjeant GR (1985) Sickle cell disease. Oxford University Press, Oxford
Sessa M, Lorioli L, Fumagalli F, Acquati S, Redaelli D, Baldoli C, Canale S, Lopez ID, Morena F, Calabria A, Fiori R, Silvani P, Rancoita PM, Gabaldo M, Benedicenti F, Antonioli G, Assanelli A, Cicalese MP, Del Carro U, Sora MG, Martino S, Quattrini A, Montini E, Di Serio C, Ciceri F, Roncarolo MG, Aiuti A, Naldini L, Biffi A (2016) Lentiviral haemopoietic stem-cell gene therapy in early-onset metachromatic leukodystrophy: an ad-hoc analysis of a non-randomised, open-label, phase 1/2 trial. Lancet 388(10043):476–487
Shapiro E, Krivit W, Lockman L, Jambaque I, Peters C, Cowan M, Harris R, Blanche S, Bordigoni P, Loes D, Ziegler R, Crittenden M, Ris D, Berg B, Cox C, Moser H, Fischer A, Aubourg P (2000) Long-term effect of bone-marrow transplantation for childhood-onset cerebral X-linked adrenoleukodystrophy. Lancet 356:713–718
Slatter MA, Gennery AR (2013) Advances in hematopoietic stem cell transplantation for primary immunodeficiency. Expert Rev Clin Immunol 9:991–999
Stein S, Ott MG, Schultze-Strasser S, Jauch A, Burwinkel B, Kinner A, Schmidt M, Kramer A, Schwable J, Glimm H, Koehl U, Preiss C, Ball C, Martin H, Gohring G, Schwarzwaelder K, Hofmann WK, Karakaya K, Tchatchou S, Yang R, Reinecke P, Kuhlcke K, Schlegelberger B, Thrasher AJ, Hoelzer D, Seger R, von Kalle C, Grez M (2010) Genomic instability and myelodysplasia with monosomy 7 consequent to EVI1 activation after gene therapy for chronic granulomatous disease. Nat Med 16:198–204
Steinberg MH, Forget BG, Higgs DR, Nagel RL (2001a) In: Forget BG (ed) Molecular mechanism of β thalassemia. Cambridge University Press, Cambridge
Steinberg MH, Forget BG, Higgs DR, Nagel RL (2001b) Disorders of hemoglobin: genetics, pathophysiology and clinical management. Cambridge University Press, Cambridge
Stephan V, Wahn V, Le Deist F, Dirksen U, Broker B, Muller-Fleckenstein I, Horneff G, Schroten H, Fischer A, de Saint Basile G (1996) Atypical X-linked severe combined immunodefi-

ciency due to possible spontaneous reversion of the genetic defect in T cells. N Engl J Med 335:1563–1567
Sugamura K, Asao H, Kondo M, Tanaka N, Ishii N, Ohbo K, Nakamura M, Takeshita T (1996) The interleukin-2 receptor gamma chain: its role in the multiple cytokine receptor complexes and T cell development in XSCID. Annu Rev Immunol 14:179–205
Tabebordbar M, Zhu K, Cheng JK, Chew WL, Widrick JJ, Yan WX, Maesner C, Wu EY, Xiao R, Ran FA, Cong L, Zhang F, Vandenberghe LH, Church GM, Wagers AJ (2016) In vivo gene editing in dystrophic mouse muscle and muscle stem cells. Science 351:407–411
Tebas P, Stein D, Tang WW, Frank I, Wang SQ, Lee G, Spratt SK, Surosky RT, Giedlin MA, Nichol G, Holmes MC, Gregory PD, Ando DG, Kalos M, Collman RG, Binder-Scholl G, Plesa G, Hwang WT, Levine BL, June CH (2014) Gene editing of CCR5 in autologous CD4 T cells of persons infected with HIV. N Engl J Med 370:901–910
Thornhill SI, Schambach A, Howe SJ, Ulaganathan M, Grassman E, Williams D, Schiedlmeier B, Sebire NJ, Gaspar HB, Kinnon C, Baum C, Thrasher AJ (2008) Self-inactivating gamma-retroviral vectors for gene therapy of X-linked severe combined immunodeficiency. Mol Ther 16:590–598
Thrasher AJ, Hacein-Bey-Abina S, Gaspar HB, Blanche S, Davies EG, Parsley K, Gilmour K, King D, Howe S, Sinclair J, Hue C, Carlier F, von Kalle C, de Saint Basile G, le Deist F, Fischer A, Cavazzana-Calvo M (2005) Failure of SCID-X1 gene therapy in older patients. Blood 105:4255–4257
Touzot F, Hacein-Bey-Abina S, Fischer A, Cavazzana M (2014) Gene therapy for inherited immunodeficiency. Expert Opin Biol Ther 14:789–798
Urnov FD, Rebar EJ, Holmes MC, Zhang HS, Gregory PD (2010) Genome editing with engineered zinc finger nucleases. Nat Rev Genet 11:636–646
Vierstra J, Reik A, Chang KH, Stehling-Sun S, Zhou Y, Hinkley SJ, Paschon DE, Zhang L, Psatha N, Bendana YR, O'Neil CM, Song AH, Mich AK, Liu PQ, Lee G, Bauer DE, Holmes MC, Orkin SH, Papayannopoulou T, Stamatoyannopoulos G, Rebar EJ, Gregory PD, Urnov FD, Stamatoyannopoulos JA (2015) Functional footprinting of regulatory DNA. Nat Methods 12:927–930
Waseem Qasim PJA, Samarasinghe S, Ghorashian S, Zhan H, Stafford S, Butler K, Gilmour GAK, Adams S, Pinner D, Chiesa R, Chatters S, Swift S, Goulden N, Peggs K, Thrasher AJ, Veys P, Pule M (2015) First clinical application of Talen engineered universal CAR19 T cells in B-ALL. In: ASH 57th Annual Meeting & Exposition. American Society of Hematology, Orlando, FL
Williams DA, Thrasher AJ (2014) Concise review: lessons learned from clinical trials of gene therapy in monogenic immunodeficiency diseases. Stem Cells Transl Med 3:636–642
Zhou S, Mody D, DeRavin SS, Hauer J, Lu T, Ma Z, Hacein-Bey Abina S, Gray JT, Greene MR, Cavazzana-Calvo M, Malech HL, Sorrentino BP (2010) A self-inactivating lentiviral vector for SCID-X1 gene therapy that does not activate LMO2 expression in human T cells. Blood 116:900–908
Zychlinski D, Schambach A, Modlich U, Maetzig T, Meyer J, Grassman E, Mishra A, Baum C (2008) Physiological promoters reduce the genotoxic risk of integrating gene vectors. Mol Ther 16:718–725

MIX
Papier aus verantwortungsvollen Quellen
Paper from responsible sources
FSC® C105338

If you have any concerns about our products,
you can contact us on
ProductSafety@springernature.com

In case Publisher is established outside the EU,
the EU authorized representative is:
Springer Nature Customer Service Center GmbH
Europaplatz 3, 69115 Heidelberg, Germany

Printed by Libri Plureos GmbH
in Hamburg, Germany